T0176505

# Telephone
# Triage Protocols
# for Pediatrics

**Julie K. Briggs,** MHA, BSN, RN
Quality Medical Management
Providence Health & Services
Portland, Oregon

**Mikki Meadows-Oliver,** PhD, RN, PNP-BC
Associate Professor
University of Connecticut
Mansfield, CT

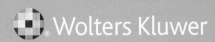 Wolters Kluwer

Philadelphia · Baltimore · New York · London
Buenos Aires · Hong Kong · Sydney · Tokyo

*Acquisitions Editor:* Nicole Dernoski
*Editorial Coordinator:* Lindsay Ries
*Marketing Manager:* Linda Wetmore
*Production Project Manager:* Bridgett Dougherty
*Design Coordinator:* Elaine Kasmer
*Manufacturing Coordinator:* Kathleen Brown
*Prepress Vendor:* S4Carlisle Publishing Services

9  8  7  6  5  4  3  2

Printed in China

**Library of Congress Cataloging-in-Publication Data**

Names: Briggs, Julie K., author. | Meadows-Oliver, Mikki, author.
Title: Telephone triage protocols for pediatrics / Julie K. Briggs, Mikki
    Meadows-Oliver.
Description: First edition. | Philadelphia: Wolters Kluwer, [2018] |
    Includes bibliographical references and index.
Identifiers: LCCN 2017016093 | ISBN 9781496363602
Subjects: | MESH: Pediatric Nursing—methods | Nursing Assessment—methods |
    Clinical Protocols | Triage—methods | Telephone | Handbooks
Classification: LCC RJ245 | NLM WY 49 | DDC 618.92/00231—dc23 LC record available at
    https://lccn.loc.gov/2017016093

# Contributors

**Gary Berg, RN, BSN, CEN**
Emergency Department
Telephone Triage Nurse
Good Samaritan Community Healthcare
Puyallup, Washington

**Julie K. Briggs, MHA, RN, BSN**
Quality Medical Management
Providence Health & Services
Portland, Oregon

**Shannon Fuller, RN**
Obstetrics Department
Good Samaritan Community Healthcare
Puyallup, Washington

**Sheila Graham, RN**
Obstetrics Department
Good Samaritan Community Healthcare
Puyallup, Washington

**Valerie G. A. Grossman, RN, BSN, MALS, NE-BC**
Nurse Manager
Medical Imaging
University of Rochester
Highland Hospital
Rochester, New York

**Elaine Keavney, RN, BSN, CEN**
Education Consultant
Portland, Oregon

**Laurie McGhee, RNC, ARNP**
Obstetrics Department
Good Samaritan Community Healthcare
Puyallup, Washington

**Mikki Meadows-Oliver, PhD, RN, PNP-BC**
Associate Professor
University of Connecticut
Mansfield, CT

**Linda Mercer, RN, CEN**
Emergency Department
Good Samaritan Community Healthcare
Puyallup, Washington

**Deborah Oakman, BSN, RN**
Obstetrics Department
Good Samaritan Community Healthcare
Puyallup, Washington

**Pat Reder, RN, CEN**
Consulting Telephonic Nurse Case Manager
Thorton, Colorado

**Sandra Velliquette, BSN, RNC**
Obstetrics Department
Good Samaritan Community Healthcare
Puyallup, Washington

# Reviewers

Chris R. Andrews, MD, FACEP
Emergency Services
Providence Health System
Portland, Oregon

Coreen Arioto, MSN, RN
Former Advice Nurse Manager
Kaiser Metropolitan Los Angeles
Los Angeles, California

Meghan Arnold, RN, BSN, MHA
Quality Medical Management
Providence Health Plans
Portland, Oregon

Stephanie H. Asher, RN, MSN
Supervisor Quality Medical Management
Providence Health Plans
Banks, Oregon

Susan Barnason, PhD, RN, CEN, CCRN, CS
Associate Professor
University of Nebraska Medical Center
College of Nursing
Lincoln, Nebraska

Michelle Birge, RN, BSN, CCM
Quality Medical Management
Providence Health Plans
Portland, Oregon

Michael Brook, MD, FACEP
Emergency Medicine
Good Samaritan Community Healthcare
Puyallup, Washington
Clinical Assistant Professor of Medicine
University of Washington Medical Center
Seattle, Washington

Nancy Church, RN, BSN, MT, CIC
Manager
Infection Control
Providence St. Vincent Medical Center
Portland, Oregon

Shelley Cohen, RN, BS, CEN
Educator/Consultant
Health Resources Unlimited
Hohenwald, Tennessee

Mary F. Condera, MS, RN, PMHNP-BC
Psychiatric Mental Health Nurse Practitioner
Northwest Catholic Counseling Center
Portland, Oregon

Sonja R. Dahl, RNC, BSN, IBCLC
Obstetric Department
Good Samaritan Community Healthcare
Puyallup, Washington

Timothy Dahlgren, MD
Emergency Medicine
Good Samaritan Community Healthcare
Puyallup, Washington

Margaret C. Dirienzo, BSN, RN, CEN
Director
Critical Care Services
North Austin Medical Center
Austin, Texas

Laura R. Favand, MS, RN
Chief
Education and Training
Army Trauma Training Center
Army Medical Department Center and School
Miami, Florida

**Vickie K. Fieler, RN, MS, AOCN**
Clinical Nurse Specialist
Oncology
Exeter Hospital
Exeter, New Hampshire

**Laura G. Genovese, RN, MSN, APRN-BC**
Assistant Clinical Manager
Network Telephone Care Program
Veterans Affairs Medical Center
Bronx, New York

**Valerie G. A. Grossman, RN, BSN, CEN, MALS, NE-BC**
Nurse Manager
Medical Imaging
University of Rochester
Highland Hospital
Rochester, New York

**Reneé S. Holleran, RN, PhD, CEN, CCRN, CFRN, FAEN**
Nurse Manager
Adult Transport Services
Intermountain Life Flight
Salt Lake City, Utah

**Elizabeth Jerabeck, RN, BSN**
Senior Nurse Counselor
ViaHealth LINK
ViaHealth System
Rochester, New York

**Diane Kamble, RNC, APRN**
Network Telephone Care Program
Veterans Affairs Medical Center
Bronx, New York

**Calvin A. Kierum, Jr., MD, FAAP**
Pediatric Medicine
Puyallup, Washington

**Bret Lambert, MD**
Emergency Physician
President of Medical Staff
Good Samaritan Hospital
Puyallup, Washington

**Eileen W. Lumb, MS, RN, CS, CEN, FNP**
Adult Nurse Practitioner
Emergency Department
Strong Memorial Hospital
University of Rochester
Rochester, New York

**Diane L. Mathews, RNC, MSN**
Urgent Care/Telephone Care Service
William S. Middleton Memorial VA Hospital
Madison, Wisconsin

**Judith McDevitt, PhD, RN, CS-FNP**
Assistant Professor of Nursing
Coordinator, Family Nurse Practitioner Option
Department of Health Maintenance, School of Nursing
University of Wisconsin–Milwaukee
Milwaukee, Wisconsin

**J. Michaelson, Jr., MD, FACOG**
Obstetrics & Gynecology Medicine
Puyallup, Washington

**Lyne Ouellet, MD**
Emergency Medicine
Good Samaritan Community Healthcare
Puyallup, Washington
Clinical Assistant Professor of Medicine
University of Washington Medical Center
Seattle, Washington

**Mary B. Passauer, BSN**
Clinical Coordinator
Saint Vincent Call Center
Erie, Pennsylvania

**Iris Reyes, MD**
Assistant Professor of Emergency Medicine
Department of Emergency Medicine
The Hospital of the University of Pennsylvania
Philadelphia, Pennsylvania

**Patty C. Seneski**
Emergency Preparedness Manager
Banner Desert Medical Center
Banner Children's Hospital at BDMC
Mesa, Arizona

**Cynthia Smith, RN**
Clinical Supervisor Specialty Clinics
Providence Medical Group
Providence Health & Services
Portland, Oregon

**Danonne R. Smith**
Project Consultant
Consumer Advocate
Portland, Oregon

**Cecil Snodgrass, MD, FACEP, MRO**
Family Practice
Puyallup, Washington

**Leeta Stoughton, MPH, RN, BC, CEN**
Regional Clinical Systems Manager
Providence Health System
Portland, Oregon

**Phyllis Straight-Millan, SPHR, CSM, MA, MPA**
Program Consultant
Senior Advocate
Workplace Violence Programs, Voluntary Protection
Programs (OSHA)
Portland, Oregon

**Rebecca Sullivan, MD**
Family Practice
Puyallup Valley Healthcare
Puyallup, Washington

**Christina Terenzi, RN, MN, CEN**
Clinical System Educator I
MultiCare Health System
Tacoma, Washington

**Lisa Utter, RNC, ASN**
Staff Nurse
Clarian Health
Indianapolis, Indiana

**Steve Weinman, RN, CEN**
Emergency Department
St. Luke's Northland Hospital
Kansas City, Missouri

**Mark A. Whitaker, MD, MMM, FAAP**
Senior Medical Director
Quality and Medical Management
Providence Health and Services
Portland, Oregon

**Addison Wilson, MD**
Medical Director
Providence Health Plans
Providence Health & Services
Portland, Oregon

**Margaret Wilson, RN, MSN, EdD**
Professor of Nursing
Cypress College
Cypress, California

# Preface

Appropriate use of health-care resources is one of the biggest challenges in today's health-care environment. The implementation of the Affordable Care Act has significantly impacted the utilization of health-care resources and the need for effective telephone triage to help people access the right level of health care at the right time. In an era of escalating health-care costs, corporate reorganization, and a surge in the number of managed care systems, consumers are forced to carefully evaluate whether and when to seek medical attention. They must contend with cost and access as key issues, and telephone triage nurses play a key role in helping consumers through this decision-making maze.

Primary care providers are increasingly called upon to control health-care costs and the use of health-care resources. However, most providers are too busy to personally answer the numerous calls from consumers who are seeking advice. The responsibility frequently falls on nurses. Standardized protocols help the nurse handle telephone questions efficiently, confidently, and in a safe and proficient manner. Telephone triage has become the entry point into the health-care system for many consumers. It is a tool to help improve access to health care.

Nurses in a variety of settings, including emergency rooms, physician offices, clinics, and schools, frequently find themselves in the position of giving health-care advice. It is important to recognize that not all nurses are equal in terms of education, experience, knowledge base, assessment skills, and communication skills. Therefore, advice based on what a nurse "thinks" is appropriate may in fact be harmful to the caller. The nurse may miss an important detail in the absence of a thorough, systematic assessment. Organized, approved protocols help to ensure that the assessment is thorough and that nothing significant is overlooked.

Telephone triage is a systematic process in which a nurse screens a caller's symptoms for urgency and advises the caller when to seek medical attention, based on the severity of the problem described. The nurse also helps direct the caller to the most appropriate health-care setting, or gives advice about home care.

Despite the potential medical–legal risks of giving telephone advice, there has been considerable interest in telephone triage as a mechanism to help control costs and resource use while still responding to the consumer's need for information. Helping a caller to make an informed decision about health care will enhance the provider's image to a much greater extent than refusing to discuss health-care options over the telephone.

As health-care delivery systems evolve and formal relationships among physician groups, hospitals, and third-party payers are cultivated, telephone triage and advice programs are rapidly emerging as a necessary service. To be successful, they must be well-organized, protocol-driven, well-documented, and evaluated for quality, accuracy, and consistency.

In this rapidly changing health-care environment, new medications, treatments, devices, and practice modalities are evolving daily. The number of FDA-approved over-the-counter medications has increased steadily and enabled individuals to effectively manage conditions at home rather than visit their care providers for a prescription. Many conditions are now treated in the outpatient setting or at home. *Telephone Triage Protocols for Pediatrics* has incorporated these considerations in the development of pediatric specific telephone triage protocols adapted from the fifth edition of *Telephone Triage Protocols for Nurses* by Julie K. Briggs.

*Telephone Triage Protocols for Pediatrics* assists health-care professionals in asking appropriate questions to quickly assess the severity of a problem and help the caller make an informed decision concerning health service utilization. The protocols are not designed to diagnose the caller's medical condition.

This manual contains 170 protocols that cover a wide range of symptoms, disorders, and medical emergencies common in the pediatric population. Although most of the protocols have "symptom-based" titles, a few have "diagnosis-based" titles for use with callers who have been previously diagnosed with a condition and are having concerns related to that condition (diabetes, sickle cell disease, asthma, etc.). Protocols are arranged alphabetically to help the health care professional quickly locate the appropriate protocol. A team of experts has extensively reviewed all of the protocols to ensure accurate and up-to-date advice.

## Key Features

- The format is easy to follow.
- Each protocol follows a standard design, which helps the nurse to utilize information efficiently.
- Questions and instructions are written in clear and concise language.
- All protocols are cross-referenced to additional protocols that may be useful in assessing the caller's problem or concern.
- The color tabs for each alphabetical section have been staggered, making it easier to locate the appropriate section of the book. The reader may also wish to purchase alphabetical stick-on tabs, which can be found at most office supply stores.
- The **Key Questions** section of the protocol prompts the nurse to ask for important information before proceeding through the protocol. This includes asking for the caller's name, age, onset of symptoms, prior history, medication usage, and questions appropriate to the complaint, such as pain scale, immunization status, or frequency of symptoms. Disease-based protocols include questions about

a known diagnosis, treatment, or known exposure to a disease.

- The **Other Protocols to Consider** section of the protocol lists related protocols, and their page numbers, serving as a quick resource for multiple symptoms or related conditions. After asking key questions, the nurse may determine that a different protocol is more appropriate, and can quickly select that protocol.
- The **Nurse Alert** section provides the nurse with additional important information to consider when choosing a specific protocol or when triaging the caller's concern. Referrals to additional resources are provided when appropriate to assist the nurse in gaining a better understanding of a specific condition.
- The **Reminder** text in the protocol ("Document caller response to advice, home care instructions, and when to call back") prompts the nurse to document the call and ensure that the caller understands the advice provided.
- The **Assessment** section of the protocol lists the symptoms, conditions, or combination of factors that should be assessed in determining urgency.
- The **Action** column of the protocol is organized around yes-or-no answers to the assessment questions. If the caller answers "no" to the question, the nurse is directed to the next category of assessment questions. If the caller answers "yes," concrete advice is given regarding when and where to receive care. This advice is prioritized so that emergency actions always appear first. The terms used in the Action section instruct the nurse or the caller how to proceed. Actions the nurse should take appear in italicized type in the list below. Instructions to the caller appear in quotation marks. Action options are as follows:
  - *Go to [a related] protocol.* The nurse is directed to a related protocol that may address an emergent problem more appropriately.
  - "Call an ambulance" (911 in many areas). Emergency first aid instructions while waiting for the ambulance are also included in this section.

- ○ "Seek emergency care now." Refer caller to the nearest emergency department. Emergency first aid instructions before going to the ED may also be included here as appropriate.
- ○ "Seek medical care within 2 to 4 hours." Refer caller to usual care provider, clinic, or emergency department for urgent conditions.
- ○ "Seek medical care within 24 hours." Refer caller to usual care provider, clinic, or emergency department for less urgent conditions.
- ○ "Seek medical care within 24 to 48 hours." Refer caller to usual care provider, clinic, or emergency department for nonurgent conditions.
- ○ "Call back or call PCP for appointment if no improvement." Refer caller to primary care provider or clinic for nonurgent problems, if no improvement occurs after following home care instructions.
- ○ *Follow home care instructions.* The nurse is directed to explain the information described in the Home Care Instructions section, which follows the Assessment/Action columns.

- The **Home Care Instructions** section explains what care should be given in the home before emergency help arrives, while waiting for an appointment, or if the problem can be managed at home. These guidelines can provide symptom relief, prevent a condition from worsening, and reassure the caller. Home and alternative remedies are included and offer less expensive options for symptom relief. Drug warnings are provided whenever over-the-counter medications are suggested to help ensure medications are used in a safe manner.

- **Emergency Instructions** are included in the beginning of **Home Care Instructions** to provide important first aid actions to take while the caller is waiting for an ambulance or before going to the emergency department.

- An **Additional Instructions** area in the protocol provides space in which the health care provider can write customized health care facility instructions.

- The **Report the Following Problems to Your PCP/ Clinic/ED** section of the protocol lists subsequent

observations, symptoms, or conditions that should be reported wherever the caller generally receives ongoing health care.

- The **Seek Emergency Care Immediately** section of the protocol lists subsequent observations, symptoms, or conditions that would require the caller to seek immediate emergency care. The caller is directed to watch for these symptoms and if they occur, either call an ambulance or go directly to the emergency department.

- The **Advice Agreement** section of the protocol prompts the nurse to ask whether or not the caller agrees with the advice given, and encourages the caller to call back or follow up with the PCP, clinic, or ED if the problem persists or worsens. This warning should be given with every call. If the caller does not agree with the advice, the nurse should reassess the advice given.

## Additional Features

- The **Table of Contents** lists each protocol alphabetically directing the reader to the appropriate page.

- The **Table of Contents by Body System** lists the protocols by body system or body part to help the user rapidly identify the appropriate protocol for a specific symptom or set of related symptoms. In addition, there are separate sections for chronic or infectious disease-related protocols, general problems, behavioral health problems, and infant-specific protocols.

- The **Appendices** include tools, forms, and information to assist in the proper and safe use of telephone triage protocols as well as maintaining a quality telephone triage program.
  - ○ Abbreviations Chart
  - ○ Sample Telephone Triage Protocol Form
  - ○ Practicing Telephone Triage Safely
    - Triage Roles and Responsibilities
    - Protocol Structure
    - Using Protocols Safely
  - ○ Documentation Guidelines
    - Telephone Triage Documentation Form

- Telephone Triage Log
  - Training Guidelines
    - Telephone Triage Training Outline
    - Practice Scenarios
    - Skills Assessment Exercise Form
  - Teaching Self-Assessment Guide
  - Quality Assurance Program
    - Call Documentation Review
    - Call Back Log
  - Community Resources Telephone List
  - Temperature and Weight Conversion Charts
  - Resources

- The **Bibliography** includes additional telephone triage and advisory resources.

- The **Index** includes all of the protocol titles as well as alternate terms to allow quick access to the correct protocol.

  *Telephone Triage Protocols for Pediatrics* is a comprehensive resource that will benefit medical offices, emergency departments, urgent care centers, clinics, schools, home health agencies, parents and caregivers, managed health care providers, and all nurses who receive calls for advice. This quick reference manual can serve as:

- A systematic screening guide to assist callers in making informed decisions about when to access health care resources.

- A ready resource for health care professionals.

- A source for community referrals.

- A tool to help reduce inappropriate utilization of emergency services.

- A telephone service to triage patients with life-threatening problems.

- A mechanism to minimize risk management difficulties through consistency and documentation.

- A resource for additional website information to learn more about specific conditions, treatments, and prevention.

# Acknowledgments

The efforts of many people are responsible for the successful completion of this book. We thank the reviewers for their consistent and thorough evaluation of the protocols for accuracy, safety, appropriateness, clarity, and completeness. Their ongoing efforts have been noteworthy and their comments invaluable.

We thank our colleagues, friends, and families for their continued support, encouragement, and suggestions throughout this time-consuming process. A special thank you to Mark A. Whitaker, MD, FAAP, MMM, for his expertise in pediatric medicine and meticulous review of the manuscript to ensure consistency with current medical practice. We want to extend a very special thank you to Shannon Magee, Senior Acquisitions Editor for making this project possible, Lindsay Reis, Editorial Assistant for assistance in moving this project smoothly through the production phase, and to Nicole Dernoski, Acquisitions Editor, for her prompt responsiveness to questions and issues, support, encouragement, and direction throughout the process.

# Contents

# Table of Contents by Body System

## Gastrointestinal Problems

## Genital/Obstetrics and Gynecologic Problems

## Chronic and Infectious Diseases

# Abdominal Pain

>> **Key Questions**  Name, Age, Onset, Medications, Pain Scale, Associated Symptoms, Prior History, Date of Last Menstrual Period

>> **Other Protocols to Consider**  Abdominal Swelling (4); Constipation (114); Diarrhea (143); Food Poisoning, Suspected (194); Menstrual Problems (299); Urination, Difficult (473); Urination, Painful (477); Vomiting (492).

> *Nurse Alert:*  Many conditions can cause abdominal pain, and some can be potentially life threatening. Err on the side of caution when triaging callers with abdominal pain.

*Reminder:*  Document caller response to advice, home care instructions, and when to call back.

| ASSESSMENT | ACTION |
| --- | --- |
| **A. Are any of the following present?** | |
| • Severe persistent pain >2 hours | **YES**  "Seek emergency care now" |
| • Rapidly increasing pain | **NO**  Go to B |
| • RLQ pain with poor appetite, nausea and/or vomiting, fever, grasping abdomen, walking bent over, screaming, grunting respirations, or lying with knees drawn toward chest | |
| • Unusually heavy vaginal bleeding and possibility of pregnancy | |
| • Ingestion of unknown chemical substance, plant, or medication | |
| • Recent abdominal trauma | |
| • Black, bloody, or jelly-like stools unrelated to hemorrhoids or iron supplements | |
| • Weight loss | |
| • Vomiting blood or dark coffee-grounds–like emesis | |
| • Weakness and inability to walk | |
| • Severe pain and swelling in testicle(s) or scrotum | |

## B. Are any of the following present?

- Severe nausea and vomiting
- Continuous pain >2 hours and unresponsive to home care
- Unexplained progressive abdominal swelling
- Painful or difficult urination
- Age <2 years and intermittent pain
- Pain interferes with activity
- Decreased urine output
- Nausea, vomiting, or diarrhea >24 hours and unresponsive to home care
- Known hernia or hydrocele and pain or crying >2 hours

**YES** "Seek medical care within 2 to 4 hours"

**NO** Go to C

## C. Are any of the following present?

- Vaginal or urethral discharge
- History of abdominal pain, and usual treatment is ineffective
- Significant increase in stress level
- Blood in urine
- Temperature >101°F (38.3°C), cough, or weakness

**YES** "Seek medical care within 24 to 48 hours"

**NO** Go to D

## D. Are any of the following present?

- Constipation
- History of a nervous stomach and increased stress level
- Intermittent mild pain associated with an empty stomach, eating certain foods, or use of pain, antibiotic, or anti-inflammatory medications
- Mild infrequent diarrhea
- Other family members are ill
- Persistent sore throat >24 hours

**YES** "Call back or call PCP for appointment if no improvement"
and
Follow **Home Care Instructions**

**NO** Follow **Home Care Instructions**

A

## Home Care Instructions
## Abdominal Pain

- Rest.
- Consume clear liquids (fruit juice diluted 50:50 with water, weak tea, broth, sports drinks, flavored ice, gelatin, clear soft drink) or bland diet (rice, potatoes, soda crackers, pretzels, dry toast, applesauce, bananas) for 12 to 24 hours. Recommend electrolyte/mineral supplement or other rehydrating fluid solution (such as Pedialyte) for small children or infants.
- If diarrhea is present, avoid fruit juice or full-strength sports drinks.
- Take medications as directed by the pharmacy. Some should be taken on an empty stomach and others with food. Avoid ibuprofen and other anti-inflammatory medications. Do not give aspirin to a child. Avoid aspirin-like products if age <20 years. Avoid acetaminophen if liver disease is present. Avoid ibuprofen if kidney disease or stomach problems exist or in the case of pregnancy. Follow the directions on the label. Use the dosing device that comes with the medication, a measuring device, or a medication syringe from the pharmacy. Household teaspoons often do not give the correct amount of medication.
- Apply a moist, hot towel or heating pad to the abdomen for cramping.

## Additional Instructions

_____

_____

_____

### Report the Following Problems to Your PCP/Clinic/ED

- Severe pain >1 hour
- Fever
- Pain worsens with heat or activity

### Seek Emergency Care Immediately If Any of the Following Occur

- Unusually firm or hard abdomen
- Persistent vomiting
- Bloody or black stools or emesis
- Weakness and inability to walk
- Severe pain and swelling in testicle(s) or scrotum

If the caller agrees with the advice given, document the call, and encourage the caller to call back or see PCP if the problem worsens. If the caller does not agree with the advice given, reevaluate and advise the caller to follow up with PCP, Clinic, or ED.

# Abdominal Swelling

 **Key Questions** Name, Age, Onset, Medications, Prior History, Pain Scale

 **Other Protocols to Consider** Abdominal Pain (1); Constipation (114); Diarrhea (143); Gas/Belching (221); Gas/Flatulence (223); Rectal Bleeding (371); Swelling (449); Vomiting (492).

*Reminder:* Document caller response to advice, home care instructions, and when to call back.

| ASSESSMENT | ACTION |
|---|---|
| **A. Is abdominal pain present?** | **YES** Go to Abdominal Pain protocol (4) |
| | **NO** Go to B |
| **B. Are any of the following present?** | |
| • History of recent trauma or abdominal surgery | **YES** "Seek emergency care now" |
| • Vomiting blood | **NO** Go to C |
| • New onset of black or bloody stools | |
| **C. Are any of the following present?** | |
| • Swelling developed suddenly within past 24 hours and is unrelieved by passing gas or vomiting | **YES** "Seek medical care within 2 to 4 hours" |
| • Fever | **NO** Go to D |
| • Painful or tender area does not disappear with pressure | |
| **D. Are any of the following present with no prior history?** | |
| • Swollen ankles | **YES** "Seek medical care within 24 hours" |
| • Difficulty breathing, especially at night | **NO** Go to E |
| • Decreased urine output | |
| • Swelling decreases after passing urine | |
| • New-onset yellow skin and eyes | |
| • Painful or tender area disappears with pressures or enlarges with coughing | |

## E. Are any of the following present?

- Persistent constipation
- Possibility of pregnancy and tender enlarged breasts, morning nausea, missed period >2 months
- Abdominal swelling in a female 1 to 5 days before or during menstruation
- Swelling associated with cramping, diarrhea, or constipation
- Swelling is slowly increasing throughout a 1-week period
- Rapid weight gain
- Increased flatus or gas

**YES** "Call back or call PCP for appointment if no improvement"
and
Follow **Home Care Instructions**

**NO** Follow **Home Care Instructions**

A

## Home Care Instructions
## Abdominal Swelling

- Drink an adequate amount of fluid each day as tolerated.
- Include fruits and high-fiber foods in daily diet.
- Establish a daily routine for bowel elimination.
- Avoid gas-producing foods such as onions, cabbage, and beans.
- Exercise regularly as tolerated.
- Eat more slowly.
- May try antacids (Di-Gel, Mylanta-II, Mylicon) to help relieve gas in child >5 years of age. Follow instructions on the label. Ask pharmacist for other product suggestions. Use the dosing device that comes with the medication, a measuring device, or a medication syringe from the pharmacy. Household teaspoons often do not give the correct amount of medication.
- Consider mild OTC laxatives, and follow the instructions on the label. Ask your local pharmacist for OTC laxative or stool softener product suggestions.

## Additional Instructions

_____

_____

_____

### Report the Following Problems to Your PCP/Clinic/ED

- Problem persists >1 week
- Sharp or severe abdominal pain
- Abdominal pain, diarrhea, constipation, vomiting, or urinary retention
- Fever

### Seek Emergency Care Immediately If Any of the Following Occur

- Black or bloody stools or emesis

If the caller agrees with the advice given, document the call, and encourage the caller to call back or see PCP if the problem worsens. If the caller does not agree with the advice given, reevaluate and advise the caller to follow up with PCP, Clinic, or ED.

# Abrasions

**>> Key Questions** Name, Age, Onset, Cause, Other Injuries, Medications, Pain Scale, Prior History

**>> Other Protocols to Consider** Foreign Body, Skin (211); Laceration (290); Puncture Wound (362); Skin Lesions: Lumps, Bumps, and Sores (414); Wound Healing and Infection (509).

***Reminder:*** Document caller response to advice, home care instructions, and when to call back.

| ASSESSMENT | ACTION |
|---|---|
| **A. Are any of the following present?** | |
| • Difficulty controlling bleeding <br> • History of hemophilia <br> • Large area of the body is affected | **YES** "Seek emergency care now" <br> **NO** Go to B |
| **B. Are any of the following present?** | |
| • Unable to remove dirt or other foreign material from the wound <br> • Source is dirty and no prior tetanus immunization or immunization was >5 years ago | **YES** "Seek medical care within 2 to 4 hours" <br> **NO** Go to C |
| **C. Are any of the following present?** | |
| • History of diabetes <br> • Difficulty moving affected part <br> • Wound is 24 to 48 hours old, and signs of infection are appearing: redness, swelling, pain, warm to touch, red streaks extending from site, drainage or pus, or fever | **YES** "Seek medical care within 24 hours" <br><br> "Call back or call PCP for appointment if no improvement" <br> **NO** Follow **Home Care Instructions** |

## Home Care Instructions
## Abrasions

- Apply direct pressure over the wound with a clean bandage or cloth to control the bleeding.
- Clean the wound daily with a soapy wash cloth and rinse thoroughly with water.
- Apply antibiotic ointment 2 to 3 times daily for several days. Follow instructions on the label.
- Cover wound with dry, clean dressing for 1 to 2 days.
- Check wound daily for signs of infection (redness, swelling, pain, warm to touch, red streaks extending from site, drainage or pus, or fever).
- If dressing sticks to the wound, soak with water.
- If wound is moist looking, allow wound to air-dry for 5 to 10 minutes, then redress each day to promote healing.

### Additional Instructions

_____

_____

_____

### Report the Following Problems to Your PCP/Clinic/ED

- Signs of infection
- Delayed healing >1 week

If the caller agrees with the advice given, document the call, and encourage the caller to call back or see PCP if the problem worsens. If the caller does not agree with the advice given, reevaluate and advise the caller to follow up with PCP, Clinic, or ED.

# Alcohol Problems

**>> Key Questions**  Name, Age, Onset, Drinking Habits (amount and frequency), Hours/Days Since Last Drink, Medications, Prior History, Other Ingested Substances; Street Drugs or Pills, History of Alcohol Withdrawal, Pain Scale (If injury occurred, see appropriate injury protocol)

**>> Other Protocols to Consider**  Anxiety (18); Confusion (107); Depression (135); Diarrhea (143); Headache (238); Heart Rate Problems (249); Vomiting (492); Seizure, Nonfebrile (397); Substance Abuse, Use, or Exposure (434).

> *Nurse Alert:* Alcohol withdrawal can be life threatening. Assess for signs of withdrawal, and refer for medical care urgently before symptoms worsen if there is a history of heavy drinking and a cessation of alcohol use >48 hours.

*Reminder:*  Document caller response to advice, home care instructions, and when to call back.

| ASSESSMENT | ACTION |
|---|---|

### A. Are any of the following present combined with a history of heavy drinking?

- Seizures
- New onset of auditory (voices, buzzing, clicks), sensory (bug crawling), or visual hallucinations or delusions
- Vomiting blood or coffee-grounds–like emesis
- 24 to 48 hours after alcohol cessation and signs of withdrawal: rapid or irregular heart rate, sweating, difficulty breathing, shakiness or tremors
- Extreme anxiety, sense of terror, agitation, or paranoia

**YES** "Call ambulance" or "Seek emergency care now"

**NO** Go to B

### B. Are any of the following present combined with a history of heavy drinking?

- History of seizures or DTs with withdrawal in the past
- Desire to hurt self or someone else
- New black or bloody stools
- Acute anxiety
- Distorted perceptions
- Persistent vomiting >24 hours and unresponsive to home measures

**YES** "Seek medical care within 2 to 4 hours"

**NO** Go to C

## C. Are any of the following present combined with a history of heavy drinking?

- Upset stomach, diarrhea, heartburn, or difficulty sleeping
- Recent abrupt cessation of alcohol
- Request for help to stop drinking

 "Seek medical care within 24 hours"
and
Follow **Home Care Instructions**

 Go to D

## D. After consuming a large quantity of alcohol, are any of the following present?

- Nausea, vomiting, or diarrhea
- Fatigue
- General ill feeling
- Headache
- 12 hours after alcohol cessation and mild tremors or anxiety, anorexia, nausea or vomiting, weakness, body aches

 "Call back or call PCP for appointment if no improvement"
and
Follow **Home Care Instructions**

NO  Follow **Home Care Instructions**

### Home Care Instructions
### Alcohol Problems

- Increase intake of fluids (nonalcoholic beverages) until urine is pale yellow, which is an indicator of proper hydration (may take as long as 2 days).
- Increase intake of fruit, vegetables, potatoes, rice, cereal, whole grains, eggs, meat, poultry, and dairy products.
- Take antacids as needed for indigestion. Follow instructions on the label.
- Take vitamin B complex supplements, and follow the directions on the label.
- Exercise daily.
- Get an adequate amount of sleep.
- Do not give aspirin to a child. Avoid aspirin-like products if age <20 years. Avoid acetaminophen if liver disease is present. Avoid ibuprofen if kidney disease or stomach problems exist or in the case of pregnancy. Follow the directions on the label. Do not take acetaminophen products with alcohol; doing so can lead to liver problems.
- If the caller requests a referral or help to stop drinking, provide telephone numbers of local resources for alcohol treatment programs; counseling; detoxification programs; inpatient and outpatient treatment programs; AA; and Al-Anon.

**Referral Phone Numbers**

_____

_____

_____

**Additional Instructions**

_____

_____

_____

A

## Report the Following Problems to Your PCP/Clinic/ED

- No improvement, or condition worsens
- Increased anxiety, agitation, or depression
- Persistent tremors

## Seek Emergency Care Immediately If Any of the Following Occur

- Seizures
- Desire to harm self or someone else
- Black or bloody stools
- Vomiting blood or coffee-grounds–like emesis
- Signs of withdrawal: rapid or irregular heart rate, sweating, difficulty breathing, shakiness or tremors
- Extreme anxiety, sense of terror, agitation, or paranoia
- Auditory, sensory, or visual hallucinations or delusions

If the caller agrees with the advice given, document the call, and encourage the caller to call back or see PCP if the problem worsens. If the caller does not agree with the advice given, reevaluate and advise the caller to follow up with PCP, Clinic, or ED.

# Allergic Reaction

**Key Questions**  Name, Age, Onset, Suspected Cause, Allergies, Prior History, Medications

**Other Protocols to Consider**  Bee Stings (42); Bites, Insect (49); Breathing Problems (68); Food Allergy (192); Hay Fever Problems (235); Hives (258); Itching (282); Piercing Problems (338); Rash (366); Swelling (449); Tattoo Problems (456); Wheezing (503).

> *Nurse Alert:*  Use this protocol only if signs of anaphylaxis or if previously diagnosed with an allergic reaction and symptoms are similar. Signs of anaphylaxis, a severe life-threatening allergic reaction, can occur within seconds to an hour after exposure to the offending substance such as food, medication, a bee sting, etc. An anaphylactic reaction involves the respiratory, cardiovascular, and central nervous systems. Sudden onset of symptoms may include: difficulty breathing, feeling faint, swelling of the tongue, throat, or lips, hives, wheezing or coughing, or a feeling of impending doom. The sooner symptoms occur after exposure to the antigen, the more severe the anaphylaxis.

*Reminder:*  Document caller response to advice, home care instructions, and when to call back.

| ASSESSMENT | ACTION |
|---|---|

### A. Are any of the following present?

- Difficulty breathing
- Difficulty swallowing
- Swelling of tongue or back of mouth
- Inability to speak
- Chest pain
- History of previous anaphylaxis to same allergen
- Used Epi-Pen as instructed by provider and symptoms have not resolved

**YES** "Call ambulance"

**NO** Go to B

### B. Are any of the following present?

- Faintness or dizziness
- Change in vision
- Confusion
- Rapid progression of symptoms
- Speaking in short words
- Sudden onset of hoarseness
- Used Epi-Pen as instructed by provider and symptoms have resolved

**YES** "Seek emergency care now"

**NO** Go to C

### C. Are any of the following present?

- Swelling in face/extremities
- Persistent nausea, vomiting, or diarrhea
- Persistent rash, fever, fatigue, or headache
- Speaking in partial sentences

**YES**    "Seek medical care within 2 to 4 hours"

**NO**    Go to D

### D. Are any of the following present?

- Cause of reaction unknown
- Controlled nausea, vomiting, or diarrhea
- Mild rash/itching
- No respiratory problems
- Normal breathing
- Suspicion of medication reaction

**YES**    "Call back or call PCP for appointment if no improvement"
and
Follow **Home Care Instructions**

**NO**    Follow **Home Care Instructions**

## Home Care Instructions
## Allergic Reaction

- Use prescribed inhalers, medications, or Epi-Pen for known allergic reaction as directed by PCP. If Epi-Pen used, should seek emergency care now as symptoms may return after the medication wears off.
- If symptoms occurred shortly after taking an OTC medication, discontinue use and contact PCP.
- Rest.
- If hives are widespread, try baking soda or oatmeal baths, or OTC preparations (Benadryl, Caladryl, Cortaid, Cortizone, Claritin) for the itching. Follow instructions on the label. Ask your local pharmacist for OTC product suggestions.
- Use the dosing device that comes with the medication, a measuring device, or a medication syringe from the pharmacy. Household teaspoons often do not give the correct amount of medication.
- Avoid hot showers. Heat can increase itching.
- Apply cold cloth or ice to small area of itchy hives.

**A**

### Additional Instructions

_____

_____

_____

### Report the Following Problems to Your PCP/Clinic/ED

- Symptoms occurred after taking medication
- Symptoms persist after taking Benadryl and following **Home Care Instructions**
- Rash worsens
- Fever

### Seek Emergency Care Immediately If Any of the Following Occur

- Difficulty breathing or swallowing
- Change in vision
- Confusion
- Chest pain
- Sudden onset of hoarseness

If the caller agrees with the advice given, document the call, and encourage the caller to call back or see PCP if the problem worsens. If the caller does not agree with the advice given, reevaluate and advise the caller to follow up with PCP, Clinic, or ED.

# Ankle Injury

 **Key Questions** Name, Age, Onset, Cause, Medications, Prior History, Pain Scale

 **Other Protocols to Consider** Extremity Injury (163); Joint Pain/Swelling (287); Swelling (449).

*Reminder:* Document caller response to advice, home care instructions, and when to call back.

| ASSESSMENT | ACTION |
|---|---|
| **A. Are any of the following present?** | |
| • Bone is protruding through the skin<br>• Obvious deformity<br>• Foot is cold or blue<br>• Difficulty controlling bleeding | **YES** "Seek emergency care now"<br>**NO** Go to B |
| **B. Are any of the following present?** | |
| • Severe pain<br>• Unable to bear weight<br>• Immediately unable to walk after injury | **YES** "Seek medical care now"<br>**NO** Go to C |
| **C. Is the following present?** | |
| • Swelling, pain, limited movement or bruising continues to increase after 24 hours, despite use of ice, elevation, compression, and rest | **YES** "Seek medical care within 2 to 4 hours"<br>**NO** Go to D |
| **D. Is the following present?** | |
| • Swelling, discomfort, bruising, limited movement, which occurred sometime after the injury<br>• Persistent limping | **YES** "Call back or call PCP for appointment if no improvement"<br>and<br>Follow **Home Care Instructions**<br>**NO** Follow **Home Care Instructions** |

## Home Care Instructions
## Ankle Injury

- Apply ice pack to injured area for 20 to 30 minutes every 2 hours for the first 24 to 48 hours after the injury. Do not place ice directly on the skin. Place a thin towel or sock between the ice pack and the skin. Unopened packages of frozen vegetables work well, as does crushed ice in a sealed plastic bag.
- Elevate the ankle as often as possible for the first 24 to 48 hours.
- When the person is up and active, the ankle should be wrapped with an elastic bandage or an air splint. If the toes begin to swell or tingle or become cold, numb, or painful, remove the bandage and rewrap loosely.
- Begin to exercise ankle after 24 hours or as tolerated.
- 48 hours after injury, apply heating pad or heat pack for 10 minutes, 3 times a day.
- Take usual pain medication for discomfort. Do not give aspirin to a child. Avoid aspirin-like products if age <20 years. Avoid acetaminophen if liver disease is present. Avoid ibuprofen if kidney disease or stomach problems exist or in the case of pregnancy. Follow the directions on the label.
- Pain should improve within 3 days, swelling within 7 days. It may take up to 2 weeks to resolve.

## Additional Instructions

_____

_____

_____

### Report the Following Problems to Your PCP/Clinic/ED

- Pain becomes intolerable
- Pain, swelling, or bruising worsens after 24 to 48 hours, despite home care measures
- Moving the joint or bearing weight becomes increasingly difficult after 24 to 48 hours
- No resolution after 1 to 2 weeks

### Seek Emergency Care Immediately If Any of the Following Occur

- Foot becomes numb, cold, blue, or symptoms persist after removing bandage

If the caller agrees with the advice given, document the call, and encourage the caller to call back or see PCP if the problem worsens. If the caller does not agree with the advice given, reevaluate and advise the caller to follow up with PCP, Clinic, or ED.

# Anxiety

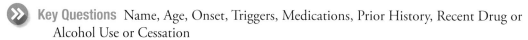 **Key Questions**  Name, Age, Onset, Triggers, Medications, Prior History, Recent Drug or Alcohol Use or Cessation

**Other Protocols to Consider**  Alcohol Problems (9); Appetite Loss (21); Chest Pain (85); Confusion (107); Depression (135); Heart Rate Problems (249); Headache (238); Substance Abuse, Use, or Exposure (434); Suicide Attempt, Threat (437).

*Reminder:*  Document caller response to advice, home care instructions, and when to call back.

| ASSESSMENT | ACTION |
|---|---|
| **A. Is chest pain present?** | |
| | **YES**  Go to Chest Pain protocol (85) |
| | **NO**  Go to B |
| **B. Are any of the following present?** | |
| • Hallucinations (auditory, tactile, or visual)<br>• Paranoia (unfounded distrust in others), new onset<br>• Confusion, new onset<br>• Suicidal threat or gesture | **YES**  "Seek emergency care now"<br><br>**NO**  Go to C |
| **C. Are any of the following present?** | |
| • Palpitations<br>• Inability to function<br>• Extreme anxiety<br>• Hyperventilation unresponsive to home care measures | **YES**  "Seek medical care within 2 to 4 hours"<br><br>**NO**  Go to D |
| **D. Are any of the following present?** | |
| • Profuse sweating<br>• Persistent upset stomach that interferes with activity<br>• Light-headedness<br>• Drug or alcohol use/abuse<br>• Recent abrupt cessation of drugs (OTC or prescription), alcohol, or caffeine | **YES**  "Seek medical care within 24 hours"<br><br>**NO**  Go to E |

### E. Are any of the following present?

- Difficulty sleeping
- History of anxiety episodes
- Chronic history of drug/alcohol abuse
- Recent onset
- Intermittent episodes
- Contributing cause, such as stress; weight loss; use of medication (including decongestants), caffeine, or tobacco; or change in job, relationships, or finances
- No physiologic or psychological symptoms

**YES** "Call back or call PCP for appointment if no improvement"
and
Follow **Home Care Instructions**

**NO** Follow **Home Care Instructions**

A

## Home Care Instructions
## Anxiety

- If the cause is known, explore ways to eliminate or reduce causative factor.
- Reduce or eliminate caffeine, tobacco, alcohol, illicit drugs, or inappropriate use of stimulants or prescription medications.
- Increase sleep, rest, and relaxation time. Rest in a dark, quiet room.
- Take a long hot bath, shower or soak in a hot tub.
- Picture yourself successfully facing and resolving the concern or conflict.
- Increase exercise, relaxation exercises, and deep breathing.
- Distract yourself watching television, a movie, reading a book, or other pleasant activity.
- Talk with a supportive person.

### Additional Instructions

_____

_____

_____

### Report the Following Problems to Your PCP/Clinic/ED
- Symptoms related to prescribed medication
- Condition persists or worsens

### Seek Emergency Care Immediately If Any of the Following Occur
- Risk of hurting self or someone else
- Hallucinations, paranoia, or confusion

If the caller agrees with the advice given, document the call, and encourage the caller to call back or see PCP if the problem worsens. If the caller does not agree with the advice given, reevaluate and advise the caller to follow up with PCP, Clinic, or ED.

# Appetite Loss

>> **Key Questions**  Name, Age, Onset, Allergies, Weight, Medications, Street Drugs, Prior History, Eating Disorder Concerns or Treatment

>> **Other Protocols to Consider**  Abdominal Pain (1); Anxiety (18); Confusion (107); Dehydration (132); Depression (135); Dizziness (147); Fainting (178); Fatigue (181); Fever (184); Heart Rate Problems (249); Vomiting (492).

***Reminder:***  Document caller response to advice, home care instructions, and when to call back.

| ASSESSMENT | ACTION | |
|---|---|---|
| **A. Is the following present?** | | |
| ● Abdominal pain | **YES** | Go to Abdominal Pain protocol (1) |
| | **NO** | Go to B |
| **B. Are any of the following present?** | | |
| ● Altered mental status | **YES** | "Seek emergency care now" |
| ● Fainting | **NO** | Go to C |
| ● Vomiting, drowsiness, irritability, and headache or stiff or painful neck | | |
| **C. Are any of the following present?** | | |
| ● Child refuses to eat or drink and looks ill | **YES** | "Seek medical care within 2 to 4 hours" |
| ● Known or suspected eating disorder, and persistent increase in dizziness and heart rate with sitting or standing | **NO** | Go to D |
| ● Signs of dehydration: | | |
|   ● decreased urination | | |
|   ● no urine for >8 hours in child <1 year of age | | |
|   ● no urine for >12 hours in child >1 year of age | | |
|   ● crying without tears | | |
|   ● sunken fontanelle | | |
|   ● excessive thirst, dry mouth | | |

## D. Are any of the following present?

- Unusual frequent urination or bed-wetting
- Nausea at sight of food, vomiting, yellow skin, fever, fatigue
- Skin persistently pale
- Dark urine and pale stools
- Persistent decrease in appetite, swollen glands, and fatigue
- Poor weight gain
- Sudden weight loss
- Severe dieting or excessive exercise and distorted body image in a teenager
- Rash or fever

**YES** "Seek medical care within 24 hours"

**NO** Go to E

## E. Are any of the following present?

- Poor eating habits
- Increased stress/anxiety
- Dry skin, brittle hair
- Recent onset of appetite loss

**YES** "Call back or call PCP for appointment if no improvement" and Follow **Home Care Instructions**

**NO** Follow **Home Care Instructions**

## Home Care Instructions
## Appetite Loss

- Encourage a balanced meal.
- Do not force child to eat when sore throat makes swallowing difficult. Encourage consumption of ice cream, flavored ice, and cold fluids.
- Avoid putting too much emphasis on food when child is ill.
- Understand that it is normal for the child's appetite to decrease around 2 years of age.
- Slowly increase amount of food after surgery or illness.
- Give acetaminophen for fever. Do not give aspirin to a child. Avoid aspirin-like products if age <20 years. Avoid acetaminophen if liver disease is present. Avoid ibuprofen if kidney disease or stomach problems exist or in the case of pregnancy. Follow the directions on the label. Use the dosing device that comes with the medication, a measuring device, or a medication syringe from the pharmacy. Household teaspoons often do not give the correct amount of medication.

## Additional Instructions

_____

_____

_____

### Report the Following Problems to Your PCP/Clinic/ED

- Nausea and vomiting
- Persistent appetite loss
- Persistent weight loss

### Seek Emergency Care Immediately If Any of the Following Occur

- Altered mental status
- Fainting
- Vomiting, drowsiness, irritability, and headache or stiff or painful neck
- Known or suspected eating disorder, and persistent increase in dizziness and heart rate with sitting or standing

If the caller agrees with the advice given, document the call, and encourage the caller to call back or see PCP if the problem worsens. If the caller does not agree with the advice given, reevaluate and advise the caller to follow up with PCP, Clinic, or ED.

# Arm/Hand Problems

>> **Key Questions**  Name, Age, Onset, Cause, Medications, Tetanus Immunization Status, Pain Scale, History

>> **Other Protocols to Consider**  Cast/Splint Problems (83); Extremity Injury (163); Numbness and Tingling (325); Weakness (496).

> *Nurse Alert:*  Immediate first aid for hand or finger amputation: Wrap amputated part in gauze moistened with saline (if available) or water and place in plastic bag. Place bag in ice bath. Do not allow to freeze.

*Reminder:*  Document caller response to advice, home care instructions, and when to call back.

| ASSESSMENT | ACTION |
|---|---|
| **A. Are any of the following present?** | |
| • Amputation | **YES**  "Call ambulance" |
| • Unable to control bleeding with pressure or spurting blood | **NO**  Go to B |
| • Bone protrudes through the skin | |
| • Altered mental status | |
| • No pulse distal to injury | |
| • Difficulty breathing | |
| • Chest pressure and pain radiates to neck, jaw, or shoulder | |
| **B. Are any of the following present?** | |
| • Fingers of affected limb cold, blue, and numb | **YES**  "Seek emergency care now" |
| • Crushing trauma | **NO**  Go to C |
| • Penetrating injury: bullet, knife, nail, etc. | |
| • High-pressure injection injury | |
| • Obvious deformity and distal pulse present | |
| • Sudden onset of arm or hand pain following physical exertion | |
| • Unable to move part of arm or hand beyond deep cut | |
| • Sudden onset of weakness in one arm | |

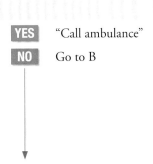
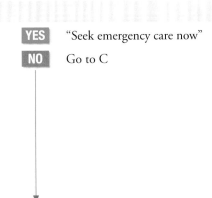

### C. Are any of the following present?

- Sudden severe swelling
- Cast or splint, and decreased color, sensation, or movement
- Deep laceration, bleeding controlled
- Sudden severe pain
- Casted extremity and pain with movement of finger

**YES** "Seek medical care immediately"

**NO** Go to D

### D. Are any of the following present?

- Moderate pain
- Swelling
- Unable to remove dirt or other foreign body from the wound
- Pain with movement
- Fever, swelling, drainage, red streaks from a wound
- Inability to make a fist
- Inability to move joint above or below injured area
- Inability to use fingers or hand
- Suspicious explanation for injury
- Gaping laceration

**YES** "Seek medical care within 2 to 4 hours"

**NO** Go to E

### E. Are any of the following present?

- Pain increasing with repetitive movement
- Gradual swelling
- Gradual bruising
- Pain with joint movement
- Laceration or puncture wound and tetanus immunization >10 years ago or >5 years if contaminated wound
- No improvement in pain or swelling >3 days and unresponsive to home care measures
- Persistent pain or swelling >2 weeks

**YES** "Seek medical care within 24 hours"

**NO** Go to F

### F. Are any of the following present?

- Chronic pain
- No known injury and pain or decreased movement >3 days
- Painful or swollen joint and limited movement
- Swelling or bruising occurred within 30 minutes of injury
- Numbness or tingling in hand at night

**YES** "Call back or call PCP for appointment if no improvement"
and
Follow **Home Care Instructions**

**NO** Follow **Home Care Instructions**

## Home Care Instructions
## Arm and Hand Problems

- Remove all rings from affected limb.
- Elevate hand higher than the heart to help reduce swelling.
- Apply ice pack (for 20 minutes at a time) to injured area to reduce swelling and pain for the first 24 hours. After that, alternate ice and heat. Do not apply ice directly to the skin; use a washcloth or other cloth barrier between ice and the skin.
- Apply compression bandage to wrist and hand and immobilize first 24 to 48 hours for swelling. If numbness or tingling occurs after application, loosen bandage.
- Rest the affected area.
- Wash wounds with antimicrobial soap and running water and cover with a sterile dressing.
- Take usual pain medication for discomfort. Do not give aspirin to a child. Avoid aspirin-like products if age <20 years. Avoid acetaminophen if liver disease is present. Avoid ibuprofen if kidney disease or stomach problems exist or in the case of pregnancy. Follow the directions on the label. Use the dosing device that comes with the medication, a measuring device, or a medication syringe from the pharmacy. Household teaspoons often do not give the correct amount of medication.

## Additional Instructions

_____

_____

_____

A

### Report the Following Problems to Your PCP/Clinic/ED

- Increasing pain
- Decreasing range of motion
- Onset of numbness or tingling
- No improvement in pain or swelling >3 days and unresponsive to home care measures
- Persistent pain or swelling >2 weeks
- Cast or splint, and decreased color, sensation, or movement
- Fever, swelling, drainage, red streaks from a wound
- Condition worsens

### Seek Emergency Care If Any of the Following Occur

- Altered mental status
- No pulse distal to injury
- Difficulty breathing
- Chest pressure and pain radiates to neck, jaw, or shoulder
- Fingers of affected limb cold, blue, and numb
- Sudden-onset arm or hand pain following physical exertion
- Unable to move part of arm or hand beyond deep cut
- Sudden onset of weakness in one arm

If the caller agrees with the advice given, document the call and encourage the caller to call back or see PCP if the problem worsens. If the caller does not agree with the advice given, reevaluate and advise the caller to follow up with PCP, Clinic, or ED.

# Asthma Problems

» **Key Questions** Name, Age, Onset, Prior Asthma History, Severity, Peak Flow Measurement, Prior Treatment, Medications, Prior History, Suspected or Known Triggers

» **Other Protocols to Consider** Breathing Problems (68); Congestion (110); Fever (184); Hay Fever Problems (235); Wheezing (503).

> *Nurse Alert:* Use this protocol only if previously diagnosed with asthma. Peak flow meters measure how well air is moving out of the lungs and help to gauge the severity of an asthma attack. Peak flow values are divided into three zones:
> Green: 80% of baseline or higher (Mild attack)
> Yellow: 50% to 80% of baseline (Moderate attack)
> Red: less than 50% of baseline (Severe attack)

*Reminder:* Document caller response to advice, home care instructions, and when to call back.

| ASSESSMENT | ACTION |
|---|---|
| **A. Are any of the following present?** | |
| • Persistent wheezing after a treatment <br> • Difficulty breathing <br> • Inability to breathe lying down; must sit up to breathe <br> • Dusky or blue lips, tongue, or face <br> • Sudden onset of wheezing after medication, food, bee sting, or exposure to known allergen <br> • Weakness, listlessness <br> • Speaking in short words <br> • Peak flow rate <50% baseline <br> • Severe wheezing or cough, and nebulizer or inhaler not available | **YES** "Seek emergency care now" "If breathing difficulty is severe, call ambulance" <br><br> **NO** Go to B |

## B.  Are any of the following present?

- Vomiting and inability to retain medication
- Upper respiratory infection symptoms and history of:
  - steroid treatment
  - prior hospitalization for same symptoms
  - intubations
- Speaking in partial sentences
- Peak flow rate 50% to 80% of baseline and no improvement using nebulizer or inhaler
- Nebulizer or inhaler used < every 4 hours

**YES**  "Seek medical care within 2 to 4 hours"

**NO**  Go to C

## C.  Are any of the following present?

- Fever >100.5°F (38.1°C)
- Cough unresponsive to asthma medication
- Minimal or temporary relief of asthma symptoms with current medications
- Yellow or green sputum
- Peak flow rate >50% to 80% of baseline

**YES**  "Seek medical care within 24 hours"

**NO**  Follow **Home Care Instructions**

A

## Home Care Instructions
## Asthma

- Increase fluid intake; consume water and clear fluids.
- Treat symptoms early to decrease severity of asthma attack. Use preventive medication as prescribed by PCP.
- Use a vaporizer, steamy bathroom, or cool damp air to help relieve symptoms.
- Follow treatment plan as prescribed by PCP.
- Avoid aspirin products and decongestants.
- Shower every night to reduce pollen exposure.
- Limit exposure to pets, particularly in sleeping areas.
- Avoid smoky and dusty areas. Encourage smokers in the home to smoke outside.
- Avoid known triggers, i.e., animal dander, body and hair products, and cleaning solvents
- If asthma symptoms are induced by strenuous exercise, take medication 90 minutes before activity (use inhaler 30 minutes before activity).

## Additional Instructions

_____

_____

_____

### Report the Following Problems to Your PCP/Clinic/ED

- No improvement after medication
- Difficulty breathing
- Prescribed treatment plan is unclear
- Peak flow rate 50% to 80% of baseline
- Nebulizer or inhaler used < every 4 hours

### Seek Emergency Care Immediately If Any of the Following Occur

- Breathing difficulty worsens
- Face, tongue, or lips become dusky or blue
- Weakness, listlessness
- Peak flow rate <50% of baseline

If the caller agrees with the advice given, document the call, and encourage the caller to call back or see PCP if the problem worsens. If the caller does not agree with the advice given, reevaluate and advise the caller to follow up with PCP, Clinic, or ED.

# Back/Neck Injury

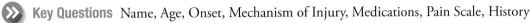

>> **Key Questions** Name, Age, Onset, Mechanism of Injury, Medications, Pain Scale, History

>> **Other Protocols to Consider** Back Pain (34); Breathing Problems (68); Headache (238); Numbness and Tingling (325); Stool, Incontinence (427); Urine, Incontinence (482); Weakness (496).

*Reminder:* Document caller response to advice, home care instructions, and when to call back.

| ASSESSMENT | ACTION |
|---|---|

### A. Did the injury result from a new traumatic event, and are any of the following present?

- Difficulty breathing or swallowing
- Severe back or neck pain
- Inability to move fingers or toes
- Numbness, tingling, or weakness in arms, legs, fingers, or toes
- Incontinence

**YES** "Call ambulance"
"Support breathing"
"Do not move person"
Follow **Emergency Home Care Instructions**

**NO** Go to B

### B. Are any of the following present?

- Traumatic event within past week and the following:
  - worsening or radiating pain
  - incontinence or impaired ability to pass urine
  - blood in urine
  - increasing or persistent weakness, numbness, or tingling

**YES** "Seek medical care within 2 to 4 hours"

**NO** Go to C

### C. Are any of the following present?

- History of cancer or bleeding disorder
- Large area of swelling or bruising >2 inches
- Impaired ability to move back or neck normally

**YES** "Seek medical care within 24 hours"
and
Follow **Home Care Instructions**

**NO** Go to D

31

## D. Are any of the following present?

- Continued mild to moderate neck or back pain unresponsive to rest, heat, ice, and pain medications
- Mild to moderate neck or back pain and home care measures not initiated

**YES**    "Call back or call PCP for appointment if no improvement"
and
Follow **Home Care Instructions**

**NO**    Follow **Home Care Instructions**

# Home Care Instructions
## Back/Neck Injury

### Emergency Instructions

- Do not move injured person; keep person warm.
- Apply sandbags, books, rolled magazines, sheets, or towels to both sides of the neck if a neck injury is suspected. Secure with tape from one support, across the forehead, to the opposite support.
- If the victim is in the water, support the body and neck as one unit until medical help arrives. Positioned at the head of the victim, the rescuer should extend his/her arms under the victim's head, neck, and shoulders, keeping the back and neck in a straight line. Do not allow the neck to bend forward, backward, or side to side.
- Apply ice packs to affected area for 20 minutes every 2 to 4 hours for as long as 48 hours after injury.
- After 48 hours, apply heat to the area for discomfort.
- Take your usual pain medication. Do not give aspirin to a child. Avoid aspirin-like products if age <20 years. Avoid acetaminophen if liver disease is present. Avoid ibuprofen if kidney disease or stomach problems exist or in the case of pregnancy. Follow the directions on the label. Use the dosing device that comes with the medication, a measuring device, or a medicine syringe from the pharmacy. Household teaspoons often do not give the correct amount of medication.
- Rest; limit activities until medically evaluated or pain subsides.

## Additional Instructions

_____

_____

_____

### Report the Following Problems to Your PCP/Clinic/ED

- Shooting pain into leg, buttocks, or arms
- Pain worsens
- No improvement in 3 days

### Seek Emergency Care Immediately If Any of the Following Occur

- Severe headaches
- Tingling, weakness, or numbness in the extremities
- Bowel or urine incontinence or inability to pass urine

If the caller agrees with the advice given, document the call and encourage the caller to call back or see PCP if the problem worsens. If the caller does not agree with the advice given, reevaluate and advise the caller to follow up with PCP, Clinic, or ED.

# Back Pain

**Key Questions**  Name, Age, Onset, Cause, Location, Medications, Pain Scale, History

**Other Protocols to Consider**  Abdominal Pain (1); Back/Neck Injury (31); Chest Pain (85); Numbness and Tingling (325); Pregnancy Problems (358); Stool, Incontinence (427); Urination, Incontinence (482); Urination, Painful (477); Abnormal Color (480); Weakness (496).

*Reminder:*  Document caller response to advice, home care instructions, and when to call back.

---

| ASSESSMENT | ACTION |
|---|---|

### A. Are any of the following present?

- Progressive weakness in legs
- New sudden onset of numbness or tingling in legs or feet or loss of bladder or bowel control
- New onset of numbness in groin or rectal area
- Dizziness, light-headedness, or abdominal fullness
- Inability to urinate for >8 hours
- Cool, moist skin

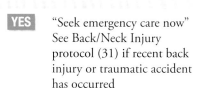 **YES** "Seek emergency care now" See Back/Neck Injury protocol (31) if recent back injury or traumatic accident has occurred

**NO** Go to B

### B. Are any of the following present?

- Severe pain
- Blood in urine
- Difficulty moving legs, feet, or toes
- Fever with nausea or vomiting in a female
- Sudden pain after a prolonged period of time in bed or a wheelchair
- New-onset, rapidly increasing pain
- Pain radiates to groin or genitals

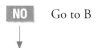 **YES** "Seek medical care immediately"

**NO** Go to C

### C. Are any of the following present?

- Pain radiates to buttocks or limbs
- Persistent severe pain
- Frequent urination or pain with urination
- Some difficulty walking because of discomfort
- No relief with OTC medications
- Fever
- History of trauma >48 hours
- History of diabetes, a weakened immune system, or steroid use
- History of cancer or unexplained weight loss
- Intravenous drug abuse
- Pain worse at night or when lying down
- Persistent loss of bowel or bladder control
- Persistent numbness or tingling in legs or feet

**YES**   "Seek medical care within 24 hours"

**NO**   Go to D

B

### D. Are any of the following present?

- History of chronic back pain, back problems, back surgery, kidney stones, or renal disease
- Mild pain without radiation or limited movement
- Fever with flu-like symptoms

**YES**   "Call back or call PCP for appointment if no improvement"
and
Follow **Home Care Instructions**

**NO**   Follow **Home Care Instructions**

## Home Care Instructions
## Back Pain

- Restrict to light activities for 2 to 3 days.
- Use a firm mattress or place a board under a soft mattress.
- Avoid activities such as prolonged sitting, lifting, or jumping until the pain is resolved (do not stay in bed).
- Take your usual pain medication for discomfort. Do not give aspirin to a child. Avoid aspirin-like products if age <20 years. Avoid acetaminophen if liver disease is present. Avoid ibuprofen if kidney disease or stomach problems exist or in the case of pregnancy. Follow the directions on the label. Use the dosing device that comes with the medication, a measuring device, or a medicine syringe from the pharmacy. Household teaspoons often do not give the correct amount of medication.
- If pain is related to an injury, apply ice packs for 20 minutes every 2 to 4 hours the first 24 hours, then moist heat.
  - Use moist heat (shower, tub, or moist hot towels) for 20 to 30 minutes every 2 hours for 48 hours, but only while person is awake.
- Sleep in a fetal position with a pillow between the knees or on the back, with one to two pillows under the knees to help reduce discomfort.
- For intermittent or chronic back discomfort, use a heating pad on the affected area 20 to 30 minutes every 2 to 4 hours. Do not sleep on a heating pad. Do not apply heating pad directly to the skin without a cloth barrier between heating pad and skin.

**Additional Instructions**

_____

_____

_____

### Report the Following Problems to Your PCP/Clinic/ED

- No improvement in 3 days
- Pain worsens
- Pain radiates into a limb, groin, or genitals
- Painful urination, frequent urination, fever, or blood in the urine

### Seek Emergency Care Immediately If Any of the Following Occur

- New onset of persistent numbness or tingling in legs or feet, or loss of bowel or bladder control, or inability to urinate for >8 hours
- Weakness in the limbs
- New-onset cool, moist skin

If the caller agrees with the advice given, document the call and encourage the caller to call back or see PCP if the problem worsens. If the caller does not agree with the advice given, reevaluate and advise the caller to follow up with PCP, Clinic, or ED.

# Bedbug Exposure or Concerns

**Key Questions**  Name, Age, Onset, Cause, Allergies, Medications, Suspect Bedbug Infestation by Presence of Bites, Shed Skins, Brown Specks or Blood Smears on Bedding, Furniture, or Carpet

**Other Protocols to Consider**  Allergic Reaction (13); Itching (282); Lice (296); Rash (366).

**B**

*Reminder:* Document caller response to advice, home care instructions, and when to call back.

| ASSESSMENT | ACTION |
|---|---|
| **A. With bedbugs visible, are any of the following also present?** | |
| • Severe itching, blisters, or hives<br>• Persistent rash and itch that interfere with sleep<br>• Rash persists after 1 week of treatment<br>• Sores spread or show signs of infection<br>• Rash clears, then returns<br>• Fever, malaise, or enlarged nodes<br>• Allergic reaction to OTC or prescribed treatment medication | **YES** "Seek medical care within 24 hours"<br>See Allergic Reaction protocol (13) if suspected allergic reaction to medication<br><br>**NO** Go to B |
| **B. With no bedbugs visible, are any of the following present?** | |
| • Red or brown spots with darker or red center<br>• Itching<br>• Multiple spots on the skin in a line or cluster<br>• New onset of flat or raised spots on the face, neck, arms, or hands<br>• Undergoing treatment for bedbugs and has questions regarding medication or preventing the spread of bedbug exposure to others<br>• Known or suspected exposure to bedbug infestation | **YES** "Call back or call PCP for appointment if no improvement"<br>and<br>Follow **Home Care Instructions**<br><br>**NO** Follow **Home Care Instructions** |

## Home Care Instructions
## Bedbug Exposure or Concerns

- If bedbug bites are suspected:
  - Inspect for insects at night when they are most active. Examine cracks or crevices in the walls, look between the mattress and box spring, and inspect upholstered furniture and behind the headboard of the bed.
  - Look for dark specks (bedbug excrement), empty light brown skins (shed before becoming an adult), and bloody smears on sheets (after bites).
- Treating the itch:
  - Apply topical hydrocortisone 1% cream sparingly for short periods of time. Do not use longer than 3 days. Ask your pharmacist for product suggestions.
  - Apply cool compresses to the area. Soak cloth in ice water then apply to skin.
  - Take OTC antihistamine (Benadryl) for severe persistent itching. Follow the instructions on the label. Ask pharmacist for additional product suggestions. Use the dosing device that comes with the medication, a measuring device, or a medicine syringe from the pharmacy. Household teaspoons often do not give the correct amount of medication.
  - Apply baking soda paste, calamine lotion, or Aveeno to the affected area.
- Treating the home environment:
  - Hire a professional exterminator. More than one treatment may be necessary as bedbugs disappear into their hiding places after consuming a blood meal.
  - Vacuum furniture, carpets, mattresses, and box springs. Vacuum thoroughly all cracks and crevices in rooms and immediately throw away the vacuum bag in a sealed plastic bag and dispose of it outside in the trash.
  - Wash clothing and linens in hot water >120°F (49°C) to kill the bedbugs. Dry the wash on medium to high heat for 20 minutes to kill bedbugs and their eggs.
  - During warm weather months, place clothing and items that cannot be washed in a plastic bag outdoors or in a car parked in the sun with the windows closed for 24 hours.
  - Place infected items in a bag in the freezer or outside when temperature is below freezing for several days.
  - Consider discarding heavily infested items such as mattress, box spring, or couch.
- Preventing bedbug infestation:
  - Cover up as much skin as possible when sleeping.
  - Inspect second-hand items before bringing them into the home.
  - Take hotel precautions: Check the mattress seams for dark specks, bloody smears, and shed skins. Check the back of the headboard and cracks in the walls. Keep unneeded clothes in zipped luggage placed on top of dressers. Do not put luggage or clothes on the floor. For further protection, zipped luggage can be kept in the bathtub overnight since bedbugs cannot climb over the side of the tub.
  - Remember that bedbugs are most commonly found in crowded lodgings with high turnover such as dormitories, hotel rooms, homeless shelters.
  - Provide reassurance that there is no known evidence that bedbugs can transmit disease.

## Additional Instructions

_____

_____

_____

### Report the Following Problems to Your PCP/Clinic/ED

- The rash disappears and then returns
- Signs of infection: redness, pain, drainage, or fever
- Questions concerning the medication for the ill, infants, children, or pregnant women
- Mild allergic reaction to the medication
- Rash itching >1 week after treatment

### Seek Emergency Care Immediately If the Following Occur

- Severe allergic reaction to medication

If the caller agrees with the advice given, document the call and encourage the caller to call back or see PCP if the problem worsens. If the caller does not agree with the advice given, reevaluate and advise the caller to follow up with PCP, Clinic, or ED.

B

# Bed-Wetting

 **Key Questions**  Name, Age, Onset, Frequency, Medications, History

 **Other Protocols to Consider**  Fever (184); Urination, Excessive (475); Urine, Incontinence (482); Weakness (496).

*Reminder:*  Document caller response to advice, home care instructions, and when to call back.

| ASSESSMENT | ACTION |
|---|---|

### A. New onset of bed-wetting and are any of the following present?

- Temperature >101°F (38.3°C)
- Pain or burning sensation with urination
- Urgency or frequency with urination
- Abdominal pain or back pain
- Blood or pus in the urine
- Nausea or vomiting

**YES** "Seek medical care within 24 hours"

**NO** Go to B

### B. Are any of the following present?

- Bed-wetting has become more frequent
- The child has previously been dry for several months or years
- Child >3 years has daytime bladder control problems
- Child >3 years soils underwear with stool during bed-wetting
- Family history of bed-wetting

**YES** "Call back or call PCP for appointment if no improvement"
and
Follow **Home Care Instructions**

**NO** Follow **Home Care Instructions**

## Home Care Instructions
## Bed-Wetting

- Encourage daytime fluids, but limit what the child drinks 2 hours before bedtime.
- Do not punish child or force child to wear diapers at night. Use waterproof underwear and thick pads or plastic cover to protect the mattress.
- Reward the child verbally or by use of a "dry night" calendar or sticker chart.

**B**

### Additional Instructions

_____

_____

_____

### Report the Following Problems to Your PCP/Clinic/ED

- Bed-wetting occurs more frequently or becomes more severe
- Child is older than 6 years and shows no improvement after following **Home Care Instructions** for 1 month
- Temperature >101°F (38.3°C)
- Urgency, frequency, or pain/burning sensation with urination
- Abdominal or back pain
- Blood or pus in urine
- Nausea or vomiting

If the caller agrees with the advice given, document the call and encourage the caller to call back or see PCP if the problem worsens. If the caller does not agree with the advice given, reevaluate and advise the caller to follow up with PCP, Clinic, or ED.

# Bee Stings

>> **Key Questions**  Name, Age, Onset, Prior Allergic Reactions, Prior Treatments, Medications, History, Allergies, Pain Scale, Prescribed an Emergency Anaphylaxis Kit

>> **Other Protocols to Consider**  Allergic Reaction (13); Bites, Insect (49); Itching (282); Rash (366); Wound Healing and Infection (509).

> *Nurse Alert:* Signs of anaphylaxis, a severe life-threatening allergic reaction, can occur within seconds to an hour after exposure to the bee sting. Sudden onset of symptoms may include difficulty breathing, feeling faint, swelling of the tongue, throat, or lips, hives, wheezing or coughing, or a feeling of impending doom. The sooner the symptoms occur after exposure to the antigen, the more severe the anaphylaxis.
>
> ● If prescribed an emergency anaphylaxis kit, instruct to use as directed by provider. Injections into outer upper thigh are usually most effective. See Emergency Home Care Instructions for additional information.

*Reminder:* Document caller response to advice, home care instructions, and when to call back.

---

| ASSESSMENT | ACTION |
|---|---|

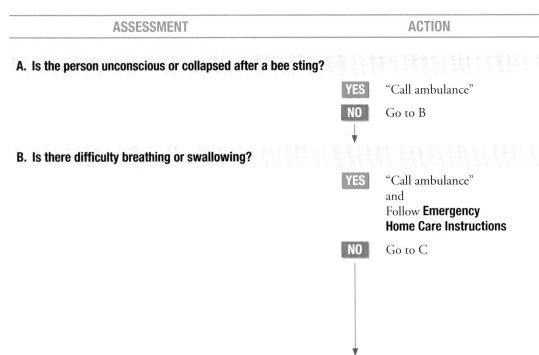

**A. Is the person unconscious or collapsed after a bee sting?**

| | |
|---|---|
| **YES** | "Call ambulance" |
| **NO** | Go to B |

**B. Is there difficulty breathing or swallowing?**

| | |
|---|---|
| **YES** | "Call ambulance" and Follow **Emergency Home Care Instructions** |
| **NO** | Go to C |

## C. Are any of the following present?

- A history of a serious bee sting reaction, such as difficulty breathing or loss of consciousness
- Bee sting in the mouth
- Swelling of tongue, throat, or lips

 "Seek emergency care now" and
Follow **Emergency Home Care Instructions**

**NO**   Go to D

## D. Are any of the following present?

- Generalized hives unresponsive to home care measures
- Itching or a rash on parts of the body other than the area surrounding the sting site, and condition is unresponsive to home care measures
- Abdominal pain, nausea, vomiting, or weakness
- More than 10 stings
- Signs of infection (drainage, fever, red streaks, or pus) >24 hours after the sting

**YES**   "Seek medical care within 2 to 4 hours" and
Follow **Home Care Instructions**

**NO**   Go to E

## E. Is there a localized reaction, such as swelling, pain, or itching around the sting site?

**YES**   Follow **Home Care Instructions**

**NO**   Follow **Home Care Instructions**

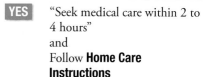

## Home Care Instructions
## Bee Stings

### Emergency Instructions

- Use emergency bee sting kit if previously instructed in use and call an ambulance.
- Take OTC antihistamine (Benadryl) to reduce allergic reaction and itching. Follow instructions on the label.
- Remove all jewelry on the affected extremity.
- If hands or feet swell because of a local sting, keep the extremities elevated to help decrease swelling.
- Try to remove the stinger if still present. Removal methods include the following:
  - Scrape the site until all of stinger is removed using a credit card, finger nails, or other flat surface.
  - Apply adhesive tape over the site and quickly pull up and off.
  - DO NOT squeeze the stinger and push more venom into the wound.
  - Wash the site with soap and water.
- Make a paste of water and meat tenderizer and apply to the wound for 20 minutes. Do not apply meat tenderizer near eyes.
- Apply cold or ice pack to the sting site for 20 minutes every 2 to 4 hours during the first 24 to 48 hours, then apply warm soaks. (Swelling may be worse on the second day.) Pain, redness, swelling, and warmth are expected immediate reactions.
- Take your usual pain medication and follow instructions on the label. Do not give aspirin to a child. Avoid aspirin-like products if age <20 years. Avoid acetaminophen if liver disease is present. Avoid ibuprofen if kidney disease or stomach problems exist or in the case of pregnancy. Follow the directions on the label. Use the dosing device that comes with the medication, a measuring device, or a medicine syringe from the pharmacy. Household teaspoons often do not give the correct amount of medication.
- Take OTC antihistamine (Benadryl) for itching, rash, or hives and follow instructions on the label. May cause drowsiness. Ask pharmacist for other product suggestions. Hydrocortisone 1% cream may also be applied topically to the area where the sting occurred.
- Apply underarm deodorant or witch hazel to the site to help reduce itching.
- Watch for signs of infection during the next few days.

Prevention: To help keep bees away from outdoor dining areas, place fabric softener towels or wasp or yellow jacket traps around the perimeter of the area.

### Additional Instructions

_____

_____

_____

### Report the Following Problems to Your PCP/Clinic/ED

- Nausea, vomiting, or weakness occurs within 24 hours
- Fever, headache, hives, swollen glands, spreading or streaking redness, or joint pain occurs after 24 hours
- Persistent pain and swelling at the sting site or foul-smelling drainage from wound after 48 hours
- No tetanus immunization, immunization status unknown, or last tetanus immunization >5 years ago
- Itching or a rash on parts of the body other than the area surrounding the sting site occurs within 24 hours

If the caller agrees with the advice given, document the call and encourage the caller to call back or see PCP if the problem worsens. If the caller does not agree with the advice given, reevaluate and advise the caller to follow up with PCP, Clinic, or ED.

**B**

# Bites, Animal/Human

**»** **Key Questions**  Name, Age, Onset, Cause, Location of Bite, Tetanus Status, Type of Animal, Immunization Status of the Animal, Medications, Pain Scale, History

**»** **Other Protocols to Consider**  Immunization, Tetanus (264); Laceration (290); Puncture Wound (362); Wound Healing and Infection (509).

> *Nurse Alert:*  Large dogs can inflict the most serious wounds, resulting in a crushing-type wound causing damage to vessels, tendons, muscles, nerves, and bones. Cat bites are at high risk for infection due to puncture wounds caused by sharp pointed teeth, pushing bacteria deep into the tissue. Hand bites have the highest rate of infection due to the relatively poor blood supply of many structures in the hand. Local infections and cellulitis are the leading causes of morbidity from bite wounds and can potentially lead to sepsis, particularly in immunocompromised individuals. Unprovoked bites from wild or sick-appearing animals (dogs, cats, skunks, bats, and raccoons) raise concern for rabies exposure.

*Reminder:*  Document caller response to advice, home care instructions, and when to call back.

| ASSESSMENT | ACTION |
|---|---|
| **A. Is the following present?** | |
| • Difficulty breathing | **YES**  "Call ambulance" |
| | **NO**  Go to B |
| **B. Are any of the following present?** | |
| • Difficulty controlling bleeding with direct pressure | **YES**  "Seek emergency care now" |
| • Deformity or inability to use affected limb | **NO**  Go to C |
| • Head, face, neck, or hand laceration | |
| • History of hemophilia | |

## C. Are any of the following present?

- Animal is not immunized for rabies or is at high risk for rabies concern (bats, skunks, raccoons)
- Animal is not available for observation
- Laceration to arms, legs, or trunk
- Signs of infection: redness, pain, swelling, red streaks from the wound, drainage, or pus
- Cat bite
- Puncture wound

 **YES**  "Seek medical care within 2 to 4 hours"

**NO**  Go to D

## D. Are any of the following present?

- Tetanus immunization status unknown or last dose was >5 years ago
- Fever
- History of diabetes or immunosuppression

 **YES**  "Seek medical care within 24 hours"

**NO**  Go to E

## E. Are any of the following present?

- Small laceration/abrasion/puncture wound

**YES**  "Call back or call PCP if no improvement within 24 to 48 hours"
and
Follow **Home Care Instructions**

**NO**  Follow **Home Care Instructions**

B

## Home Care Instructions
## Bites, Animal/Human

- Clean the area daily with a soapy cloth and rinse well with water.
- Apply your usual antibiotic ointment (e.g., Mycitracin Triple Antibiotic [bacitracin, neomycin, and polymyxin B], Neosporin, Polysporin) 2 to 3 times a day, following instructions on the label. Ask pharmacist for additional product suggestions.
- Cover the wound with a clean, dry dressing for 2 days (cleaning the wound and changing the dressing twice daily), then leave the wound open to the air, unless it is oozing blood.
- If the dressing sticks to the wound, rinse with water.
- If the wound looks moist, allow the wound to air-dry for 5 to 10 minutes, then redress it to promote healing.
- Apply ice pack for 20 minutes every 2 to 4 hours to reduce swelling during the first 24 hours. Apply heat to the area after 24 hours. Do not place ice directly on the skin; place a cloth barrier between the ice and the skin.
- Check wound daily for signs of infection. Cat and human bites become infected easily.
- Observe animal for 2 weeks for signs of rabies or illness.
- Report animal bites to animal control or appropriate authority.
- Report all bat, raccoon, and skunk bites.
- Report dog and cat bites when the following occurs:
  - Animal is sick;
  - Bite is unprovoked;
  - Animal is a stray;
  - There is no indication of rabies vaccination; or
  - Circumstances surrounding the injury are suspicious or unclear/uncertain.

## Additional Instructions

_____

_____

_____

### Report the Following Problems to Your PCP/Clinic/ED

- Signs of infection: increased pain, redness, swelling, fever, red streaks from wound, or drainage
- No improvement in 24 to 48 hours
- Sensation of foreign matter in the wound

If the caller agrees with the advice given, document the call and encourage the caller to call back or see PCP if the problem worsens. If the caller does not agree with the advice given, reevaluate and advise the caller to follow up with PCP, Clinic, or ED.

# Bites, Insect

B

>> **Key Questions**  Name, Age, Onset, Type of Insect, Allergies, Location of Bite, Medications, Pain Scale, History, Prescribed an Emergency Anaphylaxis Kit

>> **Other Protocols to Consider**  Allergic Reaction (13); Bedbug Exposure or Concerns (37); Bee Stings (42); Bites, Tick (57); Hives (258); Itching (282); Rash (366); West Nile Virus (499); Wound Healing and Infection (509).

*Nurse Alert:*  Signs of anaphylaxis, a severe life-threatening allergic reaction, can occur within seconds to an hour after a sting/bite and include difficulty breathing, feeling faint, swelling of the tongue, throat, or lips, hives, wheezing or coughing, or a sense of impending doom. The sooner symptoms occur after exposure to the antigen, the more severe the anaphylaxis.

- If prescribed an emergency anaphylaxis kit, instruct to use as directed by provider. Injections into outer upper thigh are usually most effective. See Emergency Home Care Instructions for additional information.
- If stinger is present, remove as quickly as possible to decrease toxin exposure.

*Reminder:*  Document caller response to advice, home care instructions, and when to call back.

| ASSESSMENT | ACTION |
|---|---|
| **A. Are any of the following present?** | |
| • Chest tightness or difficulty breathing or swallowing | **YES** "Call ambulance" |
| | **NO** Go to B |
| **B. Are any of the following present?** | |
| • History of severe allergic reaction to same insect<br>• Bite is from a brown recluse or black widow spider<br>• Altered mental status<br>• Sudden onset of sweating and pale skin after the bite or sting<br>• Swollen tongue, throat, or lips<br>• Bee sting in the mouth<br>• Scorpion bite | **YES** "Seek emergency care now"<br>or<br>"If the person has collapsed, is unconscious, or is in severe respiratory distress, call ambulance"<br>and<br>Follow **Emergency Home Care Instructions** |
| | **NO** Go to C |

### C. Are any of the following present?

- Sudden onset of hives, rash, itching, or swelling in areas other than the sting site
- Muscle stiffness, abdominal pain, and restlessness
- Nausea, vomiting, or abdominal cramping
- Multiple stings
- Drainage, fever, red streaks, or pus in addition to redness and swelling
- Severe pain

**YES** "Seek medical care within 2 to 4 hours"

**NO** Go to D

### D. Are any of the following present?

- Headache, chills, fever, or sweating
- Unable or unwilling to remove stinger or tick
- Peeling skin at or near the site
- Increasing redness/swelling at the site >48 hours after bite
- Diabetic and bite or sting on foot

**YES** "Seek medical care within 24 hours"

**NO** Go to E

### E. Are any of the following present?

- Persistent discomfort, itching, redness, swelling, or rash
- No tetanus immunization, immunization status unknown, or last dose was >5 years ago

**YES** "Seek medical care within 24 to 48 hours"
and
Follow **Home Care Instructions**

**NO** Follow **Home Care Instructions**

## Home Care Instructions
## Bites, Insect

### Emergency Instructions for Known Allergic Reaction

- Use emergency epinephrine kit if previously instructed in use of kit, take OTC antihistamine (Benadryl), and go to emergency department now.
- Remove entire tick promptly. Avoid crushing or squeezing. (See Bites, Tick (57) for tick removal instructions.)
- If stinger is still present, quickly remove by scraping the site until all of stinger is removed, applying adhesive tape and pulling up and off the site, or using fingernails to grasp and pull the stinger out. Wash the site with soap and water. Do not pluck or squeeze the stinger.
- Apply meat tenderizer paste to the site for 10 minutes. Do not use meat tenderizer near the eyes.
- Wash the site with mild soap and water.
- Expect initial swelling at the site. Apply cold compresses or ice packs for 20 minutes every 2 to 4 hours during the first 24 hours, then warm soaks as needed.
- Apply underarm deodorant or witch hazel to the site to help decrease itching.
- Try home remedy for itching: Apply baking soda paste mixed with white vinegar to the itchy area.
- Take usual OTC pain reliever (acetaminophen, ibuprofen) for discomfort. Do not give aspirin to a child. Avoid aspirin-like products if age <20 years. Avoid acetaminophen if liver disease is present. Avoid ibuprofen if kidney disease or stomach problems exist or in the case of pregnancy. Follow the directions on the label. Use the dosing device that comes with the medication, a measuring device, or a medicine syringe from the pharmacy. Household teaspoons often do not give the correct amount of medication.
- Take an OTC antihistamine (Benadryl) for itching, rash, or hives and follow instructions on the label. Hydrocortisone 1% cream may be applied sparingly to bites. Ask pharmacist for additional product suggestions.
- Observe for signs of allergic reaction, such as increased rash, swelling in other areas of the body, difficulty breathing, or swelling of throat.
- Watch for signs of infection: increased pain, redness, swelling, warmth, red streaks, drainage, or fever occurring approximately 48 hours after the bite or sting.
- Remember that pain, redness, swelling, and warmth immediately after the bite or sting usually are a reaction to the venom and should be expected.
- If black widow or brown recluse spider bite is suspected, collect the spider in a jar and present it for proper identification.
- If black widow or scorpion bite is suspected, apply ice pack to site for 20 minutes to reduce the spread of venom. Do not place ice directly on the skin; place a cloth barrier between the ice and the skin.

## Additional Instructions

_____

_____

_____

### Report the Following Problems to Your PCP/Clinic/ED

- No improvement or condition worsens
- Signs of infection or allergic reaction
- Rash, fever, headache, or joint pain after a tick bite
- Hives, muscle spasms, muscle weakness, or abdominal cramping

### Seek Emergency Care Immediately If Any of the Following Occur

- Altered mental status
- Difficulty breathing or swallowing (call ambulance)
- Chest tightness
- Swollen lips/tongue/throat

If the caller agrees with the advice given, document the call and encourage the caller to call back or see PCP if the problem worsens. If the caller does not agree with the advice given, reevaluate and advise the caller to follow up with PCP, Clinic, or ED.

# Bites, Marine Animal

>> **Key Questions**  Name, Age, Onset, Cause, Type of Animal, Allergies, Prior Treatment, Location of Bite, Tetanus Immunization Status, Medications, Pain Scale, History

>> **Other Protocols to Consider**  Allergic Reaction (13); Laceration (290); Puncture Wound (362); Wound Healing and Infection (509).

**B**

*Reminder:*  Document caller response to advice, home care instructions, and when to call back.

| ASSESSMENT | ACTION |
|---|---|

### A. In addition to a jellyfish or other marine animal sting, are any of the following present?

- Faintness, dizziness, or confusion
- Changes in vision
- Chest tightness, difficulty breathing or swallowing, and swollen lips or tongue
- Previous history of severe systemic allergic reaction to the same animal sting or bite
- Sudden onset of sweating and pale skin after the bite or sting
- Fast/irregular heartbeat

 **YES**  "Seek Emergency Care now" or "If the person has collapsed, is unconscious, or is in severe respiratory distress, call ambulance"

**NO**  Go to B

### B. Are any of the following present?

- Sudden onset of hives
- Stung by a Portuguese man-of-war jellyfish or stingray
- Entire arm or leg is swollen
- Severe pain interferes with activity
- Dirty or serious wound and no tetanus immunization, immunization status unknown, or if last dose was >5 years ago

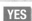 **YES**  "Seek medical care within 2 to 4 hours"

**NO**  Go to C

### C. Are any of the following present?

- Pain, redness, swelling at the sting site
- Stinger still present
- No tetanus immunization, immunization status unknown, or if last dose was >5 years ago or unknown status

**YES**  "Call back or call PCP if no improvement" and Follow **Home Care Instructions**

 **NO**  Follow **Home Care Instructions**

## Home Care Instructions
## Bites, Marine Animal

- Rinse area immediately with salt water. Do not use freshwater. For the following marine spine punctures, immerse injured part in hot salt water for 30 to 90 minutes for pain relief:
  - Catfish, coneshells, scorpion fish, sea urchins, sharks, stingrays, certain starfish, stone fish, and surgeonfish.
- Man-of-war and jellyfish: Wash site with seawater for 15 to 20 minutes. Do not use freshwater or ice.
- Leeches: Apply salt, alcohol, or vinegar to remove.
- Do not rub area.
- Apply to the sting site a solution of vinegar, alcohol, baking soda, or meat tenderizer dissolved in salt water.
- Scrape the stingers off with a towel, edge of a credit card, or sand.
- Do not touch stinger with bare hand.
- Apply a paste of sand or baking soda to help draw out the poison.
- Apply calamine lotion or hydrocortisone cream to help relieve pain and itching. Follow instructions on the label.

## Additional Instructions

_____

_____

_____

### Report the Following Problems to Your PCP/Clinic/ED
- Signs of infection, including increased or spreading redness, pain, swelling, drainage, or warmth
- No improvement or condition worsens

### Seek Emergency Care Immediately If Any of the Following Occur
- Faintness, dizziness, or confusion
- Changes in vision
- Chest tightness or difficulty breathing or swallowing
- Sudden onset of sweating and pale skin after the bite or sting
- Fast/irregular heart beat

If the caller agrees with the advice given, document the call and encourage the caller to call back or see PCP if the problem worsens. If the caller does not agree with the advice given, reevaluate and advise the caller to follow up with PCP, Clinic, or ED.

# Bites, Snake

B

**Key Questions** Name, Age, Onset, Type of Snake, Location of Bite, Prior Treatment, Medications, Pain Scale, History

**Other Protocols to Consider** Allergic Reaction (13); Laceration (290); Puncture Wound (362); Wound Healing and Infection (509).

*Reminder:* Document caller response to advice, home care instructions, and when to call back.

| ASSESSMENT | ACTION |
|---|---|
| **A. Are any of the following present?** | |
| • Bite from a poisonous snake: rattlesnake, copperhead, water moccasin, or coral snake <br> • Chest tightness or difficulty breathing or swallowing <br> • Purple rash, fever, numbness and tingling around the mouth, pale skin, or sweating after the bite |  "Call ambulance" <br>  Go to B |
| **B. Are any of the following present?** | |
| • Puncture wound or fang marks from an unidentified snake <br> • History of a reaction to a snake bite <br> • Change in mental status | **YES** "If the person has collapsed or is unconscious, call ambulance" <br> or <br> "Seek emergency care now" and Follow **Home Care Instructions** <br><br> **NO** Go to C |
| **C. Are any of the following present?** | |
| • Sudden onset of hives, rash, itching, or swelling in areas other than the bite site <br> • Multiple bites from a nonpoisonous snake <br> • Signs of infection at the bite site: redness, swelling, drainage, fever, red streaks, or warmth <br> • Severe pain and swelling around the wound <br> • No tetanus immunization, immunization status unknown, or last dose was >5 years ago | **YES** "Seek medical care within 2 to 4 hours" and Follow **Home Care Instructions** <br><br>  Follow **Home Care Instructions** and call PCP now |

55

## Home Care Instructions
## Bites, Snake

- Use emergency snake bite kit per instructions if in a remote area and medical attention is unavailable.
- Remain calm. Do not run.
- Identify snake if possible.
- Elevate and splint the affected part and seek emergency care immediately.
- Restrict movement of the affected part.
- Remove jewelry or other constricting items.
- Take your usual pain medication (acetaminophen, ibuprofen) for discomfort. Do not give aspirin to a child. Avoid aspirin-like products if age <20 years. Avoid acetaminophen if liver disease is present. Avoid ibuprofen if kidney disease or stomach problems exist or in the case of pregnancy. Follow the directions on the label. Use the dosing device that comes with the medication, a measuring device, or a medicine syringe from the pharmacy. Household teaspoons often do not give the correct amount of medication.
- Do not apply ice or a tourniquet to area.
- Expect initial swelling and pain at the site. Apply cold compresses or ice packs the first 24 hours, then warm soaks as needed. Do not place ice directly on the skin; place a cloth barrier between the ice and the skin.
- Watch for signs of infection: increased pain, redness, swelling, warmth, red streaks, drainage, or fever.

## Additional Instructions

_____

_____

_____

### Report the Following Problems to Your PCP/Clinic/ED

- No improvement or condition worsens
- Signs of infection or allergic reaction
- Purple rash, fever, headache, numbness and tingling around the mouth, bruising, or excessive sweating

### Seek Emergency Care Immediately If Any of the Following Occur

- Altered mental status
- Chest tightness
- Difficulty breathing or swallowing

If the caller agrees with the advice given, document the call and encourage the caller to call back or see PCP if the problem worsens. If the caller does not agree with the advice given, reevaluate and advise the caller to follow up with PCP, Clinic, or ED.

# Bites, Tick

**»** **Key Questions**  Name, Age, Onset, Type of Tick if Known, Location of Tick Bite, Allergies, Medications, History

**»** **Other Protocols to Consider**  Allergic Reaction (13); Foreign Body, Skin (211); Rash (366).

*Reminder:*  Document caller response to advice, home care instructions, and when to call back.

B

| ASSESSMENT | ACTION |
|---|---|

### A. Are any of the following present?

- Sudden onset of hives, rash, itching, or swelling in areas other than the bite site
- Chest tightness or difficulty breathing or swallowing

**YES** "Seek emergency care now"

**NO** Go to B

### B. Are any of the following present?

- Widespread rash, flu-like symptoms such as fever, chills, sore throat, or headache 2 to 14 days after tick bite
- Signs of infection such as redness, pain, swelling, drainage from the wound, or warmth
- History of allergic reaction to tick bites

**YES** "Seek medical care within 2 to 4 hours"

**NO** Go to C

### C. Are any of the following present?

- Unwillingness or inability to remove tick, and tick head is embedded in the skin
- No tetanus immunization, immunization status unknown, or last dose was >5 years ago
- Rash or flu-like symptoms such as fever, chills, sore throat, or headache >14 days after tick bite
- Bull's-eye rash develops around tick bite

**YES** "Seek medical care within 24 hours" and Follow **Home Care Instructions**

**NO** Go to D

### D. Is the following present?

- No attempt to remove the tick

**YES** "Call back or call PCP for appointment if no improvement" and Follow **Home Care Instructions**

**NO** Follow **Home Care Instructions**

57

## Home Care Instructions
## Bites, Tick

- Using tweezers, apply steady upward traction until the tick releases its grip (try to get a grip on its head as close to the skin as possible). If tweezers are unavailable, use fingers, plastic wrap, or paper in the same manner or tie a thread around the tick jaws and firmly pull upward.
- Tiny ticks may be removed by scraping them off with a knife edge or credit card.
- Try to avoid crushing the tick during removal or afterward. Crushing increases the chance of disease transmission.
- If the tick body is removed but the head remains, remove it with a sterile needle.
- Wash the wound and hands with soap and water and apply antibiotic ointment.
- Watch for signs of infection such as redness, swelling, pain, warmth, drainage, or fever.
- Recent studies show that ticks do not back out with the application of a hot match or when covered with petroleum jelly, fingernail polish, or rubbing alcohol.

## Additional Instructions

_____

_____

_____

### Report the Following Problems to Your PCP/Clinic/ED

- Unable to remove the tick or its head
- Rash or flu-like symptoms >14 days and up to 4 weeks after the tick bite
- Deer tick, from areas where Lyme disease is prevalent, attached >18 hours
- Signs of wound infection such as redness, swelling, pain, warmth, drainage, or fever
- Sudden onset of hives, rash, itching, or swelling in areas other than the bite site

If the caller agrees with the advice given, document the call and encourage the caller to call back or see PCP if the problem worsens. If the caller does not agree with the advice given, reevaluate and advise the caller to follow up with PCP, Clinic, or ED.

# Bottle-Feeding Problems

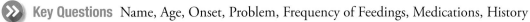

>> **Key Questions**  Name, Age, Onset, Problem, Frequency of Feedings, Medications, History

>> **Other Protocols to Consider**  Breast-Feeding Problems (63), Crying, Excessive, in Infants (128); Postpartum Problems (354); Spitting Up Infant (424).

*Reminder:*  Document caller response to advice, home care instructions, and when to call back.

**B**

| ASSESSMENT | ACTION |
|---|---|

### A. Is the bottle-feeding infant having any of the following problems?

- Respiratory distress
- Acting abnormally, extreme lethargy, or unresponsiveness
- Projectile vomiting
- Fever of ≥100.4°F in an infant less than 8 weeks of age

**YES** "Call ambulance"
or
"Seek emergency care now"

**NO** Go to B

### B. Are any of the following present?

- Infant refuses to bottle-feed because of intermittent lethargy or irritability
- Newborn jaundice (yellow skin)
- Signs of dehydration:
- fewer than six wet diapers per day by age 5 days
- fewer than three wet diapers per day after birth per day before day 5
- sunken fontanelle
- dry mouth
- more than three brick dust urinations
- Fewer than three yellow stools per day after day 5

**YES** "Seek medical care within 2 to 4 hours"

**NO** Go to C

### C. Are any of the following present?

- Infant has not urinated in ≥8 hours or passed stool in ≥24 hours
- Infant seems consistently hungry after feeding

**YES** "Seek medical care within 24 hours"

**NO** Go to D

## D. Are any of the following present?

- Parent wants to change formulas
- Infant pulls away from bottle and cries during feeding

**YES**  "Call back or call PCP for appointment if no improvement" and Follow **Home Care Instructions**

**NO**  Follow **Home Care Instructions**

## Home Care Instructions
## Bottle-Feeding Problems

- Remember that six wet diapers per 24 hours is adequate output.
- Infant should have a minimum of three yellow stools per 24 hours until the age of 6 to 8 weeks.
- Stooling decreases at 6 to 8 weeks.
- Cluster feedings (every 1 to 1½ hours) occur often during growth spurts.
- Do not give solids before infant is 4 months old and once solids are started, do not feed the infants solids from the bottle.
- Ensure that parent is mixing the formula correctly. Ready-to-feed formulas do not require that any additional water be added. Concentrated formulas are mixed in a one-to-one ratio: 1 ounce of water for every 1 ounce of formula. Powdered formulas are mixed with 2 ounces of water for every scoop of powdered formula. Use cold water to mix the formula. Warm/hot water may leach lead from pipes.
- Cow's milk and other milks not formulated for infants should not be given to infants less than 12 months of age.
- May give low-fat milk during second year of life if weight is appropriate.
- Do not give juice if age <6 months and do not give juice from a bottle.
- Babies should receive iron-fortified formula.
- Formula is supplemented with additional vitamins and minerals, so supplements are not typically needed for formula-fed infants. The exception is fluoride. If the water supply near the infant's home is not fluoridated, the parent should check with the PCP to determine if fluoride supplementation is needed.
- If infant is feeding often at night, gently stimulate and awaken the infant every 2 to 3 hours during the day.

### Sleepy Infant
- Unwrap blankets and undress infant to change diaper.
- Massage infant's legs, back, and arms.
- Give infant a back rub by walking your fingers down his/her spine.
- Try infant "sit-ups" by holding the infant away from you and gently lift him/her toward your face.
- Infant should not be allowed to fall asleep with a bottle of milk or juice. This is a choking hazard and puts the infants at risk for developing cavities or tooth decay.

**B**

## Additional Instructions

_____

_____

_____

### Report the Following Problems to Your PCP/Clinic/ED

- Condition persists or worsens
- Signs of thrush (white patches in the mouth of the infant)
- Infant has a fever or shows signs of dehydration
- Infant refuses to bottle-feed, has jaundice, or fewer than three yellow stools per day after day 5

### Seek Emergency Care Immediately If the Following Occur

- Infant has respiratory distress, extreme lethargy, or projectile vomiting

If the caller agrees with the advice given, document the call and encourage the caller to call back or see PCP if the problem worsens. If the caller does not agree with the advice given, reevaluate and advise the caller to follow up with PCP.

# Breast-Feeding Problems

 **Key Questions**  Name, Age, Onset, Problem, Frequency of Feedings, Medications, History

 **Other Protocols to Consider**  Bottle-Feeding Problems (59), Crying, Excessive, in Infants (128); Spitting Up, Infant (424).

**Reminder:**  Document caller response to advice, home care instructions, and when to call back.

B

| ASSESSMENT | ACTION |
|---|---|
| **A. Is the breast-feeding infant having any of the following problems?** | |
| • Respiratory distress <br> • Extreme lethargy or unresponsiveness <br> • Projectile vomiting <br> • Fever of ≥100.4°F in an infant less than 8 weeks of age | **YES**  "Call ambulance" <br> or <br> "Seek emergency care now" <br><br> **NO**  Go to B |
| **B. Are any of the following present?** | |
| • Infant refuses to breast-feed because of intermittent lethargy or irritability <br> • Newborn jaundice (yellow skin) <br> • Signs of dehydration: <br>   • fewer than six wet diapers per day by age 5 days <br>   • fewer than three wet diapers per day after birth per day before day 5 <br>   • sunken fontanelle <br>   • dry mouth <br>   • more than three brick dust urinations <br> • Fewer than three yellow stools per day after day 5 <br> • Pus-like drainage from the woman's nipple <br> • Woman has temperature >100°F (37.7°C), muscle aches, chills, fatigue, or headache | **YES**  "Seek medical care within 2 to 4 hours" <br><br> **NO**  Go to C |

## C. Are any of the following present?

- Mother's milk not in by day 5
- Swelling and soreness of breast that is unresponsive to home care measures
- Hard, red, warm area of breast
- Red streak on the breast tissue
- Swollen node on the same side as painful breast
- Unable to get infant to latch on for feeding
- Sudden searing, stabbing, or burning or radiating pain in breasts
- Infant seems consistently hungry after feeding
- Infant has not urinated in ≥8 hours or passed stool in ≥24 hours

**YES** "Seek medical care within 24 hours"

**NO** Go to D

## D. Are any of the following present?

- Breasts are engorged (hardness, swelling, and tenderness)
- Nipples are cracked, red, or sore
- Infant has difficulty grasping nipple and maintaining vacuum while sucking
- Infant pulls away or pushes off breast and cries during feeding
- Insufficient milk supply for breast-feeding
- Painful breasts during weaning
- Uterine cramping and increased vaginal bleeding in new mother during breast-feeding

**YES** "Call back or call PCP for appointment if no improvement" and Follow **Home Care Instructions**

**NO** Follow **Home Care Instructions**

## Home Care Instructions
## Breast-Feeding Problems

### Signs of Infection
- Apply moist hot packs to affected area 10 to 15 minutes, 4 times a day.
- Express milk manually or pump to help prevent engorgement.
- Breast-feed frequently (every 1 to 3 hours, even on affected side).
- Limit activity (encourage others to help with housework).
- Do not wean at this time.

### Engorgement
- Apply warm water compress to breast or shower before feeding.
- Massage breast toward nipple.
- Manually express milk or use a breast pump immediately before a feeding to soften the area around the nipple/areola.
- Breast-feed on both sides at each feeding.
- Wear a supportive bra.
- Apply ice packs after breast-feeding (frozen vegetable bags covered in a lightweight towel can be used).

### Sore, Cracked Nipples
- Establish rooting reflex by stroking infant's cheek and compress as much breast tissue as possible into the infant's mouth.
- Wait until the infant has a wide open mouth, like a yawn. The lips should be flanged.
- If only the nipple is in the infant's mouth, the nipple may become sore, bruised, cracked, or irritated.
- Break suction by putting a finger in the corner of the infant's mouth. Do not pull the nipple out of the infant's mouth without first breaking the suction.
- Clean the breast with plain water only. Do not use soap or antiseptic on the breast.
- A thin layer of lanolin or breast milk can be applied to the nipples after feedings. Allow nipples to air-dry briefly after each feeding.
- Rotate breast-feeding positions (cradle, football, side-lying).
- Start each feeding on the least sore side.

### Infant Has Difficulty Grasping Breast, Pulls Away, Pushes Off
- Express breast milk before feeding if breast is too full. This also helps aid letdown.
- Encourage rooting reflex and wait until the infant's mouth is wide open.
- Compress and hold the breast tissue until the infant has a good latch and starts suckling for a minute.
- Massage breast while infant's swallowing is slowing down.
- Try different breast-feeding positions (cradle, football, side-lying).

### Insufficient Milk Supply
- Remember that frequent breast-feeding stimulates milk supply.
- Try breast-feeding every 2 to 3 hours (minimum of eight breast-feedings per 24 hours).

B

- May need to awaken infant and offer breast-feeding.
- Offer both breasts at one feeding.
- Massage breast and use a warm water compress before breast-feeding.
- Encourage nutritive (active swallowing) feeding by stimulating the infant during feedings (rub back, tickle toes, touch under jaw).
- Remember that six wet diapers per 24 hours after day 5 is adequate output.
- Infant should have a minimum of three yellow stools per 24 hours from day 5 until the age of 6 to 8 weeks.
- Stooling decreases at 6 to 8 weeks.
- Sudden softening of breast at 6 to 8 weeks after delivery is normal because milk supply is adjusting and becoming efficient.
- Cluster feedings (every 1 to 1½ hours) occur often during growth spurts.
- Avoid emotional stress and anxiety and estrogen-containing birth control pills.
- Do not give solids before infant is 4 months old because solids reduce the infant's sucking and the mother's milk supply.
- Minimize use of pacifiers.
- Contact PCP or obstetrics/gynecology provider if taking estrogen-containing birth control pills.

### Uterine Cramping and Increased Vaginal Bleeding
- Cramping is normal with breast-feeding in the early postpartum period.
- Call PCP if saturating one pad per hour (bright red bleeding).
- Breast-feeding helps the uterus return to normal state faster.

### Exhaustion
- Remember that taking care of an infant is hard work.
- Try to nap while the infant naps.
- Take care of yourself by eating a well-balanced diet.
- Drink enough fluids to keep your urine light yellow.
- Take vitamins and iron supplements as directed by your PCP. Your baby may need daily vitamin D supplements starting in the first week of life.
- Avoid drugs, smoking, and drinking alcohol, and limit caffeine consumption.
- Postpartum depression may contribute to exhaustion. If depression lasts longer than 2 weeks, contact your PCP.
- If infant is feeding often at night, gently stimulate and awaken the infant every 2 to 3 hours during the day.

### Painful Breasts During Weaning
- Wear a supportive bra.
- Avoid weaning too rapidly; lengthen weaning time if needed.
- Decrease one to two feedings (at same time each day) every 2 to 4 days.
- Wait until breasts become accustomed to the change before decreasing another feeding.
- Use ice packs to reduce swelling.
- Manually express small amounts of milk or use a breast pump until a little relief is felt.

### Sleepy Infant
- Unwrap blankets and undress infant to change diaper.
- Massage infant's legs, back, and arms.
- Give infant a back rub by walking your fingers down his/her spine.
- Try infant "sit-ups" by holding the infant away from you and gently lift him/her toward your face.
- If newborn has not eaten in 6 hours and is unable to feed from the breast, feed infant pumped breast milk or formula.

**B**

## Additional Instructions

_____

_____

_____

### Report the Following Problems to Your PCP/Clinic/ED
- Condition persists or worsens
- Signs of breast infection develop
- Symptoms of breast infection persist >2 to 3 days or fever suddenly rises
- Signs of thrush (sudden breast pain in mother or white patches in the mouth of the infant)
- Infant has a fever or shows signs of dehydration
- Infant refuses to breast-feed, has jaundice, or fewer than three yellow stools per day after day 5

### Seek Emergency Care Immediately If the Following Occur
- Infant has respiratory distress, extreme lethargy, or projectile vomiting

If the caller agrees with the advice given, document the call and encourage the caller to call back or see PCP if the problem worsens. If the caller does not agree with the advice given, reevaluate and advise the caller to follow up with PCP, Clinic, or ED.

# Breathing Problems

 **Key Questions**  Name, Age, Onset, Cause, Medications, History

 **Other Protocols to Consider**  Allergic Reaction (13); Asthma (28); Chest Pain (85); Congestion (110); Cough (121); Foreign Body, Inhaled (203); Wheezing (503).

> *Nurse Alert:* Listen to the child breathing over the phone. If known respiratory problems and prescribed inhalers, $O_2$ or peak flow meters (to measure how well air is moving out of the lungs). Assess baseline functioning, $O_2$ saturation level (if caller has home oximetry device and regularly measures $O_2$ saturation levels), % oxygen delivery amount and method. Peak flow values are divided into three zones:
> Green: 80% of baseline or higher (mild attack)
> Yellow: 50% to 80% of baseline (moderate attack)
> Red: <50% of baseline (severe attack)

*Reminder:*  Document caller response to advice, home care instructions, and when to call back.

| ASSESSMENT | ACTION |
|---|---|
| **A. Are any of the following present?** | |
| • Chest pain in a child with a cardiac history <br> • Blue lips, tongue, or nail beds <br> • Slow, weak, shallow, or no respiratory effort <br> • Confusion, lethargic, decreased responsiveness <br> • Sudden severe shortness of breath <br> • History of pulmonary embolus, blood clots, or lung collapse <br> • Severe wheezing and history of asthma not relieved with inhaler <br> • Inability to speak or cry or grunting with each breath <br> • Drooling and inability to swallow <br> • Difficulty breathing after inhalation of smoke, flames, or fumes <br> • Inhalation of a foreign body and difficulty breathing | **YES**  "Call ambulance" <br><br> **NO**  Go to B |

## B. Are any of the following present?

- Difficulty taking a deep breath because of severe pain
- Severe SOB, wheezing, or noisy breathing started within past 2 hours
- Recent trauma, surgery, or childbirth
- Persistent coughing or wheezing >30 minutes after clearing an inhaled foreign body
- Exposure to something that previously caused a significant reaction (sting, medication, plant, chemical, food, or animal)
- Speaking in short words
- Inability to breathe lying down or need to sit up to breathe
- Immunosuppressed, history of sickle cell anemia or diabetes, or bedridden and temperature >101°F (38.3°C)
- Peak flow rate <50% of baseline
- Progressively worsening shortness of breath

 **YES**   "Seek emergency care now"

**NO**   Go to C

**B**

## C. Are any of the following present?

- Speaking in partial sentences
- Tight cough
- Mild audible wheezes at rest
- Pain increasing with breathing
- Upper respiratory infection and prior hospitalizations for same symptoms
- Inability to sleep >1 to 2 hours due to coughing or difficulty breathing
- Suprasternal or intercostal retractions, nasal flaring or using accessory muscles (neck muscles) to breathe
- Peak flow rate 50% to 80% of baseline

 **YES**   "Seek medical care within 2 to 4 hours"

**NO**   Go to D

## D. Are any of the following present?

- Fever
- Productive cough with gray, green, or yellow sputum
- Peak flow rate >80% of baseline

 **YES**   "Seek medical care within 24 hours"

**NO**   Go to E

## E. Are any of the following present?

- Numbness or tingling in the fingers or face
- Recent exposure to a stressful event or situation
- Exposure to environmental irritants, allergies, or recent cold or flu symptoms
- Nasal congestion
- Productive cough with clear sputum

**YES**   "Call back or call PCP for appointment if no improvement" and Follow **Home Care Instructions**

 **NO**   Follow **Home Care Instructions**

## Home Care Instructions
## Breathing Problems

- Use routine prescriptions as directed.
- If child is greater than 1 year of age, rest or sleep with head elevated on a couple of pillows if lying flat increases breathing difficulty.
- Increase fluid intake unless your physician has prescribed a fluid-restricted regimen.
- Avoid environmental irritants (smoke, smog, garden cuttings, chemicals, animals) and other irritants that seem to worsen your symptoms.
- If rapid breathing, tingling in the face or hands, and anxiety are present and patient cannot slow breathing on their own, breathe into a small paper bag held loosely around the mouth and nose for 1 minute. The problem should resolve within that time period. If it does not resolve or recurs quickly, child should be examined by PCP.
- Child should rest and relax as much as possible.
- If the problem is caused by excitement, heavy exertion (and resolved within a few minutes and there are no cardiac risk factors), or nasal congestion, there is no real cause for concern. Normal breathing should resume in a short period of time.
- Monitor peak flow rates.

## Additional Instructions

_____

_____

_____

## Report the Following Problems to Your PCP/Clinic/ED

- Condition worsens or no improvement in 2 days
- Temperature >101°F (38.3°C)
- Peak flow rate 50% to 80% of baseline

## Seek Emergency Care Immediately or Call Ambulance If Any of the Following Occur

- Chest pain in a child with a cardiac history
- Blue lips or tongue, pale or gray face
- Clammy skin
- Feeling of suffocation
- Frothy pink or copious white sputum
- Decreased level of consciousness
- Inability to speak
- Drooling, unable to swallow saliva
- Peak flow rate <50% of baseline

If the caller agrees with the advice given, document the call and encourage the caller to call back or see PCP if the problem worsens. If the caller does not agree with the advice given, reevaluate and advise the caller to follow up with PCP, Clinic, or ED.

# Bruising

**Key Questions**  Name, Age, Onset, Cause, Size and Color of Bruise, Medications (Coumadin or Aspirin History), History, Pain Scale

**Other Protocols to Consider**  Child Abuse (94); Extremity Injury (163); Eye Injury (166); Scrotal Problems (390); Swelling (449).

B

*Nurse Alert:*  Stages of Bruising:

- <24 hours since injury—red or reddish-blue skin color
- 1 to 4 days since injury—dark blue or dark purple skin color
- 5 to 7 days since injury—green or yellow-green skin color
- 7 to 10 days since injury—yellow or brown skin color
- 1 to 3 weeks since injury—normal skin color

*Reminder:*  Document caller response to advice, home care instructions, and when to call back.

| ASSESSMENT | ACTION |
|---|---|

### A. Are any of the following present?

- Severe pain and bruising on the lower back, pelvis, chest, or abdomen
- Bruising caused by a blow to the eye and
  - severe bleeding in the colored part of the eye
  - reduced or double vision
  - difficulty moving eye in all directions
  - severe pain in the eye

**YES** "Seek emergency care now"

**NO** Go to B

### B. Are any of the following present?

- Severe pain and bruising on extremities
- Severe swelling at the site
- Multiple bruises of unknown cause
- Suspected child abuse
- History of bleeding problems or use of blood thinners

**YES** "Seek medical care within 2 to 4 hours"

**NO** Go to C

**C. Are any of the following present?**

- Movement is limited
- Signs of infection: increased pain, swelling, redness, drainage, fever, heat, or red streaks extending from the area
- Frequent falls

**YES** "Seek medical care within 24 hours"

**NO** Go to D

**D. Are any of the following present?**

- Slight swelling
- Slight discomfort

**YES** "Call back or call PCP for appointment if no improvement" and Follow **Home Care Instructions**

**NO** Follow **Home Care Instructions**

## Home Care Instructions
## Bruising

- Rest involved area.
- Do not massage or rub area; this may increase bruising.
- Apply ice pack to the injured area to reduce swelling and pain for the first 24 to 48 hours. Do not apply ice directly to the skin; use a washcloth or other cloth barrier between ice and the skin.
- Elevate the affected part to help reduce swelling and bleeding.
- Apply warm moist packs for 20 minutes, 4 times a day, beginning 48 hours after injury.

**B**

### Additional Instructions

_____

_____

_____

### Report the Following Problems to Your PCP/Clinic/ED

- Severe pain
- Restricted movement
- Frequent bruising
- No improvement or condition worsens after 48 hours

If the caller agrees with the advice given, document the call and encourage the caller to call back or see PCP if the problem worsens. If the caller does not agree with the advice given, reevaluate and advise the caller to follow up with PCP, Clinic, or ED.

# Burns, Chemical

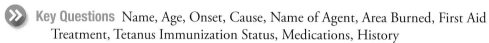

>> **Key Questions** Name, Age, Onset, Cause, Name of Agent, Area Burned, First Aid Treatment, Tetanus Immunization Status, Medications, History

>> **Other Protocols to Consider** Burns, Electrical (77); Thermal (80); Eye Injury (166); Skin Lesions: Lumps, Bumps, and Sores (414); Wound Healing and Infection (509).

> *Nurse Alert:* Important to remove substance causing the burn as quickly as possible to stop the burning process and prevent exposing other areas of the body to the causative agent.

*Reminder:* Document caller response to advice, home care instructions, and when to call back.

| ASSESSMENT | ACTION |
|---|---|
| **A. Are any of the following present?** | |
| • Difficulty breathing<br>• Altered mental status<br>• Chest pain or rapid or irregular heartbeat | **YES** "Call ambulance" and "Flush eye or skin"<br>Follow **Home Care Instructions** |
| | **NO** Go to B |
| **B. Are any of the following present?** | |
| • Eye exposed to an acid such as battery acid or caustic substance (drain cleaner, lye)<br>• Severe pain and the burned area is red, blistered, white, or charred<br>• Burns larger than the size of a hand to the face, ears, genitals, neck, hands, feet, or over a major joint<br>• Burn circles the neck or an extremity<br>• Exposed to methamphetamine lab chemicals and symptomatic | **YES** "Seek emergency care now"<br>**NO** Go to C |

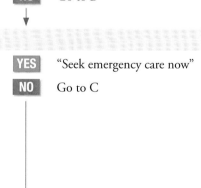

## C. Are any of the following present?

- Persistent pain >20 minutes after following home care measures
- Persistent redness, discharge, or watering of eye
- Vision changes
- Colored part of the eye appears white or cloudy
- Signs of infection develop: increased redness, pain, swelling, drainage, or warmth
- Moderate to severe pain after home treatment
- Suspected abuse
- History of impaired peripheral circulation and burn on extremity
- History of diabetes

**YES** — "Seek medical care within 2 to 4 hours" and Follow **Home Care Instructions**

**NO** — Go to D

## D. Are any of the following present?

- No tetanus immunization, immunization status unknown, or last dose >5 years ago
- Multiple open blisters

**YES** — "Seek medical care within 24 hours" and Follow **Home Care Instructions**

**NO** — "Call back or call PCP for appointment if no improvement" and Follow **Home Care Instructions**

B

## Home Care Instructions
## Burns, Chemical

### Eye

- Remove contact lens if present. Flush the eye for 15 to 20 minutes in a basin of water or under a running faucet. Position head under faucet so that water drains from inner eye to outer eye while holding lids open with fingers. Flush until pain subsides.
- After flushing, cover both eyes with a dressing or clean cloth and seek medical attention.
- Do not rub eyes.

### Skin

- Remove jewelry or shoes from burned limb before limb begins to swell. Remove clothing and flush the area with cool water for 20 minutes. Do not rub area. Cover with a dressing or clean cloth.
- Watch for signs of infection.
- Do not apply ointments, grease, butter, or pain-killing lotions.
- Take your usual pain medication (acetaminophen, ibuprofen) for discomfort. Do not give aspirin to a child. Avoid aspirin-like products if age <20 years. Avoid acetaminophen if liver disease is present. Avoid ibuprofen if kidney disease or stomach problems exist or in the case of pregnancy. Follow the directions on the label. Use the dosing device that comes with the medication, a measuring device, or a medicine syringe from the pharmacy. Household teaspoons often do not give the correct amount of medication.
- Do not puncture and drain blisters.

## Additional Instructions

_____

_____

_____

### Report the Following Problems to Your PCP/Clinic/ED

- Signs of infection
- Blisters break open
- Swelling
- No improvement in 48 hours or condition worsens
- No tetanus immunization, immunization status unknown, or last dose was >5 years ago

### Seek Emergency Care Immediately If Any of the Following Occur

- Difficulty breathing
- Chest pain
- Rapid or irregular heartbeat

If the caller agrees with the advice given, document the call and encourage the caller to call back or see PCP if the problem worsens. If the caller does not agree with the advice given, reevaluate and advise the caller to follow up with PCP, Clinic, or ED.

# Burns, Electrical

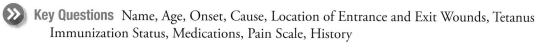

B

>> **Key Questions**  Name, Age, Onset, Cause, Location of Entrance and Exit Wounds, Tetanus Immunization Status, Medications, Pain Scale, History

>> **Other Protocols to Consider**  Burns, Thermal (80); Child Abuse (94); Confusion (107); Electrical Injury (160); Seizure, Nonfebrile (397); Wound Healing and Infection (509).

*Reminder:*  Document caller response to advice, home care instructions, and when to call back.

| ASSESSMENT | | ACTION |
|---|---|---|

### A. Are any of the following present?

- High-voltage shock
- Unconsciousness or no pulse or respirations
- Chest pain
- Rapid or irregular heart rate
- Difficulty breathing
- Burns above the neck
- Obvious entrance and exit wounds
- Burns caused by lightning

**YES** "Call ambulance" and "Start CPR or rescue breathing if no pulse or respirations"

**NO** Go to B

### B. Are any of the following present?

- Burn caused by arc or flash
- Hair singed or missing but no burn to the skin
- Burn in mouth or lip, particularly in infant or toddler
- Burn circles the neck or an extremity
- Burn over a joint
- Amnesia or any period of unconsciousness
- Thrown from electrical source and difficulty breathing, chest or abdominal pain
- Numbness, tingling, or paralysis; vision, hearing, or speech problems
- Burn to head, face, neck, hands, feet, or genital area

**YES** "Seek emergency care now"

**NO** Go to C

## C. Are any of the following present?

- Low-voltage small burn
- Pregnancy >20 weeks

**YES** — "Seek medical care immediately"

**NO** — Go to D

## D. Are any of the following present?

- >5 years since last tetanus booster or immunization status unknown
- Burns are not healing well
- Signs of infection: redness, streaks, swelling, drainage
- No other symptoms, but person or parent concerned

**YES** — "Seek medical care within 24 hours"

**NO** — Follow **Home Care Instructions**

# Home Care Instructions
## Burns, Electrical

- Stop the burning process. Remove any clothing on fire and jewelry.
- Cool the burned area with moist, clean, cool cloths.
- Do not apply ointments, grease, butter, or pain-killing lotions.
- Keep area clean and cover with clean, dry nonstick dressing.
- Watch for signs of infection.
- Take your usual pain medication. Do not give aspirin to a child. Avoid aspirin-like products if age <20 years. Avoid acetaminophen if liver disease is present. Avoid ibuprofen if kidney disease or stomach problems exist or in the case of pregnancy. Follow the directions on the label.
- Use the dosing device that comes with the medication, a measuring device, or a medicine syringe from the pharmacy. Household teaspoons often do not give the correct amount of medication.
- Do not puncture or drain blisters.
- If electrical burn is caused by an appliance, do not use until repaired. Install GFCIs to ground outlets, especially in bathrooms, kitchens, and outside. If no GFCI outlets, use GFCI extension cord.

**B**

### Report the Following Problems to Your PCP/Clinic/ED

- Burns are not healing well
- Signs of infection: redness, streaks, swelling, drainage
- Muscle pain or weakness
- Postlightning strike headache, ear pain, or memory loss
- Condition worsens or no improvement

### Seek Emergency Care Immediately If Any of the Following Occur

- Seizure
- Difficulty breathing
- Chest pain
- Numbness, tingling, or paralysis; vision, hearing, or speech problems

If the caller agrees with the advice given, document the call and encourage the caller to call back or see PCP if the problem worsens. If the caller does not agree with the advice given, reevaluate and advise the caller to follow up with PCP, Clinic, or ED.

# Burns, Thermal

**Key Questions**  Name, Age, Onset, Cause (see Burns, Chemical protocol (74) for chemical burns), Area of Burn, First Aid Treatment, Medications, History

**Other Protocols to Consider**  Breathing Problems (68); Burns, Electrical (77); Child Abuse (94); Electric Injury (160); Foreign Body, Inhaled (203); Skin (414); Sunburn (439); Wound Healing and Infection (509).

> **Nurse Alert:**  Estimate percentage of body affected. One percent of the body surface area is about the size of the palm of the hand. Instruct to remove jewelry, clothing, or other constricting clothing on affected part.

**Reminder:**  Document caller response to advice, home care instructions, and when to call back.

| ASSESSMENT | ACTION |
|---|---|
| **A. Are any of the following present?** | |
| • Extensive burn is white and painless | **YES**  "Call ambulance" |
| • Severe pain and extensive burn area is red and blistered | **NO**  Go to B |
| • Difficulty breathing | |
| • Altered mental status | |
| • Chest pain or rapid or irregular heartbeat | |
| • Singed facial or nasal hairs | |
| • Soot near nares or in mouth | |
| • Swelling at back of throat | |
| **B. Are any of the following present?** | |
| • Burn area charred | **YES**  "Seek emergency care now" |
| • Blistered or white painless burn area larger than the size of a hand | **NO**  Go to C |
| • Burn circles the neck or an extremity | |
| • Smoke inhalation | |
| • Burn over a joint | |
| • >10% body surface burned | |
| • Burn >1 square inch and located on face, eyes, ears, neck, hands, feet, or genital area | |

## C. Are any of the following present?

- Recent burn and increased redness, pain, swelling, red streaks, thick drainage, warmth, or fever
- History of diabetes
- Moderate to severe pain after home treatment and OTC medications

 "Seek medical care within 2 to 4 hours"

 Go to D

## D. Are any of the following present?

- No tetanus immunization, immunization status unknown, or last dose was >5 years ago
- Pain for >48 hours
- Multiple open blisters

**YES** "Seek medical care within 24 hours"
and
Follow **Home Care Instructions**

**NO** Follow **Home Care Instructions**

**B**

## Home Care Instructions
## Burns, Thermal

- Apply cool packs to area until pain is relieved when cool packs are removed (may take several hours). May submerge in cool water. Do not apply ice directly to the burned area.
- Do not apply ointments, grease, butter, or pain-killing lotions.
- May apply milk of magnesia, aloe vera, or yogurt for soothing effect. Ask pharmacist for additional OTC products. Follow instructions on the label.
- Keep area clean and cover with clean, dry, nonstick dressing.
- Watch for signs of infection.
- Take your usual pain medication (acetaminophen or ibuprofen). Do not give aspirin to a child. Avoid aspirin-like products if age <20 years. Avoid acetaminophen if liver disease is present. Avoid ibuprofen if kidney disease or stomach problems exist or in the case of pregnancy. Follow the directions on the label. Use the dosing device that comes with the medication, a measuring device, or a medicine syringe from the pharmacy. Household teaspoons often do not give the correct amount of medication.
- Use your usual antibiotic ointment (Mycitracin, Neosporin, Polysporin) after burn begins to heal to help prevent infection. Follow instructions on the label.
- Do not puncture and drain blisters.

## Additional Instructions

_____

_____

_____

### Report the Following Problems to Your PCP/Clinic/ED

- Increased redness, pain, swelling, red streaks, pus or cloudy drainage, or fever
- Multiple blisters break open
- No improvement after 48 hours
- Tetanus immunization unknown or last dose was >5 years ago

### Seek Emergency Care Immediately If Any of the Following Occur

- Significant decrease in urine
- Significant swelling
- Difficulty breathing
- Chest pain or rapid or irregular heartbeat

If the caller agrees with the advice given, document the call and encourage the caller to call back or see PCP if the problem worsens. If the caller does not agree with the advice given, reevaluate and advise the caller to follow up with PCP, Clinic, or ED.

# Cast/Splint Problems

>> **Key Questions**  Name, Age, Onset, Cause, Type of Cast or Splint, Location and Date Applied, Type of Injury or Surgery, History, Medications

>> **Other Protocols to Consider**  Extremity Injury (163); Itching (282); Leg Pain/ Swelling (293); Wound Healing and Infection (509).

*Reminder:*  Document caller response to advice, home care instructions, and when to call back.

| ASSESSMENT | | ACTION |
|---|---|---|
| **A. Are any of the following present?** | | |
| • Signs of poor circulation: fingers or toes cold, blue, or numb | **YES** | "Seek emergency care now" |
| | **NO** | Go to B |
| **B. Are any of the following present?** | | |
| • Severe pain, swelling, or tightness unrelieved by elevation or home care measures | **YES** | "Seek medical care within 2 hours" |
| • Signs of infection: pain, swelling, drainage, warmth, or red streaks from the wound | **NO** | Go to C |
| **C. Are any of the following present?** | | |
| • Some relief in swelling, pain, or tightness with home care measures | **YES** | "Seek medical care within 24 hours" |
| • Cracked or unstable cast/splint | **NO** | Go to D |
| **D. Are any of the following present?** | | |
| • Wet cast | **YES** | "Call back or call PCP for appointment if no improvement" and Follow **Home Care Instructions** |
| • Itching or pain without swelling in fingers or toes | | |
| • Persistent swelling or tightness that improves with home care measures | | |
| | **NO** | Follow **Home Care Instructions** |

83

## Home Care Instructions
## Cast/Splint Problems

- If cast feels too tight, elevate the part higher than the heart.
- If splint feels too tight, loosen the bandage, elevate the part, and apply ice pack to the area for 20 minutes every 2 hours for the first 24 to 48 hours.
- If cast or splint is damaged, provide support with wide adhesive tape or elastic bandage, and see PCP the next day for repairs.
- If cast or splint is wet, dry with a towel and blow dry as needed.
- If itching is present, apply a light dusting of talc powder or use blow dryer set on cold setting. Do not stick anything in the cast. Scratched skin could become infected.

**Additional Instructions**

_____

_____

_____

### Report the Following Problems to Your PCP/Clinic/ED

- Cast or splint is unstable or damaged
- New onset of pain inside the cast
- No improvement or pain worsens
- Signs of infection

### Seek Emergency Care Immediately If Any of the Following Occur

- Signs of circulation problems: fingers or toes become blue, cold, or numb
- Severe pain or swelling unrelieved by elevation or home care measures

If the caller agrees with the advice given, document the call and encourage the caller to call back or see PCP if the problem worsens. If the caller does not agree with the advice given, reevaluate and advise the caller to follow up with PCP, Clinic, or ED.

# Chest Pain

>> **Key Questions**  Name, Age, Onset, History of Cardiac Problems, Pulmonary Embolus, or Deep Vein Thrombosis, Associated Symptoms, Medications, Pain Scale

>> **Other Protocols to Consider**  Anxiety (18); Breathing Problems (68); Chest Trauma (89); Common Cold Symptoms (103); Congestion (110); Cough (121); Dizziness (147); Heartburn (245); Heart Rate Problems (249); Indigestion (273); Vomiting (492); Sweating, Excessive (446); Weakness (496).

> *Nurse Alert:*  If chest pain caused by trauma see Chest Trauma protocol (89).

*Reminder:*  Document caller response to advice, home care instructions, and when to call back.

| ASSESSMENT | ACTION |
|---|---|
| **A. Are any of the following present?** | |
| • Continuous or intermittent pain, tightness, pressure, or discomfort accompanied by: | **YES**  "Call ambulance" |
|    • shortness of breath | **NO**  Go to B |
|    • dizziness or weakness | |
|    • cool, moist skin | |
|    • nausea or vomiting | |
|    • pain in the neck, shoulders, jaw, back, or arms | |
|    • blue or gray face, lips, earlobes, or fingernails | |
|    • heart palpitations | |
| • Chest pain persists, unrelieved by rest, pain medication, antacids | |

C

### B. Are any of the following present?

- Change in chest pain pattern in known cardiac patient
- Chest pain at rest or that awakens person
- Recent period of prolonged sitting (such as traveling long distances)
- Pain, swelling, warmth, or redness of leg
- Sudden onset of swollen ankles
- Coughing up blood
- Fever, cough, congestion, and shortness of breath
- Trauma, childbirth, or surgery in past month
- History of blood clotting problems
- Recreational street drug or prescription drug abuse within past 24 hours
- Syncope

**YES** "Seek emergency care now"

**NO** Go to C

### C. Is the following present?

- Recent injury and pain increases with movement
- Chest pain with exertion that is relieved with rest
- Fracture <2 months previously

**YES** "Seek medical care within 24 hours"

**NO** Go to D

### D. Are any of the following present?

- Pain occurs with deep breathing
- Pain occurs when pressure is applied to the area
- Pain that occurs with strenuous exercise
- Intermittent mild chest discomfort with deep productive coughing

**YES** "Call back or call PCP for appointment if no improvement"
and
Follow **Home Care Instructions**

**NO** Follow **Home Care Instructions**

## Home Care Instructions
## Chest Pain

- For heartburn or GERD:
  - Take your usual liquid antacid (Maalox, Mylanta, Riopan, or other antacids) for indigestion and follow instructions on the label.
  - Liquids provide faster relief than tablets.
  - Consult with PCP if taking other medications.
  - Do not give adult Pepto-Bismol to a child. Children's Pepto-Bismol does not contain salicylates and is okay to use for heartburn.
  - Avoid eating 2 to 3 hours before bedtime.
  - Avoid activity that requires frequent bending for 2 to 3 hours after a meal.
- Take your usual pain medication (aspirin, acetaminophen, or ibuprofen). Do not give aspirin to a child. Avoid aspirin-like products if age <20 years. Avoid acetaminophen if liver disease is present. Avoid ibuprofen if kidney disease or stomach problems exist or in the case of pregnancy. Follow the directions on the label. Use the dosing device that comes with the medication, a measuring device, or a medicine syringe from the pharmacy. Household teaspoons often do not give the correct amount of medication.
- If pain is related to an injury that occurred 24 hours ago or longer and pain increases with movement, apply heat to the area for 20 minutes, 4 times a day.
- For a cough:
  - Drink 6 to 8 glasses of water daily (if no fluid restrictions prescribed).
  - Breathe steam from a shower or tea kettle with towel held over the head for 10 to 15 minutes to loosen phlegm. Younger children should be accompanied in the bathroom by a parent at all times when breathing steam from shower.
  - Elevate head of bed to reduce coughing at night.
  - Drink warm lemonade, apple cider, or tea with honey to help soothe cough. Do not give honey to children less than 1 year of age.
  - Avoid irritants such as smoking, smog, and chemicals.
  - Turn down the heat, open the windows, or go out into cooler air to help suppress cough.
  - Take cough suppressants (ask your pharmacist for product suggestions) if cough is interfering with activity, causing chest pain or vomiting, or interrupting sleep at night. Follow instructions on the label. Children with asthma should not take cough suppressants. Do not use if age <6 years.
  - Take OTC medications as needed, being sure to follow instructions on the label. Ask your pharmacist for product suggestions. Use the dosing device that comes with the medication, a measuring device, or a medicine syringe from the pharmacy. Household teaspoons often do not give the correct amount of medication.

**C**

## Additional Instructions

_____

_____

_____

## Report the Following Problem to Your PCP/Clinic/ED

- No improvement or condition worsens
- Localized area of painful blisters or rash

## Seek Emergency Care Immediately If Any of the Following Occur

- Continuous or intermittent pain, tightness, pressure, or discomfort accompanied by
  - shortness of breath
  - dizziness
  - cool, moist skin
  - nausea or vomiting
  - pain in the neck, shoulders, jaw, teeth, back, or arms
  - blue or gray face, lips, earlobes, or fingernails
  - heart palpitations
- Persistent severe pain

If the caller agrees with the advice given, document the call and encourage the caller to call back or see PCP if the problem worsens. If the caller does not agree with the advice given, reevaluate and advise the caller to follow up with PCP, Clinic, or ED.

# Chest Trauma

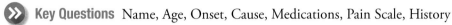 **Key Questions**  Name, Age, Onset, Cause, Medications, Pain Scale, History

**Other Protocols to Consider**  Breathing Problems (68); Chest Pain (85); Cough (121); Weakness (496).

*Reminder:*  Document caller response to advice, home care instructions, and when to call back.

| ASSESSMENT | ACTION |
|---|---|

**A. Recent injury to the chest or trunk and are any of the following present?**

- Severe shortness of breath
- Altered mental status, confusion, unresponsive
- Lips or face are blue, very pale, or gray
- Air bubbles in chest wound with inspiration
- Severe pain or bruising in chest wall or over breastbone
- Foreign object impaled in chest wall (Do not remove).
- Difficulty breathing, pain, and chest moves in with inspiration and out with expiration

**YES** "Call ambulance" and Follow **Emergency Home Care Instructions**

**NO** Go to B

**B. Are any of the following present?**

- Increasing pain with movement or breathing
- Increasing shortness of breath
- Coughing up blood or pink frothy sputum

**YES** "Seek emergency care now"

**NO** Go to C

**C. Are any of the following present?**

- Persistent pain >48 hours
- Fever
- Light-headedness develops after 24 hours

**YES** "Seek medical care within 24 hours"

**NO** Follow **Home Care Instructions**

## Home Care Instructions
## Chest Trauma

### Emergency Instructions

- For sucking chest wound, cover wound on three sides with plastic wrap or layers of tape to let air out but prevent the movement of air into the wound. Seal in place when person is exhaling.
- Do not remove objects impaled in chest.
- Take your usual pain medication (aspirin, acetaminophen, or ibuprofen). Do not give aspirin to a child. Avoid aspirin-like products if age <20 years. Avoid acetaminophen if liver disease is present. Avoid ibuprofen if kidney disease or stomach problems exist or in the case of pregnancy. Follow the directions on the label. Use the dosing device that comes with the medication, a measuring device, or a medicine syringe from the pharmacy. Household teaspoons often do not give the correct amount of medication.
- Support painful ribs with a pillow if movement increases pain.

## Additional Instructions

_____

_____

_____

### Report the Following Problems to Your PCP/Clinic/ED

- Increased difficulty breathing, fever, pain, or light-headedness

### Seek Emergency Care Immediately If Any of the Following Occur

- Altered mental status, confusion, unresponsive
- Sudden severe pain or shortness of breath
- Cool, clammy, pale skin
- Coughing up blood or pink frothy sputum

If the caller agrees with the advice given, document the call and encourage the caller to call back or see PCP if the problem worsens. If the caller does not agree with the advice given, reevaluate and advise the caller to follow up with PCP, Clinic, or ED.

# Chickenpox

**Key Questions**  Name, Age, Onset, Known Exposure to Chickenpox, Date of Exposure, Pregnancy Status, Immunization Status, Description of the Lesions and Location, History, Medications

**Other Protocols to Consider**  Breathing Problems (68); Cough (121); Fever (184); Immunization Reactions (267); Itching (282); Rash (366).

> *Nurse Alert:*
> * Use this protocol if known or suspected exposure to chickenpox or shingles within the past 3 weeks and stages of lesions have progressed from small red bumps to blisters, then brown dry scabs on several parts of the body.

*Reminder:*  Document caller response to advice, home care instructions, and when to call back.

| ASSESSMENT | ACTION |
|---|---|
| **A. Are any of the following present?** | |
| • Difficulty in awakening <br> • Confusion or delirium <br> • Difficulty breathing | **YES**  "Call ambulance" <br> or <br> "Seek emergency care now" |
| | **NO**  Go to B |

C

**B. Are any of the following present?**

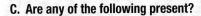

- Severe headache
- Fast breathing
- Stiff neck
- Red, painful area of skin or red streaks
- Severe pain or swelling of the face
- Child age <1 month and lesions present
- Eye pain and lesions are on the white or colored part of the eye
- Fever >104.9°F (40.5°C)
- Current/recent steroid treatment or immunocompromised

**YES**  "Seek medical care within 2 hours"

**NO**  Go to C

**C. Are any of the following present?**

- Cough or fever unresponsive to home care measures
- Vomiting more than 3 to 4 times
- Dry brown scab changes to soft and golden or drains pus
- Fever for >4 days
- Severe itching unresponsive to home care measures
- No history of chickenpox or varicella immunization and pregnant
- Secondary case within the household
- No history of chickenpox or varicella immunization and exposure to chickenpox or shingles <5 days
- Infant's mother had chickenpox <5 days before or <2 days after delivery
- Swollen and tender lymph nodes

**YES**  "Seek medical care within 24 hours"

**NO**  Go to D

**D. Are any of the following present?**

- Fever and general tiredness
- Rash with red spots and blisters

**YES**  "Call back or call PCP for appointment if no improvement"
and
Follow **Home Care Instructions**

**NO**  Follow **Home Care Instructions**

# Home Care Instructions
## Chickenpox

- Increase fluid intake. May give cold drinks to ease pain if lesions are in the mouth
- Take cool baths every 3 to 4 hours and take your usual medication (acetaminophen) for fever. Follow instructions on the label. Do not take aspirin or ibuprofen. Use the dosing device that comes with the medication, a measuring device, or a medicine syringe from the pharmacy. Household teaspoons often do not give the correct amount of medication.
- To control itching, try OTC preparations (Benadryl [oral], Caladryl, Cortaid, Cortizone [topical]) and follow instructions on the label, or take an oatmeal bath (Aveeno).
- Infected person should stay home until all lesions are dry.
- Avoid contact with pregnant women and children less than 1 year of age who have not been immunized against chickenpox.
- Keep nails short and discourage scratching of lesions
- Remember that
    - new eruptions will occur for 5 to 6 days
    - the contagious period is usually 7 days
    - symptoms occur 10 to 14 days after exposure

## Additional Instructions

_____

_____

_____

### Report the Following Problems to Your PCP/Clinic/ED

- Signs of infection: increased redness, pain, drainage, pus, red streaks
- Itching interferes with sleep
- Persistent fever >4 days
- Cough or difficulty breathing

### Seek Emergency Care Immediately If Any of the Following Occur

- Stiff neck or severe headache
- Confusion or altered mental status
- Difficulty breathing

If the caller agrees with the advice given, document the call and encourage the caller to call back or see PCP if the problem worsens. If the caller does not agree with the advice given, reevaluate and advise the caller to follow up with PCP, Clinic, or ED.

# Child Abuse

>> **Key Questions** Name, Address and Phone Number, Age, Onset, Cause, History of Abuse, Medical History, Injury Location and Description, Present Condition and Behavior of Child, Present Location of Child, Safety of Child's Present Environment, Other Children in Family or Household

>> **Other Protocols to Consider** Bruising (71); Burns, Chemical (74), Electrical (77), Thermal (80); Extremity Injury (163); Sexual Assault (400).

*Nurse Alert:*

- Children suspected of being abused should be seen immediately for an evaluation.
- Nurses are mandated by law in all 50 states to report cases of suspected child abuse.
- Stages of bruising:
  - <24 hours since injury—red or reddish-blue skin color
  - 1 to 4 days since injury—dark blue or dark purple skin color
  - 5 to 7 days since injury—green or yellow-green skin color
  - 7 to 10 days since injury—yellow or brown skin color
  - 1 to 3 weeks since injury—normal skin color

*Reminder:* Document caller response to advice, home care instructions, and when to call back.

| ASSESSMENT | ACTION |
|---|---|
| **A. Are any of the following present?** | |
| • Abuse occurring at time of call<br>• Severe injuries<br>• Unresponsive | **YES** "Call ambulance"<br>or<br>"Seek emergency care now and call police" |
| | **NO** Go to B |

## B. Are any of the following present?

- Bruises in various stages of healing or in unusual areas (such as abdomen), yellow bruises >18 hours
- Burns (such as those in a pattern [e.g., iron] or from cigarettes or hot water)
- Extremities swollen, tender, or deformed
- Suspected fractures or dislocations
- Multiple abrasions
- Bite, buckle, slap marks or any other patterned marks (e.g., belt) on face or body
- Parent wants to place child in a receiving home temporarily because of crisis or fear of abusing the child
- Caller suspects injured child is victim of abuse
- Caller or another person has thoughts about hurting the child

**YES** "Seek medical care within 2 to 4 hours"

**NO** Go to C

## C. Are any of the following present?

- Suspected child abuse but no physical signs or symptoms present
- Request to discuss suspected abuse with a health care professional

**YES** "Seek medical care within 24 hours"

**NO** Follow **Home Care Instructions**

## Home Care Instructions
## Child Abuse

- Keep in mind that a safe environment must be provided for the child.
- Refer parent or caregiver to local resources: child protective services; social services; or state health department; area housing shelters; local police; Child Abuse Registry Hotline; family services; counseling services; or crisis hotline.

## Referral Telephone Numbers

_____

_____

_____

- Follow state-mandated laws for reporting alleged abuse or neglect.
- Place a follow-up call to parent or caregiver within 1 hour.
- If caller is advised to call child protective services, place a follow-up call to the caller within 1 hour; make sure the call to child protective services was made.

## Additional Instructions

_____

_____

_____

### Report the Following Problem to Your PCP/Clinic/ED
- Child has been abused or abuse is suspected.

If the caller agrees with the advice given, document the call and encourage the caller to call back or see PCP if the problem worsens. If the caller does not agree with the advice given, reevaluate and advise the caller to follow up with PCP, Clinic, or ED.

# Circumcision Care

 **Key Questions** Name, Age, Date of Circumcision, Onset, History

 **Other Protocols to Consider** Penis Problems (331); Wound Healing and Infection (509).

*Reminder:* Document caller response to advice, home care instructions, and when to call back.

| ASSESSMENT | ACTION |
|---|---|
| **A. Are any of the following present?** | |
| • Difficulty controlling persistent bleeding at circumcision site <br> • Baby is acting weak or abnormal <br> • Head of penis dark blue or black <br> • Age <4 weeks and fever 100.4°F (38.0°C) or higher rectally | **YES** "Seek emergency care now" <br> **NO** Go to B |
| **B. Are any of the following present?** | |
| • Few drops or no urine in >8 hours <br> • Age <12 weeks and fever 100.4°F (38.0°C) or higher rectally <br> • New onset of blisters <br> • Red streaks extending down penis shaft <br> • Crying that lasts longer than 2 hours | **YES** "Seek medical care within 2 to 4 hours" <br> **NO** Go to C |
| **C. Are any of the following present?** | |
| • Swelling <br> • Discharge or drainage from the site <br> • Plastic ring remains in place >14 days <br> • Plastic ring shifted to shaft of penis | **YES** "Seek medical care within 24 hours" <br> **NO** Go to D |

C

## D. Is the following present?

- Redness at circumcision site

**YES**    "Call back or call PCP for appointment if no improvement"
and
Follow **Home Care Instructions**

**NO**    Follow **Home Care Instructions**

# Home Care Instructions
## Circumcision Care

- Apply petroleum jelly to the head of the penis every time the diaper is changed to help prevent the scab from sticking to the diaper for the first 4 days.
- Wash the penis gently with warm water and pat dry with a soft towel twice a day and when soiled. Fasten the diaper loosely to prevent friction and bleeding.
- Do not use baby wipes or alcohol to clean the circumcision site.
- Use your normal antibiotic ointments (Bacitracin or Neosporin) if the circumcision is red. Follow the instructions on the label.
- The plastic ring will fall off naturally in 7 to 14 days. Do not pull the ring off even if it is loose and barely connected.

**C**

## Additional Instructions

_____

_____

_____

### Report the Following Problems to Your PCP/Clinic/ED

- Bleeding from circumcision site
- Red streaks extending down penis shaft
- Head of penis dark blue or black
- Few drops or no urine in >8 hours
- Age <12 weeks and fever >100.4°F (38.0°C)
- New onset of blisters
- Crying that lasts longer than 2 hours

### Seek Emergency Care Immediately If Any of the Following Occur

- Age <4 weeks and fever >100.4°F (38.0°C)
- Baby is acting weak or abnormal

If the caller agrees with the advice given, document the call and encourage the caller to call back or see PCP if the problem worsens. If the caller does not agree with the advice given, reevaluate and advise the caller to follow up with PCP, Clinic, or ED.

# Cold Exposure Problems

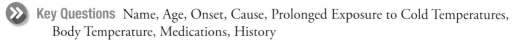 **Key Questions**  Name, Age, Onset, Cause, Prolonged Exposure to Cold Temperatures, Body Temperature, Medications, History

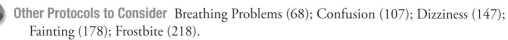 **Other Protocols to Consider**  Breathing Problems (68); Confusion (107); Dizziness (147); Fainting (178); Frostbite (218).

> *Nurse Alert:*
> - The risk of serious cold injury, especially hypothermia, is higher in people who are young, lacking in insulating body fat, abusing drugs and alcohol, smoking, suffering from cardiac disease, fatigued, or malnourished. Hypothermia can be a sign of sepsis in neonates.
> - Use Frostbite protocol (218) if there has been prolonged exposure to freezing conditions and skin changes are present.

*Reminder:*  Document caller response to advice, home care instructions, and when to call back.

| ASSESSMENT | ACTION |
|---|---|

**A. Prolonged exposure to the cold (indoors or outdoors), and are any of the following present?**

- Altered mental status or loss of consciousness
- Persistent rigid muscles
- Persistent purple fingers, toes, and nail beds
- Stumbling, poor coordination
- Impaired judgment, confusion, incoherence
- Difficulty breathing
- Temperature: <94°F (34.4°C) oral; <95°F (35°C) rectal

 **YES**  "Call ambulance"
or
"Seek emergency care now"
and
Follow **Home Care Instructions**

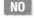 **NO**  Go to B

## B. Prolonged exposure to the cold, and are any of the following present?

- Infant, disabled, or immunosuppressed person
- Persistent pain or shivering after warming
- Cold pale skin after exposure and unresponsive to home care measures
- Faintness
- Unable to raise body temperature to normal after 4 hours of home care

**YES** "Seek medical care within 2 to 4 hours"
and
Follow **Home Care Instructions**

**NO** Go to C

## C. Prolonged exposure to the cold, and are any of the following present?

- Cold skin
- Shivering
- Wet
- Able to talk and drink fluids

**YES** "Call back or call PCP for appointment if no improvement"
and
Follow **Home Care Instructions**

**NO** Follow **Home Care Instructions**

C

## Home Care Instructions
## Cold Exposure Problems

- Remove from the cold exposure and avoid reexposure, if possible.
- Do not walk on frozen feet.
- If severe exposure is less than 24 hours, rewarm affected part in warm water for 10 to 30 minutes or apply warm wet packs. Avoid dry heat such as a heating pad or heat lamp. Stop rewarming when part is warm, red, and pliable.
- Do not place frozen part in the snow.
- Remove wet clothing and change into warm, dry clothing.
- Warm with own body and/or blankets or a sleeping bag.
- Drink warm fluids if alert and oriented.
- Eat high-energy food, such as candy, fruit, health bars.
- Do not drink alcoholic beverages.
- Do not massage frozen areas.
- Do not put cold-exposed person in front of a fireplace.

## Additional Instructions

_____

_____

_____

## Report the Following Problems to Your PCP/Clinic/ED

- Body temperature does not return to normal after 4 hours of warming
- Symptoms persist or worsen

If the caller agrees with the advice given, document the call and encourage the caller to call back or see PCP if the problem worsens. If the caller does not agree with the advice given, reevaluate and advise the caller to follow up with PCP, Clinic, or ED.

# Common Cold Symptoms

>> **Key Questions**  Name, Age, Onset, Runny or Stuffy Nose, Sore Throat, Fever, Cough, Headache, Medications, History

>> **Other Protocols to Consider**  Asthma (28); Breathing Problems (68); Chest Pain (85); Congestion (110); Cough (121); Earache (150); Fever (184); Hay Fever Problems (235); Sore Throat (420); Swine Flu (H1N1 Virus) Exposure (452); West Nile Virus (499); Wheezing (503).

*Reminder:*  Document caller response to advice, home care instructions, and when to call back.

C

| ASSESSMENT | ACTION |
|---|---|

**A. Is there difficulty breathing for reasons other than nasal congestion?**

| | |
|---|---|
| YES | Go to Breathing Problems protocol (68) |
| NO | Go to B |

**B. Is chest pain present unrelated to deep breathing or coughing?**

| | |
|---|---|
| YES | Go to Chest Pain protocol (85) |
| NO | Go to C |

## C. Are any of the following present?

- Signs of dehydration:
  - decreased urine
  - sunken eyes or fontanelle
  - pinched skin does not spring back
  - excessive thirst or dry mouth
  - crying without tears
- Fever and neck pain bending head forward
- Altered mental status, change in behavior or responsiveness
- Immunosuppressed, history of cystic fibrosis, diabetes or sickle cell anemia, or bedbound with temperature >101°F (38.3°C)
- Infant <3 months with temperature >100.4°F (38.0°C) rectally
- Child with temperature >105°F (40.6°C)
- Fever and child appears very ill
- Drooling because unable to swallow saliva
- Change in child's breathing pattern: labored, noisy, wheezing, or chest retractions >30 minutes
- Persistent wheezing unrelieved by home care measures

**YES**  "Seek emergency care now"

**NO**  Go to D

## D. Are any of the following present?

- Sore throat or fever >2 days
- Wheezing and age <4 years
- Ear pain or drainage
- Sinus pain with fever >24 hours
- Temperature <101°F (38.3°C) and history of asthma, cancer, diabetes, heart disease, or renal disease
- Honey-colored crusts in nostril or ear canal or around the mouth

**YES**  "Seek medical care within 24 hours"

**NO**  Go to E

## E. Are any of the following present?

- Blood streaks in sputum
- History of asthma, cancer, diabetes, heart disease, or renal disease
- Yellow eye drainage

**YES**  "Call back or call PCP for appointment if no improvement"
and
Follow **Home Care Instructions**

**NO**  Follow **Home Care Instructions**

# Home Care Instructions
## Common Cold Symptoms

- Do not give cold or cough medications to a child <12 years old.
- Rest.
- Drink six to eight glasses of liquids daily, especially warm liquids, such as tea with lemon and honey. Do not give honey to a child <1 year old.
- Take pain reliever of choice (acetaminophen, ibuprofen) for discomfort and fever. Do not give aspirin to a child. Avoid aspirin-like products if age <20 years. Avoid acetaminophen if liver disease is present. Avoid ibuprofen if kidney disease or stomach problems exist or in the case of pregnancy. Follow the directions on the label. Use the dosing device that comes with the medication, a measuring device, or a medication syringe from the pharmacy. Household teaspoons often do not give the correct amount of medication.
- Take decongestant of choice for congestion (unless there is a history of hypertension or the child <12 years old).
- Take expectorant of choice for cough. For child >12 years of age, give ½ tsp lemon juice or honey.
- Suction secretions from infant's nose with soft rubber suction bulb.
- Use saline nose drops as needed for nasal congestion. (For homemade saline nasal drops, add ¼ tsp regular salt to ½ cup warm water.) Place three drops in each nostril and wait 1 minute, then attempt to blow nose or suction with a soft rubber suction bulb.
- Apply petroleum jelly to nasal opening to protect from irritation.
- Use a vaporizer or humidifier to keep air moist, especially at night, and change the water daily.
- If the throat is sore, gargle several times a day with warm water. Use frozen cough drops or hard candy, if age >6 years, or sip warm chicken broth for additional relief.
- Use water to rinse red eyes and wipe with moistened cotton balls. Discard cotton ball after use in each eye.
- Clear nose of child before breast- or bottle-feeding.
- Remember that colds are very contagious and have an incubation period of 2 to 5 days. Use good hygiene, wash hands, dispose of used tissues, and cover mouth when sneezing or coughing.
- Avoid smoking and exposure to second-hand smoke.

**Additional Instructions**

_____

_____

_____

### Report the Following to Your PCP/Clinic/ED

- Persistent fever >3 days or temperature of 105°F (40.6°C)
- Nasal discharge >10 days
- Persistent earache, sinus pain, or yellow eye drainage
- Formation of honey-colored crusts under nostrils
- Productive cough or fever
- Condition persists or worsens

### Seek Emergency Care Immediately If Any of the Following Occur

- Difficulty breathing for reasons other than nasal congestion
- Severe chest pain
- Drooling because unable to swallow saliva
- Persistent wheezing unrelieved by home care measures
- Signs of dehydration

If the caller agrees with the advice given, document the call and encourage the caller to call back or see PCP if the problem worsens. If the caller does not agree with the advice given, reevaluate and advise the caller to follow up with PCP, Clinic, or ED.

# Confusion

 **Key Questions**  Name, Age, Onset, Cause, Medications, History, Pain Scale

**Other Protocols to Consider**  Alcohol Problems (9); Fever (184); Headache (238); Head Injury (242); Seizure, Nonfebrile (397); Seizure, Febrile (393); Substance Abuse, Use, or Exposure (434).

> **Nurse Alert:**  Signs of confusion may include irritability; less responsive to voice or touch; drowsiness; combative, uncooperative, nonsensical verbalizing; sudden change in behavior, thinking process, or ability to communicate; auditory (voices, buzzing, clicks), sensory (bug crawling), or visual hallucinations.
>
> • Confusion may be one of the first indicators of a fever, dehydration, an insulin reaction in a diabetic, poisoning, rapidly progressing meningitis, drug abuse, hypoxia or a head injury after trauma.

**Reminder:**  Document caller response to advice, home care instructions, and when to call back.

| ASSESSMENT | ACTION |
|---|---|
| **A. Are any of the following present?** | |
| • History of recent head trauma<br>• Exposure to chemicals or drug ingestion<br>• Diabetes<br>• Disorientation to name, date, place, or situation<br>• Fruity breath<br>• Flushing or dry skin<br>• Severe vomiting<br>• Temperature >102°F (38.9°C)<br>• Stiff neck, severe headache, rigidity<br>• Sudden weakness on one side of body<br>• Facial drooping on one side when smiling or crying<br>• Difficulty speaking<br>• Sudden change in vision<br>• Pale, diaphoretic, and light-headed or weak<br>• Ill child and sudden change in behavior; combative, uncooperative, nonsensical verbalizing | **YES**  "Call ambulance" or "Seek emergency care now"<br><br>**NO**  Go to B |

## B. Are any of the following present?

- New onset of hallucinations or paranoia
- History of drug or alcohol abuse
- Temperature >101°F (38.3°C)
- Seizure disorder
- Confusion recurs after resolving fully

**YES** "Seek medical care within 2 hours"

**NO** Go to C

## C. Are any of the following present?

- Currently taking medications known to cause confusion
- Recently taking a new medication
- Temperature >101°F (38.3°C)
- Recent abrupt cessation of drugs (OTC or prescription), alcohol, or caffeine

**YES** "Seek medical care within 24 hours"

**NO** Go to D

## D. Is the following present?

- Confusion resolved, has not returned and no change in status

**YES** "Call back or call PCP for appointment if no improvement"
and
Follow **Home Care Instructions**

**NO** Follow **Home Care Instructions**

## Home Care Instructions
## Confusion

- If taking medications that can cause delirium (antihistamines, belladonna, alkaloids), discontinue use and call back or call PCP if no improvement within 1 hour.
- Give usual medication (acetaminophen, ibuprofen) for discomfort and fever. Do not give aspirin to a child. Avoid aspirin-like products if age <20 years. Avoid acetaminophen if liver disease is present. Avoid ibuprofen if kidney disease or stomach problems exist or in the case of pregnancy. Follow the directions on the label. Use the dosing device that comes with the medication, a measuring device, or a medication syringe from the pharmacy. Household teaspoons often do not give the correct amount of medication.
- Keep person comfortable in a well-lighted room in familiar surroundings and with someone in attendance.

**C**

## Additional Instructions

_____

_____

_____

### Report the Following Problems to Your PCP/Clinic/ED
- Persistent confusion >1 hour
- Persistent confusion after fever is controlled
- Other symptoms are present after delirium clears

### Seek Emergency Care Immediately If Any of the Following Occur
- Severe headache or stiff neck or rigidity
- Sudden weakness on one side of body
- Difficulty speaking
- Pale, diaphoretic, and light-headed or weak
- Hallucination, paranoia, or suicidal threat or attempt
- Ill child and sudden change in behavior
- Severe vomiting
- Fruity breath
- Flushing or dry skin

If the caller agrees with the advice given, document the call and encourage the caller to call back or see PCP if the problem worsens. If the caller does not agree with the advice given, reevaluate and advise the caller to follow up with PCP, Clinic, or ED.

# Congestion

 **Key Questions** Name, Age, Onset, Prior Treatment, Medications, History

 **Other Protocols to Consider** Asthma (28); Breathing Problems (68); Chest Pain (85); Common Cold Symptoms (103); Cough (121); Earache, Drainage (150); Fever (184); Hay Fever Problems (235); Influenza (276); Sinus Problems (411); Sore Throat (420); Swine Flu (H1N1 Virus) Exposure (452); Wheezing (503).

*Reminder:* Document caller response to advice, home care instructions, and when to call back.

| ASSESSMENT | ACTION |
|---|---|
| **A. Is there difficulty breathing for reasons other than nasal congestion?** | |
| | **YES** Go to Breathing Problems protocol (68) |
| | **NO** Go to B |
| **B. Is chest pain present?** | |
| | **YES** Go to Chest Pain protocol (85) |
| | **NO** Go to C |
| **C. Is wheezing present?** | |
| | **YES** Wheezing protocol (503) |
| | **NO** Go to D |

## D. Are any of the following present?

- Fever >101°F (38.3°C) and bedridden, or weakened immune system
- Fever >100.4°F (38.0°C) rectally and age <3 months
- Child appears very ill
- Young child with signs of dehydration:
  - sunken eyes or fontanelle
  - pinched skin that does not spring back
  - infant cries without tears
- severe pain, swelling, or redness of the upper part of the face

**YES**  "Seek emergency care now"

**NO**  Go to D

## E. Are any of the following present?

- Several signs of dehydration:
  - infrequent urination
  - dark yellow urine
  - sunken eyes
  - pinched skin that does not spring back
  - excessive thirst
  - dry mouth or mucous membranes
- Severe pain, swelling, or redness of the upper part of the face

**YES**  "Seek medical care within 2 to 4 hours"

**NO**  Go to F

## F. Are any of the following present?

- Sore throat or fever >2 days
- Persistent fever >100.4°F (38.0°C) >3 days
- Weakness and listlessness
- Wheezing and younger than 4 years
- Ear pain or drainage
- History of asthma, cancer, diabetes, renal disease, or weakened immune system
- Persistent pain >24 hours after home care

**YES**  "Seek medical care within 24 hours"

**NO**  Go to G

## G. Are any of the following present?

- Blood streaks in sputum
- Persistent sinus congestion >7 days after home care

**YES**  "Call back or call PCP for appointment if no improvement"
and
Follow **Home Care Instructions**

**NO**  Follow **Home Care Instructions**

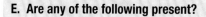

## Home Care Instructions
## Congestion

- Do not give cold or cough medications to a child <12 years old.
- Rest and drink six to eight glasses of water a day. Warm liquids, such as tea with lemon and honey, are also soothing. Do not give honey to a child <1 year old.
- Give usual medication (acetaminophen, ibuprofen) for discomfort and fever. Do not give aspirin to a child. Avoid aspirin-like products if age <20 years. Avoid acetaminophen if liver disease is present. Avoid ibuprofen if kidney disease or stomach problems exist or in the case of pregnancy. Follow the directions on the label. Use the dosing device that comes with the medication, a measuring device, or a medication syringe from the pharmacy. Household teaspoons often do not give the correct amount of medication.
- Try a vaporizer, a humidifier, or a hot steamy shower and saline nose drops; if no relief occurs, try decongestants if age >12 years (ask the pharmacist for product suggestions) for congestion. Follow the instructions on the label. (Many decongestants are contraindicated if there is a history of hypertension, asthma, heart disease, glaucoma, or enlarged prostate.)
- For sinus pain, inhale the vapor of peppermint tea. Peppermint has anti-inflammatory compounds and pain relievers like menthol that relax constricted sinuses.
- Take an expectorant if age >12 years (ask your pharmacist for product suggestions) for cough. Follow the instructions on the label.
- Try antihistamine if congestion is due to allergy.
- Use saline nose drops as needed for nasal congestion. (For homemade saline nasal drops, add ¼ tsp of regular salt to ½ cup of warm water.) Blow each nostril separately.
- Use a vaporizer or humidifier to keep the air moist, especially at night, and change the water daily.
- If the throat is sore, gargle several times a day with warm water. Use frozen cough drops for additional relief if age >6 years.
- Remember that infants <3 months old often have congestion. Use saline nose drops and a humidifier to reduce congestion. Suction secretions from the infant's nose with a soft rubber suction bulb.
- Apply petroleum jelly to the nasal opening to protect it from irritation.
- Clear the child's nose before breast- or bottle-feeding.
- Remember, colds are contagious; use good hygiene, wash hands, and dispose of used tissues. Cover the mouth with a tissue or inside the elbow sleeve when sneezing or coughing.
- Avoid smoking or exposure to second-hand smoke.

## Additional Instructions

_____

_____

_____

### Report the Following to Your PCP/Clinic/ED

- Persistent temperature >101°F (38.3°C) and age >4 months
- Sore throat >2 days
- Persistent earache, sinus pain, or yellow eye drainage
- Chest pain
- Severe pain, swelling, or redness of the upper part of the face
- Difficulty breathing
- Fever >100.4°F (38.0°C) rectally and age <3 months

### Seek Emergency Care Immediately If Any of the Following Occur

- Chest pain unrelated to coughing or deep breathing
- Difficulty breathing for reasons other than congestion
- Young child with signs of dehydration

C

If the caller agrees with the advice given, document the call and encourage the caller to call back or see PCP if the problem worsens. If the caller does not agree with the advice given, reevaluate and advise the caller to follow up with PCP, Clinic, or ED.

# Constipation

>> **Key Questions**  Name, Age, Onset, Last Bowel Movement, Medications, History, Pain Scale

>> **Other Protocols to Consider**  Abdominal Pain (1); Abdominal Swelling (4); Diarrhea (143); Foreign Body, Rectum (209); Vomiting (492); Rectal Bleeding (371); Rectal Problems (374).

***Reminder:***  Document caller response to advice, home care instructions, and when to call back.

| ASSESSMENT | ACTION |
|---|---|

### A. Is the following present?

- Severe abdominal pain, swelling, or vomiting

**YES** "Seek emergency care now"

**NO** Go to B

### B. Are any of the following present?

- Persistent vomiting and progressive abdominal swelling
- Severe pain or cramping
- Vomiting brown, yellow, or green bitter-tasting emesis
- Significant rectal bleeding with no history of hemorrhoids or bleeding with constipation
- Infant <1 month, breast-feeding, and signs of dehydration

**YES** "Seek medical care within 2 to 4 hours"

**NO** Go to C

### C. Are any of the following present?

- No bowel movement in 3 days and constipation unresponsive to home care measures
- Recent surgery, injury, or childbirth
- Exclusively breast-fed infant (greater than 1 month of age) has no stool for >6 days
- Child/infant crying, bloating, passing hard stools, and not responding to home care measures
- Fever for 24 to 48 hours, cause unknown
- Infant younger than 2 months had first stool after 24 hours and is now constipated

**YES** "Seek medical care within 24 hours"

**NO** Go to D

## D. Are any of the following present?

- Dry hard stools
- Pain with bowel movements
- Recent change in stools or bowel habits
- Chronic constipation
- Small, frequently occurring, liquid or hard stools
- Intermittent constipation
- Recent decrease in activity or bed rest
- Taking pain medications with codeine or other medications that increase constipation
- Blood on tissue or surface of stool
- Leaking stool

**YES** "Call back or call PCP for appointment if no improvement"
and
Follow **Home Care Instructions**

**NO** Follow **Home Care Instructions**

C

## Home Care Instructions
## Constipation

- Make sure diet is adequate in volume (quantity), bulk (high fiber), and fluids (6 to 8 [8 ounce] glasses a day, unless on a restricted fluid diet).
- Drink a hot beverage each morning, such as tea, or hot water with lemon.
- Establish a regular time for privacy and elimination each day.
- Increase exercise as tolerated.
- Infants:
  - For infants >1 month, if the infant is drinking juice, give prune or apricot juice mixed with water to help relieve constipation (no more than 1 ounce per day). Do not give enemas or laxatives.
  - For infants >2 months, give fruit juice (1 ounce per month of age, each day).
  - For infants >4 months, add baby foods high in fiber such as prunes, plums, peaches, pears, or sweet potatoes.
- Children: Increase fruit juice and decrease milk to 16 ounces a day. Increase high-fiber foods, such as bran cereals, oatmeal, bran muffins, or popcorn (if child >4 years).
- May use an OTC laxative such as Miralax, which can be mixed with any fluid. (Read directions on container label before administering.)
- For rectal pain due to constipation, sit in a warm bath for 20 minutes.
- For painful and bleeding hemorrhoids, sit in a warm tub of water after each bowel movement. Try OTC medications for hemorrhoids.

## Additional Instructions

_____

_____

_____

## Report the Following Problems to Your PCP/Clinic/ED

- Condition persists or worsens
- Fever, vomiting, and pain
- Home care measures are ineffective

## Seek Emergency Care Immediately If Any of the Following Occur

- Severe abdominal pain, swelling, or vomiting

If the caller agrees with the advice given, document the call and encourage the caller to call back or see PCP if the problem worsens. If the caller does not agree with the advice given, reevaluate and advise the caller to follow up with PCP, Clinic, or ED.

# Contraception, Emergency

>> **Key Questions**  Name, Age, Onset (number of hours since last unprotected intercourse), Cause, Medications, Birth Control History, Other Symptoms

>> **Other Protocols to Consider**  Foreign Body, Rectum (209), Foreign Body, Vagina (216); Sexual Assault (400); Sexually Transmitted Disease (STD); Vaginal Bleeding (484); Vaginal Discharge/Pain/Itching (486).

*Reminder:*  Document caller response to advice, home care instructions, and when to call back.

C

| ASSESSMENT | ACTION |
|---|---|
| **A. Are any of the following present?** | |
| • Recently taken emergency contraception (EC) pills and signs of allergic reaction (difficulty breathing or swallowing, sudden throat or tongue swelling, inability to speak, or chest pain) | **YES** "Go to Allergic Reaction protocol (13)"  <br> **NO** Go to B |
| **B. Has sexual assault occurred with any of the following present?** | |
| • Vaginal or anal tears or bleeding <br> • Request for sexual assault examination and evidence collection <br> • Victim is a minor | **YES** "Seek emergency care now" and "Do not shower or change clothes to allow for evidence collection"  <br> **NO** Go to C |
| **C. Are any of the following present?** | |
| • Sexual assault or forced sex occurred and medical examination without collection of evidence has been requested <br> • Unprotected intercourse occurred <120 hours (5 days) and person requests protection for sexually transmitted disease and pregnancy <br> • Copper IUD as EC has been requested; unprotected intercourse has occurred within past 5 days | **YES** "Seek medical care within 24 hours"  <br> **NO** Go to D |

## D. Are any of the following present?

- Questions or concerns about EC
- Unprotected sex >120 hours and person has concerns about pregnancy
- EC pills taken and concerns about side effects exist; or person has nausea/vomiting, abdominal pain, dizziness, fatigue, headache, menstrual changes, or breast tenderness

**YES** "Call back or call PCP for appointment if no improvement"
and
Follow **Home Care Instructions**

**NO** Follow **Home Care Instructions**

## Home Care Instructions
## Emergency Contraception

- Provide reassurance and general information:
  - Emergency contraception (EC) pills are for emergencies and should not be used for ongoing contraception.
  - EC pills do not protect against sexually transmitted diseases.
  - EC pills are most effective in the first 72 hours but can be taken up to 120 hours after unprotected sex. (The EC product "Next Choice" is taken within 72 hours [telephone 866-9WATSON]. "Plan B" is taken within 120 hours. [1-888-not-2-late or 1-668-2-5283].)
  - EC can be obtained without a prescription from select pharmacies if age is 16 years or older (some states may vary in age restrictions). If age <16 years or younger, a prescription is required. Check with your pharmacy for any age requirements.
  - Additional information about EC can be located at http://ec.princeton.edu or at the hotline 1-888-not-2-late (1-668-2-5283).
  - If pregnancy is a concern, advice a urine pregnancy test be taken. Urine pregnancy tests can be purchased at most drug stores and many markets with pharmacy products.
- To prevent nausea and vomiting, Dramamine II or Benadryl may be taken 1 hour before the first EC dose.
- Provide reassurance; nausea usually passes in a short period of time.
- If vomiting occurs within 1 hour of taking EC pills, repeat the dose along with an antinausea medication.
- If side effects such as nausea/vomiting, abdominal pain, dizziness, fatigue, or breast tenderness persist >24 hours after taking EC pills, contact the PCP.
- After taking EC pills within 120 hours and having had no menses within 21 days, take a urine pregnancy test. If positive, follow up with the PCP. If negative, wait another 7 days. If no menses occur, take another urine pregnancy test and follow up with the PCP with results.

**Additional Instructions**

_____

_____

_____

C

### Report the Following Problems to Your PCP/Clinic/ED

- Persistent nausea/vomiting, abdominal pain, dizziness, fatigue, or breast tenderness >24 hours
- Pelvic pain with or without fever
- Concerns about pregnancy or sexually transmitted disease
- Vaginal drainage

### Seek Emergency Care Immediately If Any of the Following Occur After Taking EC Pills

- Signs of allergic reaction; difficulty breathing, sudden throat or tongue swelling, rash, or hives
- Skin or lips turn gray, blue, or pale
- Sudden onset of profuse sweating
- Decrease in level of consciousness

If the caller agrees with the advice given, document the call and encourage the caller to call back or see PCP if the problem worsens. If the caller does not agree with the advice given, reevaluate and advise the caller to follow up with PCP, Clinic, or ED.

# Cough

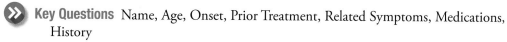

**Key Questions** Name, Age, Onset, Prior Treatment, Related Symptoms, Medications, History

**Other Protocols to Consider** Asthma (28); Breathing Problems (68); Chest Pain (85); Common Cold Symptoms (103); Congestion (110); Foreign Body, Inhaled (203); Foreign Body, Swallowing of (214); Influenza (276); Pertussis (334); Sore Throat (420); Wheezing (503).

***Reminder:*** Document caller response to advice, home care instructions, and when to call back.

| ASSESSMENT | ACTION |
|---|---|
| **A. Is coughing caused by choking on a foreign body, food, or vomit?** | |
| | **YES** Go to Foreign Body, Inhaled (203), or Foreign Body, Swallowing of (214) |
| | **NO** Go to B |
| **B. For reasons other than nasal congestion, is the following present?** | |
| • Sudden shortness of breath, rapid breathing, or wheezing | **YES** Go to Breathing Problems protocol (68) |
| | **NO** Go to C |
| **C. Is chest pain present?** | |
| | **YES** Go to Chest Pain protocol (85) |
| | **NO** Go to D |

## D. Are any of the following present?

- Blue face, lips, or tongue
- Feeling of suffocation
- Difficulty breathing and inability to speak
- Difficulty breathing after smoke, flame, or fume inhalation
- Sudden onset after exposure to something that previously caused a significant reaction (sting, medication, plant, chemical, food, or animal)
- Drooling
- Potential that child has swallowed a foreign object
- Infant less than 3 months old with a temperature ≥100.4°F rectally
- Fever and immunocompromised or has a chronic illness (sickle cell disease, diabetes, cystic fibrosis)

**YES** "Call ambulance"
or
"Seek Emergency Care Now"

**NO** Go to E

## E. Are any of the following present?

- Cough is unrelated to cold symptoms and person has a history of
  - chest trauma >48 hours
  - blood clots or recent long sedentary period
  - recent surgery
  - recent childbirth
  - asthma and unresponsiveness to home care measures or medication
- Coughing up blood
- Child younger than 6 months with rapid breathing and persistent cough
  - Child appears very ill
- Change in child's breathing pattern: labored, noisy, wheezing, or chest retractions

**YES** "Seek medical care within 2 hours"

**NO** Go to F

## F. Are any of the following present?

- Persistent fever >72 hours that is unresponsive to fever-reducing measures
- Child has a "barking" cough that is unrelieved by exposure to cool air, humidifier, or steam

**YES** "Seek medical care within 24 hours"

**NO** Go to G

## G. Are any of the following present?

- Cough caused by exercise
- Persistent or worsening cough during a period of several weeks or months
- Intermittent mild chest discomfort with deep productive coughing
- Child with temperature >101°F (38.3°C) for >24 hours
- Cough with weight loss

**YES** "Call back or call PCP for appointment if no improvement" and Follow **Home Care Instructions**

**NO** Follow **Home Care Instructions**

C

## Home Care Instructions
## Cough

- Drink six to eight glasses of water daily.
- Warm mist may help improve conditions. Sit in a steam-filled bathroom. Ensure that an adult is with the child at all times in the bathroom.
- Elevate head of bed to reduce coughing at night.
- For children younger than 1 year, give ½ tsp lemon mixed with ½ tsp corn syrup to soothe cough.
- Give older children ½ tsp lemon mixed with ½ tsp honey or corn syrup. (DO NOT give honey to a child <1 year old.)
- Drink warm lemonade, apple cider, or tea to help soothe cough.
- Avoid irritants such as smoking, smog, and chemicals.
- Turn down the heat, open the windows, or go out into cooler air to help suppress cough.
- Take cough suppressants (ask your pharmacist for product suggestions) if cough is interfering with activity, causing chest pain or vomiting, or interrupting sleep at night. Do not give cough suppressants to a child <12 years of age. Follow instructions on the label.
- Take usual pain medication (acetaminophen, ibuprofen) for discomfort and fever. Do not give aspirin to a child. Avoid aspirin-like products if age <20 years. Avoid acetaminophen if liver disease is present. Avoid ibuprofen if kidney disease or stomach problems exist or in the case of pregnancy. Follow the directions on the label. Use the dosing device that comes with the medication, a measuring device, or a medication syringe from the pharmacy. Household teaspoons often do not give the correct amount of medication.

## Additional Instructions

_____

_____

_____

### Report the Following Problems to Your PCP/Clinic/ED

- No improvement or condition worsens
- Fever for >72 hours
- Coughing up blood (more than streaks or flecks)

### Seek Emergency Care Immediately If Any of the Following Occur

- Blue face, lips, or tongue
- Feeling of suffocation
- Difficulty breathing and inability to speak

If the caller agrees with the advice given, document the call and encourage the caller to call back or see PCP if the problem worsens. If the caller does not agree with the advice given, reevaluate and advise the caller to follow up with PCP, Clinic, or ED.

# Croup

>> **Key Questions**  Name, Age, Onset, Description of Cough, Prior Treatment, Medications, Associated Symptoms, History

>> **Other Protocols to Consider**  Breathing Problems (68); Congestion (110); Cough (121); Fever (184); Influenza (276); Pertussis (334); Sore Throat (420).

*Reminder:*  Document caller response to advice, home care instructions, and when to call back.

| ASSESSMENT | ACTION |
|---|---|
| **A. Are any of the following present?** | |
| • Drooling, difficulty swallowing, and child looks ill <br> • Lips blue or dusky <br> • Severe difficulty breathing <br> • Chest caves in when breathing <br> • Child is unresponsive | **YES** "Call ambulance" <br> **NO** Go to B |
| **B. Are any of the following present?** | |
| • Crowing sound when breathing in that does not clear after 20 minutes of steam, or more than three episodes during the last 24 hours <br> • Child appears very ill <br> • Child may have swallowed a foreign body | **YES** "Seek emergency care now" <br> **NO** Go to C |
| **C. Are any of the following present?** | |
| • History of pneumonia or other lung problems <br> • History of asthma and no improvement after home breathing treatment and usual bronchodilator | **YES** "Seek medical care within 2 hours" <br> **NO** Go to D |
| **D. Are any of the following present?** | |
| • Condition worsens when lying down <br> • Condition interferes with sleep <br> • Temperature >104°F (40°C) | **YES** "Seek medical care within 24 hours" <br> **NO** Go to E |

C

## E. Are any of the following present?

- Barking cough >5 days
- Cough worse at night
- Barking cough heard during daytime hours

**YES**    "Call back or call PCP for appointment if no improvement"
and
Follow **Home Care Instructions**

**NO**    Follow **Home Care Instructions**

## Home Care Instructions
## Croup

- Warm mist may help improve condition: Sit in a steam-filled bathroom for 20 to 30 minutes. Younger children should be accompanied in the bathroom by a parent at all times when breathing steam from shower.
- Continuous cool mist may help. Use a cool-mist humidifier or go out into the cool night air.
- Drink warm clear fluids to soothe cough.
- Take usual pain medication (acetaminophen, ibuprofen) for discomfort and fever. Do not give aspirin to a child. Avoid aspirin-like products if age <20 years. Avoid acetaminophen if liver disease is present. Avoid ibuprofen if kidney disease or stomach problems exist or in the case of pregnancy. Follow the directions on the label. Use the dosing device that comes with the medication, a measuring device, or a medication syringe from the pharmacy. Household teaspoons often do not give the correct amount of medication.

**C**

### Additional Instructions

_____

_____

_____

### Report the Following Problems to Your PCP/Clinic/ED

- No improvement or condition worsens
- Difficulty breathing
- Temperature >104°F (40°C)
- Condition persists in child with asthma after home breathing treatment

### Seek Emergency Care Immediately If Any of the Following Occur

- Drooling, difficulty swallowing, and child looks ill
- Lips turn blue or dusky
- Severe difficulty breathing
- Child appears very ill
- Chest caves in with breathing
- Crowing sound that does not clear after 20 minutes of home care measures or more than three episodes in a 24-hour period

If the caller agrees with the advice given, document the call and encourage the caller to call back or see PCP if the problem worsens. If the caller does not agree with the advice given, reevaluate and advise the caller to follow up with PCP, Clinic, or ED.

# Crying, Excessive, in Infants

 **Key Questions**  Name, Age, Onset, Cause, Medications, History

 **Other Protocols to Consider**  Bottle-Feeding Problems (59); Breast-Feeding Problems (63); Earache, Drainage (150); Sore Throat (420); Teething (460).

*Reminder:* Document caller response to advice, home care instructions, and when to call back.

---

| ASSESSMENT | ACTION |
|---|---|

### A. Are any of the following present?

- Respiratory distress
- Extreme lethargy or other abnormal behavioral changes
- Exhausted parent expressing fear that he or she may hurt the infant
- Temperature ≥100.4°F rectally in infant younger than 12 weeks
- Bulging fontanelle

**YES** "Call ambulance"
or
"Seek emergency care now"

**NO** Go to B

### B. Are any of the following present?

- Projectile vomiting
- Constant crying >2 hours and unresponsive to home care measures
- Intermittent lethargy or irritability
- Temperature >104°F in infant older than 12 weeks
- Signs of dehydration present
- Swelling in testicle or groin area
- Possibility of a hair tourniquet (finger or toe swollen and discolored)

**YES** "Seek medical care within 2 hours"

**NO** Go to C

### C. Are any of the following present?

- New onset of crying
- Infant appears sick to parent
- Crying accompanied by fever, vomiting, or pulling on ears
- Fussiness >48 hours
- Inability to sleep at night without feeding
- Crying when infant tries to sleep

**YES** "Seek medical care within 24 hours"

**NO** Go to D

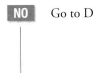

## D. Are any of the following present?

- Mother breast-feeding and has unrestricted diet
- Crying mostly at night from 6 pm to midnight in infant younger than 12 weeks
- Recent immunizations with fever
- Temperature >101°F (38.3°C)
- Teething with red gums and infant is 4 to 8 months old

**YES**  "Call back or call PCP for appointment if no improvement"
and
Follow **Home Care Instructions**

**NO**  Follow **Home Care Instructions**

C

## Home Care Instructions
## Crying, Excessive, in Infants

- When infant begins to cry, check immediate needs for food, diaper changing, holding, or fever.
- Do not feed infant every time he/she cries; try to comfort for 15 to 20 minutes. If crying persists, lay down the infant for 15 to 20 minutes and repeat the process. Look for other causes: pulling on ears, diarrhea, eyelash in eye, or hair around finger, toe, or penis. Hold, comfort, and burp the infant. Periods of irritability are normal.
- If crying mainly at evening or night, infant may have colic pain. Rhythmic soothing activities such as rocking, swinging, or cradling often help. Apply a blanket or towel warmed in the dryer to infant's stomach; give a warm bath, provide a pacifier, and play recordings of monotonous sounds. Keep infant from sleeping more than 3 hours between daytime feedings to help increase nighttime sleep. A car ride in the car seat and sounds of vacuum cleaner, dishwasher, dryer, or washing machine may help soothe infant.
- If breast-feeding, avoid excessive caffeine and smoking. Breast-feed on demand, rather than on a rigid schedule.
- Acetaminophen may be given for pain or fever. Do not give aspirin to an infant or to a child. Avoid aspirin-like products if age <20 years. Avoid acetaminophen if liver disease is present. Avoid ibuprofen if kidney disease or stomach problems exist or in the case of pregnancy. Follow the directions on the label. Use the dosing device that comes with the medication, a measuring device, or a medication syringe from the pharmacy. Household teaspoons often do not give the correct amount of medication.
- If the infant is teething, provide a cold teething ring, frozen ice wrapped in a cloth, frozen banana or frozen bagel (as appropriate for age) for the infant to chew. Avoid teething gels with benzocaine because they may numb the throat and cause choking or a drug reaction.
- Ibuprofen may be helpful in infants older than 6 months. Follow the instructions on the label.
- If taking cough or cold medications, discontinue them.

**Additional Instructions**

_____

_____

_____

### Report the Following Problems to Your PCP/Clinic/ED

- Crying becomes severe, constant, and/or interferes with infant's sleep >2 hours
- Any new signs or symptoms
- Parent/caregiver becomes exhausted

### Seek Emergency Care Immediately If Any of the Following Occur

- Respiratory distress
- Extreme lethargy
- Exhausted parent expresses fear that he or she may hurt the infant

If the caller agrees with the advice given, document the call and encourage the caller to call back or see PCP if the problem worsens. If the caller does not agree with the advice given, reevaluate and advise the caller to follow up with PCP, Clinic, or ED.

C

# Dehydration

>> **Key Questions**  Name, Age, Onset, Cause, Medications, History, Caller or Triagor Concerned about Possible Dehydration Symptoms

>> **Other Protocols to Consider**  Diabetes Problems (138); Diarrhea (143); Fever (184); Heat Exposure Problems (252); Vomiting (492); Sweating, Excessive (446).

> *Nurse Alert:* Instruct the caller how to assist in the assessment of dehydration through observations, assessing capillary refill and skin tenting. See Teaching Self Assessment (Appendix G (547)) to assist the caller in performing assessment techniques.

*Reminder:*  Document caller response to advice, home care instructions, and when to call back.

| ASSESSMENT | ACTION |
|---|---|

### A. Are several of the following present?

- Altered mental status: listlessness, unusual irritability, confusion, delirium, or difficulty arousing
- Severe headache, stiff neck, or pain bending head forward
- Vomiting bright red blood or dark coffee-grounds–like emesis
- Bloody or black stools
- Severe abdominal or chest pain
- Difficulty breathing
- Fever >103°F (39.4°C) without urination in >12 hours
- Hard or fast breathing or appears very ill
- Infant less than 3 months of age with fever >100.4°F
- Has two or more signs of dehydration
  - infrequent urination (<1 void in >12 hours) (<1 void in >8 hours in an infant)
  - dark yellow urine
  - sunken eyes or fontanelle
  - pinched skin does not spring back
  - excessive thirst
  - dry mouth or mucous membranes
  - Capillary refill >2 seconds
  - infant cries without tears

 **YES**  "Seek emergency care now"

**NO**  Go to B

## B. Are several of the following present?

- No urine in >8 hours
- Capillary refill <2 seconds
- Persistent vomiting, diarrhea, or fever >24 hours
- Diabetes and persistent vomiting, diarrhea, or fever
- Weakened immune system

 "Seek medical care within 2 to 4 hours"

 Go to C

## C. Are either of the following present?

- Dizzy when rising to a sitting or standing position
- Feeling faint
- Decreased urine production

 "Seek medical care within 24 hours," "Call back or call PCP for appointment if no improvement,"
and
Follow **Home Care Instructions**

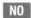 Follow **Home Care Instructions**

D

## Home Care Instructions
## Dehydration

- Cool down if dehydration is due to heat exposure. Remove excess clothing, apply damp towels, or spray mist the skin. If no air-conditioning, place person near fans or in the shade if outside.
- In infants younger than 1 year:
  - Introduce 1 tsp Lytren, Pedialyte, Infalyte, Rehydrate, Resol, Ricelyte, or KAO-Lectrolyte every 5 minutes and increase as tolerated.
  - If breast-feeding, offer breast milk for 4 to 5 minutes every 30 to 60 minutes, and offer electrolyte solution between breast-feeds, 1 tsp every 5 to 15 minutes. It is usually not necessary to discontinue breast-feeding.
- In children >1 year:
  - Do not eat or drink anything for 30 minutes after last emesis.
  - Drink 1 tbsp every 5 minutes for 4 hours (fruit juice diluted with water, weak tea with sugar, clear broth, gelatin, flavored ice, sport drink diluted 50:50 with water).
  - Slowly introduce bland foods as tolerated (rice, potatoes, soda crackers, pretzels, dry toast, applesauce, bananas) after 8 hours without vomiting.

## Additional Instructions

_____

_____

_____

## Report the Following Problems to Your PCP/Clinic/ED

- High fever, weakness, or abdominal pain >2 hours
- No improvement in 24 hours or condition worsens

## Seek Emergency Care Immediately If Any of the Following Occur

- Altered mental status
- Vomiting blood or dark coffee-grounds–like emesis
- Black or bloody stools
- Severe headache, stiff neck, or pain bending head forward
- Difficulty breathing
- Fever >103°F (39.4°C) or >100.4°F in a child <3 months of age
- Persistent signs of dehydration

If the caller agrees with the advice given, document the call and encourage the caller to call back or see PCP if the problem worsens. If the caller does not agree with the advice given, reevaluate and advise the caller to follow up with PCP, Clinic, or ED.

# Depression

>> **Key Questions**  Name, Age, Onset, Trigger; Recent Related Event, Prior Suicide Attempts and Date of Last Attempt; History, Medications

>> **Other Protocols to Consider**  Alcohol Problems (9); Anxiety (18); Appetite Loss (21); Fatigue (181); Substance Abuse, Use or Exposure (434); Suicide Attempt, Threat (437).

> *Nurse Alert:* Obtain as much history as possible with potentially high-risk individuals: Loss of a loved one, recent major life-changing event, history of prior suicide attempts, severe eating disorders, substance abuse, inability to perform daily-living activities.

*Reminder:* Document caller response to advice, home care instructions, and when to call back.

| ASSESSMENT | ACTION |
|---|---|
| **A. Are any of the following present?** | |
| • Suicidal thoughts with a plan and means to carry out the plan | **YES** "Call ambulance" or "Seek emergency care now" |
| • Intent to harm others | **NO** Go to B |
| • Suicidal thoughts and injured self | |
| • Overdose | |
| • Altered mental status: confusion, delusional, psychotic | |
| **B. Are any of the following present?** | |
| • Suicidal thoughts without a plan or means to carry out the plan | **YES** "Seek medical care within 2 to 4 hours" Call Crisis #_____ |
| • New onset of delusional ideas | |
| • Past inpatient admission for depression | **NO** Go to C |
| • Adolescent acting out, provocative or risk-taking behavior | |
| • New onset and recent change or addition of new medication | |

D

135

## C.  Are any of the following present?

- Previous suicide attempts
- Depression interfering with ability to work or function
- Loss of appetite and eating poorly
- Abrupt cessation of drugs (OTC or Rx), alcohol, or caffeine
- Drug or alcohol abuse

 "Seek medical care within 24 hours"

 Go to D

## D.  Are several of the following present?

- Difficulty concentrating
- Difficulty sleeping
- Irregular or absent menstruation
- No interest in activity
- Change in interpersonal relationships
- Increased use/abuse of alcohol or drugs
- Pregnant or recent childbirth
- Recent major life change
- History of depression

**YES** "Call back or call PCP for appointment if no improvement" and Follow **Home Care Instructions**

**NO** Follow **Home Care Instructions**

## Home Care Instructions
## Depression

- If currently in counseling, call counselor for an appointment.
- Call local crisis intervention _____
  - Community counseling services _____
  - Family services _____
  - Drug and alcohol services _____
  - AA _____
- Contact friends or family for support.
- Increase exercise and enjoyable activities.
- Eat a balanced diet, drink plenty of fluids, and rest as needed.
- Alcohol or other recreational drugs can worsen depression. If heavy use of drugs or alcohol, contact counselor or PCP for help to reduce consumption.

## Additional Instructions

_____

_____

_____

### Report the Following Problems to Your PCP/Clinic/ED

- Suicidal thoughts without a plan or means to carry out the plan
- Depression interferes with daily activities
- Persistent inability to sleep

### Seek Emergency Care Immediately If Any of the Following Occur

- Suicidal thoughts and a plan and means to carry out the plan
- Injury to self or others
- Altered mental status: confusion, delusional, psychotic

If the caller agrees with the advice given, document the call and encourage the caller to call back or see PCP if the problem worsens. If the caller does not agree with the advice given, reevaluate and advise the caller to follow up with PCP, Clinic, or ED.

D

# Diabetes Problems

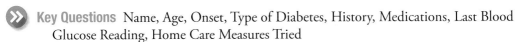 **Key Questions**  Name, Age, Onset, Type of Diabetes, History, Medications, Last Blood Glucose Reading, Home Care Measures Tried

**Other Protocols to Consider**  Confusion (107); Diarrhea (143); Fever (184); Vomiting (492); Wound Healing and Infection (509).

> *Nurse Alert:* Use this protocol only if previously diagnosed with diabetes.

**Reminder:**  Document caller response to advice, home care instructions, and when to call back.

| ASSESSMENT | ACTION |
|---|---|

### A. Are any of the following present?

- Gradual onset of high blood glucose symptoms and
  - decreased level of consciousness or confusion, excessive thirst, dry mouth, frequent urination, or dry flushed skin
  - deep and rapid breathing
  - breath smells fruity
  - weakness, fatigue, or drowsiness
- High glucose and ketones in urine
- After taking insulin or oral hypoglycemic agents:
  - weakness, pale moist skin, shallow breathing, blurred or double vision, profuse sweating, light-headedness or dizziness, headache, confusion, or irritability and no improvement 15 minutes after eating something containing glucose
- Seizure
- Severe dehydration
- Insulin overdose
- Persistent diarrhea and rapid or labored breathing

**YES**  "Seek emergency care now" or "Call ambulance"

**NO**  Go to B

## B. Are any of the following present?

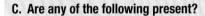

- High glucose level, some ketones, and person is alert
- Open or infected wound unresponsive to home care measures
- Persistent vomiting for >12 hours and unable to keep down medication
- Blood glucose >300
- Abdominal pain
- Blood glucose <80 and unresponsive to usual methods to raise blood glucose
- Temperature >100.4°F (38.0°C)

**YES** "Seek medical care within 2 to 4 hours"

**NO** Go to C

## C. Are any of the following present?

- Progressive fatigue
- Upper respiratory infection with fever and productive cough
- Painful urination, back pain, or cloudy or bloody urine
- Poor compliance with insulin or oral medication and feels ill

**YES** "Seek medical care within 24 hours"

**NO** Go to D

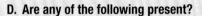

## D. Are any of the following present?

- Taking insulin or oral hypoglycemic agents, and blood glucose is 200 to 300
- Vomiting or diarrhea, no fever, and diabetes under control
- Requests dietary guidance
- Beginning signs of insulin reaction and responsive to sugar intake
- Requests blood glucose medication refill
- Slow-healing wound

**YES** "Call back or call PCP for appointment if no improvement" and Follow **Home Care Instructions**

**NO** Follow **Home Care Instructions**

D

## Home Care Instructions
## Diabetes Problems

- When first signs of insulin reaction occur, immediately drink orange juice, milk, or soda (not diet), or suck on a hard candy or a sugar cube, but only if the person is conscious.
- Person with diabetes should continue taking insulin when ill, unless he/she is not able to eat. Regularly check blood or urine for glucose and acetone during illness.
- Exercise regularly.
- Pay special attention to the feet. Avoid cuts, sores, blisters, ill-fitting shoes, or going barefoot. Promptly treat injuries to the feet.
- Take medications as directed by physician.
- Drink extra water or noncaffeinated, nonsugared drinks to prevent dehydration. If low blood glucose is a frequent problem, keep quick-sugar foods with you at all times. Examples are table sugar, fruit juice or regular soda pop, fat-free milk, honey or corn syrup, jam, raisins, gumdrops, Life Savers candy, hard candy, glucose tablets, and glucose gel. Expect the blood glucose to rise in 15 to 20 minutes.

## Additional Instructions

_____

_____

_____

## Report the Following Problems to Your PCP/Clinic/ED

- Signs of infection: increased swelling, pain, redness, drainage, or warmth
- No improvement or condition worsens
- Persistent vomiting for >12 hours and unable to keep down medication
- Blood glucose >300

## Seek Emergency Care Immediately If Any of the Following Occur

- Person with diabetes becomes unconscious; call ambulance
- Signs of high blood glucose: decreased level of consciousness or confusion, excessive thirst, dry mouth, frequent urination, or dry flushed skin
- Signs of insulin reaction with no improvement 15 minutes after eating something with sugar
- Persistent diarrhea and rapid or labored breathing
- Severe dehydration

If the caller agrees with the advice given, document the call and encourage the caller to call back or see PCP if the problem worsens. If the caller does not agree with the advice given, reevaluate and advise the caller to follow up with PCP, Clinic, or ED.

# Diaper Rash

 **Key Questions**  Name, Age, Onset, History, Medications, Description of the Rash

 **Other Protocols to Consider**  Bedbug Exposure or Concerns (37); Bed-Wetting (40); Diarrhea (143); Skin Lesions: Lumps, Bumps, and Sores (414).

**Reminder:**  Document caller response to advice, home care instructions, and when to call back.

| ASSESSMENT | ACTION |
|---|---|
| **A. Are any of the following present?** | |
| • Large painful blisters or open sores <br> • Pus, boils, pimples, or crusting <br> • Bleeding <br> • Discomfort that interferes with sleep <br> • Rash that spreads beyond the diaper area <br> • Solid bright red rash <br> • Sore or scab on end of penis <br> • Unexplained temperature of >100.4°F (38.0°C) | **YES** "Seek medical care within 24 hours" <br><br> **NO** Go to B |
| **B. Are any of the following present?** | |
| • Rash >3 days <br> • Red or weeping rash in groin and diaper area | **YES** "Call back or call PCP for appointment if no improvement" <br> and <br> Follow **Home Care Instructions** <br><br> **NO** Follow **Home Care Instructions** |

D

141

## Home Care Instructions
## Diaper Rash

- Air-dry skin as much as possible—at least 1 hour a day.
- Change diapers frequently. Check each hour for wetness or soiling.
- Clean area with warm water at every diaper change. Wash with a mild soap once a day and allow to air-dry.
- Once skin is dry, apply a protective barrier, for example, OTC A and D Ointment, Desitin, or zinc oxide. The barrier helps to protect the skin, especially if diarrhea is present.
- Apply diaper loosely. Pin diaper front and back to T-shirt and leave sides of diaper open.
- If using cloth diapers, avoid plastic pants until rash is gone.
- At night, use disposable diapers that keep wetness inside the diaper, away from the skin.
- Avoid diaper wipes.
- If red rash involves skin creases or has lasted >3 days, apply OTC Lotrimin to involved area.

## Additional Instructions

_____

_____

_____

## Report the Following Problems to Your PCP/Clinic/ED

- Rash turns bright red or raw
- Blisters, pus, pimples, or crusting
- Persistent rash >3 days that is unresponsive to home care measures
- Rash worsens
- Unexplained fever

If the caller agrees with the advice given, document the call and encourage the caller to call back or see PCP if the problem worsens. If the caller does not agree with the advice given, reevaluate and advise the caller to follow up with PCP, Clinic, or ED.

# Diarrhea

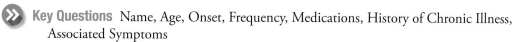

**Key Questions** Name, Age, Onset, Frequency, Medications, History of Chronic Illness, Associated Symptoms

**Other Protocols to Consider** Abdominal Pain (1); Abdominal Swelling (4); Confusion (107); Constipation (114); Dehydration (132); Fever (184); Rectal Bleeding (371); Stools, Abnormal (429); Vomiting (492).

*Reminder:* Document caller response to advice, home care instructions, and when to call back.

| ASSESSMENT | ACTION |
|---|---|

### A. Are any of the following present?

- Diarrhea and severe weakness, lethargy, listlessness, or faintness
- Vomiting with right-sided abdominal pain
- Infant younger than 3 months with diarrhea and temperature 100.4°F (38.0°C) rectally
- Cold and gray skin
- Grossly bloody stool
- Breathing fast and hard
- Severe pain, drawing knees to chest with cramping

**YES** "Seek emergency care now"

**NO** Go to B

### B. Are any of the following present?

- Signs of dehydration:
  - decreased urination
  - no urine for >8 hours
  - crying without tears
  - sunken eyes or fontanelles
  - excessive thirst, dry mouth
- Temperature >104°F (40.0°C), age >3 months, and unresponsive to fever-reducing measures
- Listlessness
- Persistent vomiting and diarrhea
- Diarrhea every hour for >8 hours
- Blood in stool
- History of cancer, sickle cell disease, diabetes, or weakened immune system and fever

**YES** "Seek medical care within 2 to 4 hours"

**NO** Go to C

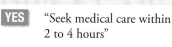

D

## C. Are any of the following present?

- Less than three diarrhea stools in 24 hours in a child younger than 1 month
- Diarrhea for >3 days or diarrhea while receiving antibiotic therapy
- Pus or mucus in stool
- No improvement with home care measures
- Temperature >103°F (39.4°C) or temperature >101°F (38.3°C) for more than 48 hours
- Fever unresponsive to fever-reducing measures

**YES** "Seek medical care within 24 hours"

**NO** Go to D

## D. Are any of the following present?

- Chronic diarrhea
- Recent change in diet
- Other family members or pets have diarrhea
- Recent travel to a foreign country
- New prescription
- Recent contact with a snake, lizard, or turtle

**YES** "Call back or call PCP for appointment if no improvement"
and
Follow **Home Care Instructions**

**NO** Follow **Home Care Instructions**

## Home Care Instructions
## Diarrhea

### Breast-Feeding Infants ≤1 Year Old
- Continue to feed every 2 hours and offer rehydration fluids (Pedialyte, Infalyte, Rehydralyte) between feedings. Stools usually follow feeding. Diarrhea is a sudden increase in the frequency of stools with loose consistency.
- Do NOT give Jell-O water mixtures or sports drinks, as these do not contain enough sodium, and the sugar content can make diarrhea worse.

### Formula-Fed Infants ≤1 Year Old
- Give Pedialyte, Infalyte, or Rehydralyte for the first 4 to 6 hours only. Each hour, give at least 2 tsp for every pound your child weighs. Then resume full-strength formula, but give more often than usual. If diarrhea is severe, use a soy formula or soy with added rice until diarrhea has been gone for 3 days, or switch to soy or lactose-free formula if diarrhea lasts longer than 3 days.
- Do NOT give Jell-O water mixtures or sports drinks, as these do not contain enough sodium, and the sugar content can make diarrhea worse.

### All Infants >4 and <12 Months
- Offer solids, such as infant cereal (especially rice), strained applesauce, carrots, bananas, mashed potatoes, or other high-fiber foods. These starchy foods are more easily digested when your child has diarrhea.
- Avoid all fruit juices, as these will make diarrhea worse.
- If your child refuses the solids, offer extra formula rather than water.

### Children >1 Year Old
- Fluids: Avoid juices, and increase water and other fluids that are caffeine free. Eat or drink less milk and milk products for 2 to 3 days. If solids are being taken well, milk products can still be used and should be well tolerated.
- Maintain regular diet if tolerated well.
- Avoid foods that would normally cause loose stools in your child, such as spicy sauces or beans.

### Additional Home Care Advice
- Acetaminophen can be given for fever. Do not give aspirin to a child. Avoid aspirin-like products if age <20 years. Avoid acetaminophen if liver disease is present. Avoid ibuprofen if kidney disease or stomach problems exist or in the case of pregnancy. Follow the directions on the label. Use the dosing device that comes with the medication, a measuring device, or a medication syringe from the pharmacy. Household teaspoons often do not give the correct amount of medication.
- Diarrhea often is very contagious. Wash hands with soap and water after using the toilet or changing a diaper.
- If diaper rash or redness occurs in the anus, wash with running water, dry, and apply petroleum jelly or other barrier ointment to protect the area, particularly at night and during naps.

## Additional Instructions

### Report the Following Problems to Your PCP/Clinic/ED

- No improvement or diarrhea worsens after 48 hours of home care measures
- Yellow, frothy, bloody, or green stool occurs more than once
- Signs of dehydration: decreased urination, dry mouth, no tears
- Fever, weakness, or lethargy
- Watery diarrhea and vomiting clear fluid >3 times

### Seek Emergency Care Immediately If Any of the Following Occur

- Rapid or labored breathing
- Severe abdominal pain, swelling, and fever
- Infant <2 months and fever ≥100.4°F (38.0°C)
- Gross bloody stools
- Cold and gray skin
- Severe listlessness or fainting

If the caller agrees with the advice given, document the call and encourage the caller to call back or see PCP if the problem worsens. If the caller does not agree with the advice given, reevaluate and advise the caller to follow up with PCP, Clinic, or ED.

# Dizziness

 **Key Questions**  Name, Age, Onset, History, Medications

 **Other Protocols to Consider**  Breathing Problems (68); Chest Pain (85); Confusion (107); Dehydration (132); Earache and Drainage (150); Fainting (178); Headache (238); Heat Exposure Problems (252); Neurologic Symptoms (312); Rectal Bleeding (371); Substance Abuse, Use, and Exposure (434); Weakness (496).

> *Nurse Alert:* Dizziness can be a minor symptom caused by inadequate fluid or food intake, heat or sun exposure, or standing up too quickly. It may also be an indication of a serious condition related to an infectious process, cardiovascular, respiratory, gastrointestinal, or neurologic disorder. Dizziness may be described as light-headedness, feeling faint, fuzzy, woozy, or a sensation of motion by the person or the environment such as spinning or whirling.

*Reminder:*  Document caller response to advice, home care instructions, and when to call back.

| ASSESSMENT | ACTION |
|---|---|
| **A. Is chest pain present?** | |
| | **YES**  Go to Chest Pain protocol (85) |
| | **NO**  Go to B |
| **B. In addition to the dizziness, are any of the following present?** | |
| • Sudden onset of weakness or numbness in the face, arms, or legs on one side of the body | **YES**  "Seek emergency care now" |
| • Difficulty speaking or walking, confusion, facial droop | **NO**  Go to C |
| • Fainting spells or loss of consciousness | |
| • Heart rate <50 or >130 bpm or irregular heart rhythm | |
| • Persistent severe headache or change in vision | |
| • Fever, pale skin, and weakness | |
| • Potential ingestion of poison or overdose of medication | |

D

## C. Are any of the following present?

- History of recent trauma or blow to the head <48 hours ago
- Recent history of severe vomiting, diarrhea, or bleeding and dizziness and pulse increase when sitting or standing
- History of diabetes
- Signs of dehydration

 **YES**    "Seek medical care within 2 to 4 hours"

**NO**    Go to D

## D. Are any of the following present?

- Earache, ringing in the ears, or loss of hearing
- Fever unresponsive to fever-reducing measures
- Persistent light-headedness >3 days
- Recent abrupt cessation of drugs (OTC or prescription), alcohol, or caffeine

**YES**    "Seek medical care within 24 hours"

**NO**    Go to E

## E. Are any of the following present?

- Dizziness interferes with activities
- History of dieting, and dizziness does not improve after eating
- Dizziness occurs after taking a new medication
- Increase in stress
- Dizziness occurs during or after drinking alcohol
- Dizziness occurs when moving the head

**YES**    "Call back or call PCP for appointment if no improvement"
and
Follow **Home Care Instructions**

**NO**    Follow **Home Care Instructions**

# Home Care Instructions
# Dizziness

- During the dizzy spell, reach out and touch something, then lie flat or sit with head down on your lap and take deep breaths for a few minutes.
- If dizziness is accompanied by anxiety, rapid breathing, and numbness in the face or fingers, have the child hold a paper bag covering the mouth and nose and breathe into the bag for 1 minute or 12 breaths. **Never use a plastic bag.** Child should be old enough to safely hold the bag to the face.
- Sit up or stand up slowly. Avoid sudden changes in posture.
- If diagnosed with labyrinthitis, consider having someone else provide transportation. Dizziness can take up to 4 weeks to resolve after starting treatment.
- In the case of persistent dizziness, avoid noisy environments.
- Limit intake of caffeinated beverages and alcohol.
- If dehydrated, drink plenty of water or sports drinks.
- Use a night light.
- Consider OTC motion sickness medications (Benadryl, Bonine) if dizziness is related to motion, and follow the instructions on the label.
- When feeling a "dizzy attack" coming on, stop moving for a few minutes. Reach out and lightly touch something solid and firm, then sit down and stay still.

**D**

## Additional Instructions

_____

_____

_____

### Report the Following Problems to Your PCP/Clinic/ED
- Problem persists >1 week or worsens
- Persistent vomiting and dizziness

### Seek Emergency Care Immediately If Any of the Following Occur
- Chest pain
- Decrease in level of consciousness
- Weakness or difficulty speaking
- Heart rate <50 or >130 bpm or irregular heart rhythm

If the caller agrees with the advice given, document the call and encourage the caller to call back or see PCP if the problem worsens. If the caller does not agree with the advice given, reevaluate and advise the caller to follow up with PCP, Clinic, or ED.

# Earache, Drainage

 **Key Questions**  Name, Age, Onset, Medications, Pain Scale

 **Other Protocols to Consider**  Common Cold Symptoms (103); Crying, Excessive, in Infants (128); Ear Injury, Foreign Body (154); Fever (184); Piercing Problems (338); Sore Throat (420).

*Reminder:*  Document caller response to advice, home care instructions, and when to call back.

---

| ASSESSMENT | ACTION |
|---|---|

### A. Are any of the following present?

- Earache, stiff neck, and fever
- Temperature 100.4°F (38.0°C) or greater rectally in infant <12 weeks old

 "Seek emergency care now"

 Go to B

### B. Are any of the following present?

- Swelling, pain, and redness on one side of the face
- Age >12 weeks and temperature >104°F (40°C) rectally
- Traumatic blow to the ear followed by severe pain, loss of hearing, bruising behind the ear, clear discharge or bleeding in the ear canal, or significant swelling
- Severe pain unresponsive to pain medication
- History of diabetes or immunosuppression
- Ear deviated outward
- Tenderness of bone behind ear
- Potential foreign body in the ear
- Child with a cochlear implant
- Bloody drainage

 "Seek medical care within 2 to 4 hours"

 Go to C

150

## C. Are any of the following present?

- Sudden hearing loss and pain, ear drainage, or dizziness
- Swelling, pain, warmth, drainage, or fever
- Increased pain when moving or touching the ear
- Blisters or sores
- Fever, congestion, or sore throat
- Light-headedness

**YES** "Seek medical care within 24 hours"

**NO** Go to D

## D. Are any of the following present?

- Unable to remove wax plug with medication and pain or decreased hearing
- Sunburned ears
- Pain after exposure to cold
- Muffled hearing but no pain
- Pain after swimming or exposure to water
- Itching
- Sudden pain with cracking or popping noise, decreased hearing and congestion
- Ringing in the ears
- Taking antibiotics for ear infection >3 days and earache persists

**YES** "Call back or call PCP for appointment if no improvement"
and
Follow **Home Care Instructions**

**NO** Follow **Home Care Instructions**

E

## Home Care Instructions
## Earache, Drainage

- Do not instill liquid drops in the ear if pain is related to an injury or a ruptured eardrum is suspected (sudden pain, hearing loss, bleeding or discharge, ringing in the ears, dizziness).
- Apply cool compresses to sunburned ears or ice packs to swollen area caused by a blow to the ear. Apply ice packs for 20 minutes, 4 times a day. Do not apply ice directly to the skin; use a washcloth or other cloth barrier between ice and the skin.
- To remove excessive ear wax, use Debrox (carbamide peroxide) as directed for as long as 3 days, or use two drops of mineral oil in the affected ear twice a day for 2 days.
- Apply warm compresses for ear pain for 15 to 20 minutes, 4 times a day, until resolved or while waiting for appointment. Fill a sock half full of rice. Knot the end. Microwave the sock until warm and apply against the ear. Check temperature against inner wrist before applying to the ear.
- Avoid swimming until ear pain and drainage subside.
- Swimmer's ear prevention: Mix equal parts of white vinegar and rubbing alcohol. Instill five drops of the mixture in each ear before and after swimming.
- Relieve ear congestion by frequent swallowing, chewing gum, and swallowing with the nose pinched closed.
- Avoid air travel when an earache or congestion is present. If travel is unavoidable, take a decongestant before flying, and if the child is older than 6 years, chew gum during takeoff and landing. A pacifier may be used for an infant and drinking fluids during takeoff and landing for toddlers.
- Take acetaminophen for earache or fever. Do not give aspirin to a child. Avoid aspirin-like products if age <20 years. Avoid acetaminophen if liver disease is present. Avoid ibuprofen if kidney disease or stomach problems exist or in the case of pregnancy. Follow the directions on the label. Use the dosing device that comes with the medication, a measuring device, or a medication syringe from the pharmacy. Household teaspoons often do not give the correct amount of medication.

## Additional Instructions

_____

_____

_____

### Report the Following Problems to Your PCP/Clinic/ED

- No improvement in 3 days or condition worsens
- Persistent fever unresponsive to fever-reducing measures
- Vomiting, diarrhea, fatigue, lethargy, or stiff neck
- Fever or swelling

### Seek Emergency Care Immediately If the Following Occur

- Earache, stiff neck, fever
- Temperature 100.4°F (38.0°C) or greater rectally in infants <12 weeks old

If the caller agrees with the advice given, document the call and encourage the caller to call back or see PCP if the problem worsens. If the caller does not agree with the advice given, reevaluate and advise the caller to follow up with PCP, Clinic, or ED.

E

# Ear Injury, Foreign Body

 **Key Questions** Name, Age, Onset, Cause, Medications, History, Pain Scale

 **Other Protocols to Consider** Earache, Drainage (150); Head Injury (242); Piercing Problems (338).

*Reminder:* Document caller response to advice, home care instructions, and when to call back.

| ASSESSMENT | ACTION |
|---|---|
| **A. After an injury to the ear, are any of the following present?** | |
| • Loss of coordination <br> • Facial paralysis or drooping <br> • Whirling vertigo | **YES** "Seek emergency care now" <br><br> **NO** Go to B |
| **B. Are any of the following present?** | |
| • Hearing loss <br> • Ear canal bleeding <br> • Dizziness <br> • Recent blow to head and clear or bloody ear canal drainage <br> • Unable to remove foreign body or embedded piercing <br> • Severe pain <br> • Persistent ringing in ear <br> • Lacerated earlobe <br> • Insect in ear canal <br> • Severe swelling of earlobe <br> • Persistent bleeding >30 minutes | **YES** "Seek medical care within 2 to 4 hours" <br><br> **NO** Go to C |

## C. Are any of the following present?

- Persistent pain >48 hours
- Earache after a blast of air, noise, or a blow to the head
- External ear red and swollen
- Recent use of Q-tips
- Minor laceration and tetanus immunization >5 years
- No improvement after 3 days of home care

**YES**  "Seek medical care within 24 hours"
"Call back or call PCP for appointment if no improvement"
and

**NO**  Follow **Home Care Instructions**

E

## Home Care Instructions
## Ear Injury, Foreign Body

- Apply ice pack to ear for 20 minutes, 4 times a day, for the first 24 to 48 hours after injury. Do not apply ice directly to the skin; use a washcloth or other cloth barrier between ice and the skin.
- Point the ear toward the light and pull up on the ear to encourage an insect to crawl out of the ear toward the light.
- Do not try to remove foreign object if unable to remove by pointing ear down toward the ground and gently shaking the head while pulling up on the ear.
- Take your usual pain medication (aspirin, acetaminophen, or ibuprofen) for discomfort. Do not give aspirin to a child. Avoid aspirin-like products if age <20 years. Avoid acetaminophen if liver disease is present. Avoid ibuprofen if kidney disease or stomach problems exist or in the case of pregnancy. Follow the directions on the label. Use the dosing device that comes with the medication, a measuring device, or a medication syringe from the pharmacy. Household teaspoons often do not give the correct amount of medication.
- Watch for signs of infection: increased pain, drainage, fever, redness, or warmth.

## Additional Instructions

_____

_____

_____

### Report the Following Problems to Your PCP/Clinic/ED

- Signs of infection: increased pain, drainage, fever, redness, or warmth
- Persistent pain >48 hours
- Dizziness
- Persistent ear canal drainage
- No improvement or condition worsens

### Seek Emergency Care Immediately If Any of the Following Occur

- Loss of coordination
- Facial paralysis or drooping
- Whirling vertigo

If the caller agrees with the advice given, document the call and encourage the caller to call back or see PCP if the problem worsens. If the caller does not agree with the advice given, reevaluate and advise the caller to follow up with PCP, Clinic, or ED.

# Ear Ringing

 **Key Questions**  Name, Age, Onset, Cause, Medications, History

 **Other Protocols to Consider**  Congestion (110); Dizziness (147); Earache, Drainage (150); Ear Injury, Foreign Body (154).

*Reminder:*  Document caller response to advice, home care instructions, and when to call back.

| ASSESSMENT | ACTION |
|---|---|

### A. Is the following present?

- Overdose or frequent ingestion of aspirin or aspirin products

**YES** "Seek emergency care now"

**NO** Go to B

### B. Are any of the following present?

- Foreign body in the ear
- Severe ear pain unresponsive to home care measures

**YES** "Seek medical care within 2 to 4 hours"

**NO** Go to C

### C. Are any of the following present?

- Recent ingestion of aspirin or medications containing aspirin, quinine, or streptomycin
- History of recent head injury or recent ear surgery
- Dizziness or vertigo
- Nausea or vomiting
- Persistent ear pain
- Ear drainage
- Persistent hearing loss

**YES** "Seek medical care within 24 hours"

**NO** Go to D

E

## D. Are any of the following present?

- Upper respiratory infection
- Congestion associated with allergies
- Feeling of fullness in one or both ears
- Excessive wax buildup
- History of Ménière disease with similar symptoms

**YES** "Call back or call PCP for appointment if no improvement"
and
Follow **Home Care Instructions**

**NO** Follow **Home Care Instructions**

## Home Care Instructions
## Ear Ringing

- Take decongestants to relieve ear congestion. Follow instructions on the label. Ask your pharmacist for product suggestions. Use the dosing device that comes with the medication, a measuring device, or a medication syringe from the pharmacy. Household teaspoons often do not give the correct amount of medication.
- If taking medications containing aspirin, quinine, or streptomycin, stop taking and notify PCP.
- Do not poke at wax or try to remove with fingers or cotton swabs. These measures worsen the problem.
- Decrease use of salt, caffeine, and alcohol if history of Ménière disease is present.

**Additional Instructions**

_____

_____

_____

### Report the Following Problems to Your PCP/Clinic/ED

- Significant hearing loss or dizziness
- Ear pain or drainage
- Persistent vomiting, increased ringing, headache

E

If the caller agrees with the advice given, document the call and encourage the caller to call back or see PCP if the problem worsens. If the caller does not agree with the advice given, reevaluate and advise the caller to follow up with PCP, Clinic, or ED.

# Electric Injury

>> **Key Questions**  Name, Age, Onset, Cause, Medications, Location of Entrance Wound and Exit Wound, Tetanus Immunization Status, History

>> **Other Protocols to Consider**  Breathing Problems (68); Burns, Electrical (77); Confusion (107); Heart Rate Problems (249); Seizure (393).

*Reminder:*  Document caller response to advice, home care instructions, and when to call back.

| ASSESSMENT | ACTION |
|---|---|
| **A. Is the victim still engaged with the source of electricity?** | |
| | **YES**   Instruct caller how to safely remove the victim from the electric source and call ambulance. Follow **Home Care Instructions** |
| | **NO**   Go to A |
| **B. After exposure to an electric shock, are any of the following present?** | |
| • Unconscious or altered mental status <br> • No pulse or respirations <br> • Rapid or irregular heart rate <br> • Difficulty breathing <br> • Burns above the neck <br> • Seizures <br> • High-voltage shock <br> • Obvious entrance and exit wounds | **YES**   "Call ambulance, and start CPR or rescue breathing if no pulse or respirations" |
| | **NO**   Go to B |

## C.  Are any of the following present?

- Numbness, tingling, paralysis
- Vision, hearing, or speech problems
- Burn to head, face, neck, hands, feet, or genital area
- Pale, sweaty, and light-headed or weak
- Thrown from electrical source and difficulty breathing, chest or abdominal pain
- Pain or deformity in hand or foot

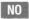 "Seek emergency care now"

 Go to C

## D.  Are any of the following present?

- Muscle pain
- Headache
- Irritability
- Fatigue
- 220-W voltage or greater

 "Seek medical care within 2 to 4 hours"

**NO** Follow **Home Care Instructions**

E

## Home Care Instructions
## Electric Injury

- Remove victim from electrical source:
  - If possible, turn off the electrical current at the breaker box.
  - Do not touch a person who is connected to an electrical source.
  - Try to break the contact between the person and the source using a dry nonmetal object, such as a broom handle.
  - Use the nonmetal object to push the electrical source away from the victim.
- If the victim is in a car near a downed power line, advise the victim to stay in the car until help arrives.
- Do not go near a victim electrocuted by a high-voltage current until the power is turned off.
- Once the victim is removed from the source, check for breathing and a pulse. Begin CPR or rescue breathing if indicated. If the caller does not know CPR, provide instruction, or call emergency dispatcher for instruction.
- Keep the victim warm.
- Observe for entrance and exit wounds.

## Additional Instructions

_____

_____

_____

### Report the Following Problems to Your PCP/Clinic/ED

- When electrical current passes through the body, internal damage can occur. Victims of electrical shock should seek medical care and evaluation.
- Signs of infection: increased redness, pain, swelling, drainage, red streaks, or fever.
- Bloody or very cloudy urine.

### Call Ambulance Immediately If Any of the Following Occur

- Altered mental status
- Seizures
- Palpitations
- Pale, sweaty, and light-headed or weak

If the caller agrees with the advice given, document the call and encourage the caller to call back or see PCP if the problem worsens. If the caller does not agree with the advice given, reevaluate and advise the caller to follow up with PCP, Clinic, or ED.

# Extremity Injury

 **Key Questions**  Name, Age, Onset, Cause of Injury, Medications, History, Pain Scale

 **Other Protocols to Consider**  Ankle Injury (16); Arm/Hand Problems (24); Finger and Toe Problems (189); Joint Pain/Swelling (287).

*Reminder:* Document caller response to advice, home care instructions, and when to call back.

| ASSESSMENT | ACTION |
|---|---|
| **A. Are any of the following present?** | |
| • Altered mental status <br> • Difficulty breathing <br> • Severe pain in the hip or thigh and unable to ambulate <br> • Bone protrudes through the skin | **YES** "Call ambulance" or "Seek emergency care now" <br><br> **NO** Go to B |
| **B. Are any of the following present?** | |
| • Affected limb is deformed <br> • Fingers or toes of the affected limb are cold, blue, and numb | **YES** "Seek emergency care now" <br> **NO** Go to C |
| **C. Are any of the following present?** | |
| • Severe pain with movement or weight bearing <br> • Difficulty moving the joint nearest the injury | **YES** "Seek medical care within 2 to 4 hours" <br> and <br> Follow **Home Care Instructions** <br><br> **NO** Go to D |

**D. Did any of the following occur within 30 minutes of the injury?**

- Pain
- Swelling
- Discoloration

**YES** "Seek medical care within 24 hours"
and
Follow **Home Care Instructions**

**NO** Go to E

**E. Did pain, swelling, or discoloration occur within 24 to 48 hours?**

**YES** Follow **Home Care Instructions**

**NO** Follow **Home Care Instructions**

## Home Care Instructions
## Extremity Injury

- Apply ice pack for 20 minutes, 4 times a day to the injured area to reduce swelling and pain for the first 24 to 48 hours. After that, alternate ice and heat. Do not apply ice directly to the skin; use a washcloth or other cloth barrier between ice and the skin.
- Elevate the affected part higher than the heart to help reduce swelling.
- For severe injuries, before going to the hospital, splint the affected limb (pillows, cardboard, or magazines can be used) above and below the injury.
- Cover open wounds with a sterile dressing.
- Take your usual medication for discomfort. Do not give aspirin to a child. Avoid aspirin-like products if age <20 years. Avoid acetaminophen if liver disease is present. Avoid ibuprofen if kidney disease or stomach problems exist or in the case of pregnancy. Follow the directions on the label. Use the dosing device that comes with the medication, a measuring device, or a medication syringe from the pharmacy. Household teaspoons often do not give the correct amount of medication.

**Additional Instructions**

_____

_____

_____

**Report the Following Problem to Your PCP/Clinic/ED**

- No improvement in pain, swelling, or ability to use extremity after ice and elevation

**Seek Emergency Care Immediately If Any of the Following Occur**

- Extremity becomes cold, blue, and numb
- No pulse in affected extremity
- Difficulty breathing

If the caller agrees with the advice given, document the call and encourage the caller to call back or see PCP if the problem worsens. If the caller does not agree with the advice given, reevaluate and advise the caller to follow up with PCP, Clinic, or ED.

E

# Eye Injury

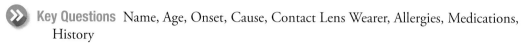

>> **Key Questions**  Name, Age, Onset, Cause, Contact Lens Wearer, Allergies, Medications, History

>> **Other Protocols to Consider**  Burns, Chemical (74); Eye Problems (169); Foreign Body, Eye (201); Head Injury (242); Piercing Problems (338); Vision Problems (489).

*Reminder:*  Document caller response to advice, home care instructions, and when to call back.

| ASSESSMENT | ACTION |
|---|---|

### A. Are any of the following present?

- Laceration or penetrating injury to the eye or eyelid
- Blow to the eye and sudden loss of vision
- Bulging eyeball
- Clear jelly-like discharge from injured eye
- Blunt trauma to the eye
- Pupils of unequal size
- Blood or cloudy fluid in the colored part of the eye
- Persistent severe pain
- Exposure to acid such as battery acid or caustic substance (drain cleaner, lye)

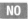 **YES** "Seek emergency care now" and for chemical exposure, flush eye with cold running water
and
Follow **Home Care Instructions**

 **NO**  Go to B

### B. Are any of the following present?

- Swelling, pain, and tearing >30 minutes
- Exposure to a strong light, such as a welder's arc or sun lamp
- Injury caused by hot water, chemical, or foreign body and pain persists after home care treatment or white part of eye becomes cloudy
- Persistent blurred or double vision
- Irritability or refusal to open eye

**YES** "Seek medical care within 2 hours" and for chemical exposure, flush eye with cold water
and
Follow **Home Care Instructions**

 **NO**  Go to C

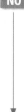

## C. Are any of the following present?

- Discomfort or irritation persists 24 hours after the injury or removal of a foreign body
- Signs of infection develop after an injury: pain, swelling, redness, drainage, or fever

**YES** "Seek medical care within 24 hours"

**NO** Go to D

## D. Are any of the following present?

- Area surrounding the eye is black and blue
- Blood on white part of the eye for >3 days

**YES** "Call back or call PCP for appointment if no improvement"
and
Follow **Home Care Instructions**

**NO** Follow **Home Care Instructions**

E

## Home Care Instructions
## Eye Injury

- Chemicals in the eye: Immediately flush eye with cold running water for 20 to 30 minutes. Tilt head under running water with injured eye down. While holding eyelids apart, allow water to run across the inner eye to the outer part of the eye.
- Do not rub eye.
- Apply ice pack or cool compresses to reduce swelling for the first 24 hours. Apply ice packs for 20 minutes, 4 times a day. Do not apply ice directly to the skin; use a washcloth or other cloth barrier between ice and the skin.
- Take acetaminophen for discomfort. Do not give aspirin to a child. Avoid aspirin-like products if age <20 years. Avoid acetaminophen if liver disease is present. Avoid ibuprofen if kidney disease or stomach problems exist or in the case of pregnancy. Follow the directions on the label. Use the dosing device that comes with the medication, a measuring device, or a medication syringe from the pharmacy. Household teaspoons often do not give the correct amount of medication.

## Additional Instructions

_____

_____

_____

### Report the Following Problems to Your PCP/Clinic/ED

- Increased pain, swelling, drainage, or fever
- Changes in vision
- No improvement in pain after 48 hours
- Bruising around the eye persists >2 weeks
- White part of eye becomes cloudy

### Seek Emergency Care Immediately If Any of the Following Occur

- Any bleeding or jelly-like discharge from the eye
- Sudden change in vision
- Persistent severe pain

If the caller agrees with the advice given, document the call and encourage the caller to call back or see PCP if the problem worsens. If the caller does not agree with the advice given, reevaluate and advise the caller to follow up with PCP, Clinic, or ED.

# Eye Problems

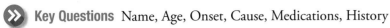

>> **Key Questions**  Name, Age, Onset, Cause, Medications, History

>> **Other Protocols to Consider**  Neurologic Symptoms (312); Stye (432); Vision Problem (489). If injury or foreign body, see Eye Injury (166) or Foreign Body, Eye (201).

*Reminder:*  Document caller response to advice, home care instructions, and when to call back.

| ASSESSMENT | ACTION |
|---|---|

### A. Are any of the following present?

- Sudden or severe pain
- Sudden vision loss or blurred or double vision
- Sudden onset of pupils of unequal size
- Curtain over field of vision
- Sudden increase in floaters
- Flashes of light
- Halos or rainbows around light
- Blood in the colored part of the eye
- Redness and unable to open eye or keep it open
- Fever, light sensitivity, bilateral swelling, and redness

**YES**  "Seek emergency care now"

**NO**  Go to B

### B. Are any of the following present?

- Pain, redness, watering, eye drainage, and wears contact lenses
- Fever and swollen red eyelids
- Pain increases with pressure to the eye or eye movement
- Lesion on the eyeball or corner of the eye
- Eye swollen shut

**YES**  "Seek medical care within 2 to 4 hours"

**NO**  Go to C

**E**

## C. Are any of the following present?

- Persistent pain unresponsive to home care measures
- Persistent itching, redness, burning, and drainage
- Persistent pain after removing contact lenses and irrigating eyes
- Swollen neck, lymph nodes, and redness around the entire eye
- Stye returns or bleeds
- Stye located on bottom eyelid near the nose is unresponsive to home care
- Eye pain or drainage and fever >100.4°F (38.0°C)
- Excessive persistent tearing of eye

**YES** "Seek medical care within 24 hours"

**NO** Go to D

## D. Are any of the following present?

- Blood in the white part of the eye >3 days
- History of eye pain late in the day
- History of wearing contact lenses too long or improper cleaning
- Tear duct area swollen and painful
- Small red, swollen, tender area on upper or lower lid
- Exposure to smoke, fumes, smog, pool water, known allergens, or sun lamp
- Eyes dry and itching
- Eyes crusted closed in the morning

**YES** "Call back or call PCP for appointment if no improvement" and Follow **Home Care Instructions**

**NO** Follow **Home Care Instructions**

## Home Care Instructions
## Eye Problems

- If drainage is present, encourage family members to use separate towels and washcloths. Eye infections are highly contagious.
- Avoid rubbing or touching eyes.
- Clean crusting or discharge with cotton ball moistened in warm water. Discard cotton ball after use. Do not use same cotton ball for both eyes. Wash your hands after cleaning.
- Apply warm compresses to eyes for 15 to 20 minutes, 4 times a day.
- Wash hands frequently.
- Instill saline drops in dry itchy eyes.
- Avoid wearing contact lenses for several days until the problem is resolved.
- For styes: See Home Care Instructions in Stye protocol (432).

## Additional Instructions

E

### Report the Following Problems to Your PCP/Clinic/ED

- Condition persists or worsens after 48 hours
- Yellow or green discharge
- Fever
- Sores
- Red and swollen eyelids

### Seek Emergency Care Immediately If Any of the Following Occur

- Severe pain
- Sudden loss of vision or blurred or double vision
- Sudden onset of unequal pupil size
- Blood or cloudy fluid in colored part of the eye
- Redness and unable to open eye or keep it open
- Fever, light sensitivity, bilateral swelling, and redness

If the caller agrees with the advice given, document the call and encourage the caller to call back or see PCP if the problem worsens. If the caller does not agree with the advice given, reevaluate and advise the caller to follow up with PCP, Clinic, or ED.

# Facial Problems

 **Key Questions**  Name, Age, Onset, Cause, Medications, History, Pain Scale

 **Other Protocols to Consider**  Congestion (110); Facial Skin Problems (175); Mouth Problems (302); Numbness and Tingling (325); Piercing Problems (338); Rash (366); Sinus Problems (411); Skin Lesions: Lumps, Bumps, and Sores (414); Tattoo Problems (456); Toothache (465).

***Reminder:***  Document caller response to advice, home care instructions, and when to call back.

| ASSESSMENT | ACTION |
|---|---|
| **A. Are any of the following present?** | |
| • Sudden loss of vision<br>• Severe pain on one side of face, over eye, blurred vision, and red eye<br>• Sudden onset of facial drooping on one side | **YES** "Seek emergency care now"<br>**NO** Go to B |
| **B. Are any of the following present?** | |
| • Sudden severe pain interferes with activity<br>• Facial paralysis<br>• Pain, swelling, redness, warmth, drainage, or fever | **YES** "Seek medical care within 2 to 4 hours"<br>**NO** Go to C |
| **C. Are any of the following present?** | |
| • Increased pain in afternoon or when bending over<br>• Green, brown, or yellow nasal discharge<br>• Pain along ridge between nose and lower eyelid<br>• Temperature >101°F (38.3°C)<br>• Persistent facial swelling<br>• Facial rash, blisters, or lesions | **YES** "Seek medical care within 24 hours"<br>**NO** Go to D |

## D. Are any of the following present?

- Recent red, blistered facial rash
- Pain, swelling, or bruising after blow to the face
- History of recent cold
- Pain follows ingestion of ice-cold foods or fluids
- Nose and eye drainage

**YES**   "Call back or call PCP for appointment if no improvement" and Follow **Home Care Instructions**

**NO**   Follow **Home Care Instructions**

F

## Home Care Instructions
## Facial Problems

- Alternate cold and warm compresses to forehead and cheeks 1 minute each for 10 minutes, 4 times a day. A sock filled with rice and heated in the microwave works well.
- Increase fluid intake.
- Apply ice pack to face injury for 10 to 20 minutes, 4 times a day for first 24 hours to help reduce swelling. Do not apply ice directly to the skin; use a washcloth or other cloth barrier between ice and the skin.
- Sit in a steamy bathroom for 20 minutes several times a day to promote sinus drainage. Younger children should be accompanied in the bathroom by a parent at all times when breathing steam from shower.
- Take OTC decongestants as needed for congestion and follow instructions on the label. Ask your pharmacist for product suggestions.
- Take usual pain medication (acetaminophen, ibuprofen) for discomfort and fever. Do not give aspirin to a child. Avoid aspirin-like products if age <20 years. Avoid acetaminophen if liver disease is present. Avoid ibuprofen if kidney disease or stomach problems exist or in the case of pregnancy. Follow the directions on the label. Use the dosing device that comes with the medication, a measuring device, or a medication syringe from the pharmacy. Household teaspoons often do not give the correct amount of medication.

## Additional Instructions

_____

_____

_____

## Report the Following Problems to Your PCP/Clinic/ED

- Persistent pain or condition worsens
- Temperature >101°F (38.3°C)
- Signs of infection: pain, swelling, redness, warmth, drainage, or red streaks
- Persistent nasal discharge
- Change in vision, hearing, smell, or taste

## Seek Emergency Care Immediately If Any of the Following Occur

- Sudden loss of vision
- Severe pain on one side of face, over eye, blurred vision, and red eye
- Sudden facial drooping on one side of the face

If the caller agrees with the advice given, document the call and encourage the caller to call back or see PCP if the problem worsens. If the caller does not agree with the advice given, reevaluate and advise the caller to follow up with PCP, Clinic, or ED.

# Facial Skin Problems

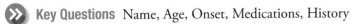

» **Key Questions**  Name, Age, Onset, Medications, History

» **Other Protocols to Consider**  Facial Problems (172); Mouth Problems (302); Rash (366); Skin Lesions: Lumps, Bumps, and Sores (414).

*Reminder:* Document caller response to advice, home care instructions, and when to call back.

| ASSESSMENT | ACTION |
|---|---|

**A. Are any of the following present?**

- Sudden onset of facial drooping
- Severe facial swelling
- Rapidly spreading red or purple rash that develops into blisters on mucous membranes (lips, mouth, eyes, genitals)
- Peeling or shedding large amount of skin
- Unexplained widespread pain

**YES** "Seek emergency care now"

**NO** Go to B

**B. Are any of the following present?**

- Signs of infection: swelling, redness, pain, warmth, temperature >100°F (37.8°C), drainage, or red streaks
- Large, open, draining lesions

**YES** "Seek medical care within 2 to 4 hours"

**NO** Go to C

**C. Are any of the following present?**

- Crusty, tender lesions around nostrils or lips
- Blisters on one side of face preceded by pain and burning 1 to 2 days before rash appearance
- Persistent flat or slightly raised lesions with irregular borders
- Recent rapid change in color, size, or shape of mole

**YES** "Seek medical care within 24 hours"

**NO** Go to D

F

## D. Are any of the following present?

- Itching rash interferes with sleep
- Persistent acne unresponsive to OTC and home care measures
- Flushed face
- Blister, or red, rough, or painful area around mouth
- Swollen, tender lump under skin
- Sudden appearance of mole or painless lump
- Persistent sore >1 week

**YES**  "Call back or call PCP for appointment if no improvement" and Follow **Home Care Instructions**

**NO**  Follow **Home Care Instructions**

## Home Care Instructions
## Facial Skin Problems

- Wash with mild soap (OTC products, i.e., Aveeno, Basis, Cetaphil, Dove, Neutrogena) and rinse well.
- For signs of infection, apply hot moist packs to area for 20 minutes, 4 to 6 times a day.
- Do not break open or squeeze lesions.
- Keep scalp hair off face.
- Apply lip protectant (Blistex) or analgesic (Campho-Phenique) to sores around mouth to reduce discomfort. Keep sores moist with petroleum jelly–based product. Follow instructions on the label. Ask your pharmacist for suggestions for other OTC products.

## Additional Instructions

_____

_____

_____

### Report the Following Problems to Your PCP/Clinic/ED
- Persistent sores around mouth >7 days
- No improvement or condition worsens
- Signs of infection
- Severe pain or itching interferes with activity

### Seek Emergency Care Immediately If Any of the Following Occur
- Sudden onset of facial drooping or numbness
- Severe facial swelling
- Rapidly spreading red or purple rash that develops into blisters on mucous membranes (lips, mouth, eyes, genitals)
- Peeling or shedding large amount of skin
- Unexplained widespread pain

F

If the caller agrees with the advice given, document the call and encourage the caller to call back or see PCP if the problem worsens. If the caller does not agree with the advice given, reevaluate and advise the caller to follow up with PCP, Clinic, or ED.

# Fainting

 **Key Questions** Name, Age, Onset, Cause, Additional Injuries, Medications, History

 **Other Protocols to Consider** Alcohol Problems (9); Confusion (107); Diabetes Problems (138); Dizziness (147); Heart Rate Problems (249); Heat-Exposure Problems (252); Weakness (496).

*Reminder:* Document caller response to advice, home care instructions, and when to call back.

| ASSESSMENT | ACTION |
|---|---|

**A. Is the person still unconscious or has slow, irregular, or noisy breathing?**

| | |
|---|---|
| **YES** | "Call ambulance" |
| **NO** | Go to B |

**B. Is chest, jaw, neck, shoulder, or arm pain present?**

| | |
|---|---|
| **YES** | Go to Chest Pain protocol (85) |
| **NO** | Go to C |

**C. Are any of the following present?**

- Loss of consciousness >1 to 2 minutes
- Loss of movement in arms or legs, confusion, difficulty speaking, numbness or tingling, or blurred vision
- History of recent head injury
- History of heart problems or diabetes
- Irregular or rapid heartbeat
- Severe headache
- Severe back or abdominal pain
- Recent bloody or black tarry stools
- Shortness of breath
- Fainted during exercise

| | |
|---|---|
| **YES** | "Call ambulance" or |
| **NO** | "Seek emergency care now" Go to D |

178

### D. Are any of the following present?

- Signs of dehydration:
  - infrequent urination
  - dark yellow urine
  - sunken eyes
  - poor skin elasticity
  - excessive thirst
  - dry mouth or mucous membranes
- Continued light-headedness or dizziness
- More than one fainting episode in the same day

**YES**   "Seek medical care within 2 to 4 hours"

**NO**   Go to E

### E. Are any of the following present?

- Pregnancy or LMP >6 weeks ago

**YES**   "Seek medical care within 24 hours"

**NO**   Go to F

### F. In addition to light-headedness, are any of the following present?

- Several hours of exposure to the sun or a hot environment
- Prolonged period of time since eating
- Feeling faint after suddenly standing from a lying, sitting, or bending position
- Recent onset of an emotional event
- Feeling faint after strenuous exercise
- Faintness after prolonged standing in one spot
- New medication
- Faintness occurred after a period of rapid breathing and numbness in hands, toes, or face

**YES**   "Call back or call PCP for appointment if no improvement"
and
Follow **Home Care Instructions**

**NO**   Follow **Home Care Instructions**

F

## Home Care Instructions
## Fainting

- For faintness, raise legs higher than the head or sit and lower head between the knees until sensation passes.
- If there has been prolonged exposure to heat, sip cool fluids and apply cold compresses to cool the body.
- Avoid sudden posture changes: slowly stand from a lying, sitting, or bending position.
- If the person has diabetes, check blood sugar and take appropriate action. For low blood sugar, drink a glass of orange juice, cola, or milk.
- Eat frequent small protein snacks. Eat a well-balanced, sensible, weight-reduction diet if overweight.
- Avoid prolonged standing in one position. Shift weight from foot to foot. Walk around if possible.

### Additional Instructions

### Report the Following Problems to Your PCP/Clinic/ED

- Frequent episodes of light-headedness
- New medication and faintness persists
- Condition persists or worsens
- New-onset, bloody or black tarry stools
- Possibility of pregnancy

### Seek Emergency Care Immediately If Any of the Following Occur

- Chest, jaw, neck, shoulder, or arm pain
- Severe headache
- Severe back or abdominal pain
- Fainting recurs
- Shortness of breath

If the caller agrees with the advice given, document the call and encourage the caller to call back or see PCP if the problem worsens. If the caller does not agree with the advice given, reevaluate and advise the caller to follow up with PCP, Clinic, or ED.

# Fatigue

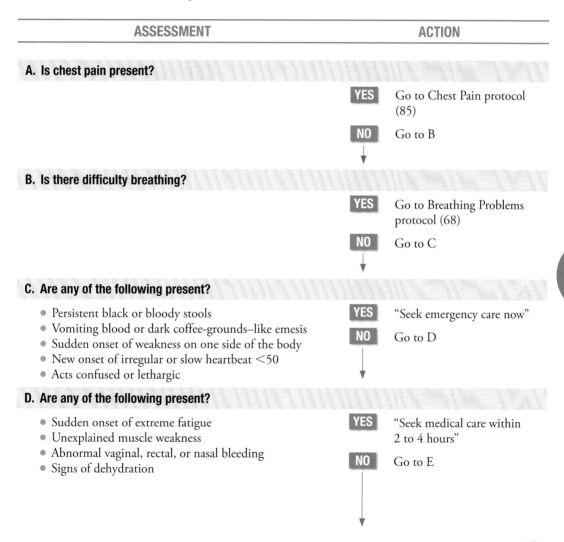

**Key Questions** Name, Age, Onset, Medications, History

**Other Protocols to Consider** Depression (135); Fever (184); Heart Rate Problems (249); Rectal Bleeding (371); Vaginal Bleeding (484); Weakness (496).

*Reminder:* Document caller response to advice, home care instructions, and when to call back.

| ASSESSMENT | ACTION |
|---|---|
| **A. Is chest pain present?** | |
| | **YES** Go to Chest Pain protocol (85) |
| | **NO** Go to B |
| **B. Is there difficulty breathing?** | |
| | **YES** Go to Breathing Problems protocol (68) |
| | **NO** Go to C |
| **C. Are any of the following present?** | |
| • Persistent black or bloody stools <br> • Vomiting blood or dark coffee-grounds–like emesis <br> • Sudden onset of weakness on one side of the body <br> • New onset of irregular or slow heartbeat <50 <br> • Acts confused or lethargic | **YES** "Seek emergency care now" <br><br> **NO** Go to D |
| **D. Are any of the following present?** | |
| • Sudden onset of extreme fatigue <br> • Unexplained muscle weakness <br> • Abnormal vaginal, rectal, or nasal bleeding <br> • Signs of dehydration | **YES** "Seek medical care within 2 to 4 hours" <br><br> **NO** Go to E |

F

### E. Are any of the following present?

- Progressive fatigue that limits usual activities
- Persistent fever unresponsive to fever-reducing measures
- Sudden unexplained loss of weight

**YES**  "Seek medical care within 24 hours"

**NO**  Go to F

### F. Are any of the following present?

- Depression or psychological problems
- Intermittent or persistent fatigue
- Difficulty sleeping
- Poor diet or eating habits
- Chronic allergies
- Recovering from an illness
- History of anemia, cardiac problems, kidney disease, diabetes, or other chronic disease
- Onset with recent increase in stress or activity

**YES**  "Call back or call PCP for appointment if no improvement"
and
Follow **Home Care Instructions**

**NO**  Follow **Home Care Instructions**

# Home Care Instructions
# Fatigue

- Eat a sensible, well-balanced diet. Avoid sweets to "boost energy."
- Take vitamin supplements as needed.
- Maintain a regular exercise routine. Take short walks if vigorous activity is too strenuous.
- Get an adequate amount of sleep. Try to establish a consistent sleeping pattern.
- Increase rest, relaxation, and recreation to decrease stress.
- Limit medications that contribute to fatigue, such as cold and allergy medications. If prescription medication is causing fatigue, contact your PCP.
- Limit use of caffeine, smoking, and alcohol consumption.

## Additional Instructions

_____

_____

_____

## Report the Following Problems to Your PCP/Clinic/ED
- Condition persists >2 weeks or worsens
- Fever

## Seek Emergency Care Immediately If Any of the Following Occur
- Chest pain or difficulty breathing
- Black or bloody stools
- Vomiting blood or dark coffee-grounds–like emesis
- Sudden onset of one-sided weakness
- New onset of irregular or slow heartbeat <50

F

If the caller agrees with the advice given, document the call and encourage the caller to call back or see PCP if the problem worsens. If the caller does not agree with the advice given, reevaluate and advise the caller to follow up with PCP, Clinic, or ED.

# Fever

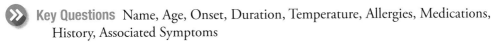

**⟫ Key Questions**  Name, Age, Onset, Duration, Temperature, Allergies, Medications, History, Associated Symptoms

**⟫ Other Protocols to Consider**  Abdominal Pain (1); Common Cold Symptoms (103); Earache, Drainage (150); Diarrhea (143); Headache (238); Heat-Exposure Problems (252); Rash (366); Sore Throat (420); Sweating, Excessive (446); Vomiting (492); Wound Care: Sutures or Staples (506).

> *Nurse Alert:* There are many conditions that cause fever; however, it can indicate a serious problem in newborns <1 month old, immunosuppressed, and frail children. Provide reassurance that the cause of the fever may not be known for 24 hours until other symptoms begin to develop. See Appendix E (545) for Temperature Conversion chart.

*Reminder:* Document caller response to advice, home care instructions, and when to call back.

| ASSESSMENT | ACTION |
|---|---|
| **A. Are any of the following present?** | |
| • Difficulty breathing (for reason other than congestion) <br> • Skin or lips turning blue <br> • New-onset drooling <br> • Unable to swallow <br> • Purple or blood-colored spots or dots on skin <br> • New seizure and no history of febrile seizure <br> • Rash, red tongue and enlarged lymph nodes <br> • Child appears very ill, confused, lethargic, or very irritable <br> • Infant <4 weeks of age and temperature >100.4°F (38.0°C) rectally <br> • Infant <12 months of age with sickle cell disease <br> • Bulging fontanelle | **YES**  "Seek emergency care now" <br><br> **NO**  Go to B |

## B. Are any of the following present?

- Neck pain when bending head forward
- Severe headache or abdominal pain
- Difficult or rapid breathing, trouble swallowing, or wheezing
- Infant 1 to 3 months of age and temperature >100.4°F (38.0°C)
- Infant 3 to 6 months of age and temperature >102.2°F (39.0°C)
- Fever occurs >48 hours after recent immunization
- Infant >6 months of age and temperature >105°F (40.6°C) or diarrhea and vomiting
- Temperature >104°F (40°C) and is unresponsive to fever-reducing measures (fever decreases 2°F to 3°F or 1°C to 1.5°C, 2 hours after medication)
- Seizure (history of febrile seizure)
- Signs of dehydration:
  - decreased urine
  - sunken eyes or fontanelle
  - pinched skin does not spring back
  - excessive thirst, dry mouth
  - crying without tears
- Difficulty drinking "adequate" amount of fluids
- Solid red rash that is tender to touch
- History of sickle cell disease, splenectomy, steroid use, cancer, AIDS, or cystic fibrosis
- Recent travel outside of the United States

**YES** "Seek medical care within 2 hours"

**NO** Go to C

## C. Are any of the following present?

- Fever >24 hours and age >2 years with no other symptoms
- Fever >72 hours that is unresponsive to fever-reducing measures or no known cause
- Yellow phlegm >72 hours
- History of diabetes, asthma, seizures
- Frequent or painful urination
- Vaginal bleeding, pain, or discharge
- Vomiting, diarrhea, or abdominal pain
- Earache, sore throat, and/or swollen glands
- Rash
- Fever lasts 2 to 3 days, 7 to 14 days after measles, mumps, and rubella (MMR) vaccine

**YES** "Seek medical care within 24 hours"

**NO** Go to D

F

## D. Are any of the following present?

- Congestion, sneezing, or achiness
- Other family members are ill
- Fever >72 hours that is responsive to self-care measures
- Parent is comfortable with advice given

**YES**   Follow **Home Care Instructions**

**NO**   "Call back or call PCP for appointment if no improvement"
and
Follow **Home Care Instructions**

## Home Care Instructions
## Fever

- Provide reassurance that children often eat less with a fever but need to consume adequate fluids.
- Encourage increased consumption of cold beverages, such as juices and gelatin, as well as warm tea and broth, which are soothing to the throat.
- Give acetaminophen (if infant is >3 months) or ibuprofen (if age >6 months) for fever >102°F and achiness. Do not give aspirin to a child. Avoid aspirin-like products if age <20 years. Avoid acetaminophen if liver disease is present. Avoid ibuprofen if kidney disease or stomach problems exist or in the case of pregnancy. Follow the directions on the label. Avoid alternating acetaminophen and ibuprofen. Do not give ibuprofen if child has abdominal pain, is vomiting, or is dehydrated. Use the dosing device that comes with the medication, a measuring device, or a medication syringe from the pharmacy. Household teaspoons often do not give the correct amount of medication.
- Dress the child in light clothing. Do not bundle baby in blankets. Keep room temperature at 70°C if possible.
- Check the child's temperature every 2 to 4 hours. If no improvement, notify PCP or call back.
- Remember that fever is a normal body reaction to fighting infections; fevers rarely go above 104°F to 105°F (40°C to 40.6°C), even without treatment.
- Recommend return to day care or school and participation in normal activities when fever subsides for 24 hours without antipyretics.
- May use spongebath with lukewarm water for high fevers. Spongebath should be discontinued if child starts to shiver. Rubbing alcohol should never be used for spongebaths. Lukewarm spongebaths are not as effective as antipyretics and may cause discomfort.

## Additional Instructions

F

## Report the Following Problems to Your PCP/Clinic/ED

- Temperature >104°F (40°C) for children 3 months of age and older and ≥100.4°F (38.0°C) rectally for children <3 months of age
- Rash, painful neck, or severe headache
- Frequent or painful urination
- Condition worsens or no improvement after 3 days
- Signs of dehydration
- Seizure
- Fever persists 48 hours and no other symptoms

## Seek Emergency Care Immediately If Any of the Following Occur

- Unresponsiveness
- Difficulty breathing
- Stiff neck or bulging fontanelle
- Purple/red spots on skin
- Skin or lips turn blue
- New onset of drooling
- Unable to swallow
- New seizure and no history of febrile seizure
- Rash, red tongue and enlarged lymph nodes

If the caller agrees with the advice given, document the call and encourage the caller to call back or see PCP if the problem worsens. If the caller does not agree with the advice given, reevaluate and advise the caller to follow up with PCP, Clinic, or ED.

# Finger and Toe Problems

 **Key Questions**  Name, Age, Onset, Contributing Cause, Allergies, Medications, History

 **Other Protocols to Consider**  Extremity Injury (163); Joint Pain/Swelling (287); Wound Healing and Infection (509).

*Reminder:* Document caller response to advice, home care instructions, and when to call back.

| ASSESSMENT | ACTION |
|---|---|
| **A. Are any of the following present?** | |
| • Amputation or near-amputation | **YES** "Seek emergency care now" |
| • Deformity with break in the skin or bone protrudes through the skin | **NO** Go to B |
| • Fingers or toes cold or blue compared with other fingers and toes | |
| • Inability to stop bleeding with pressure | |
| **B. After an injury, are any of the following present?** | |
| • Obvious deformity or dislocation | **YES** "Seek medical care within 2 hours" |
| • Severe pain | |
| • Inability to remove rings, and digit is beginning to turn pale, white, or blue | **NO** Go to C |
| • Fever or chills | |
| • Nail loose or dislodged | |
| • High-pressure nail gun injury | |
| • Puncture wound into a joint | |
| **C. Are any of the following present?** | |
| • Swollen and tender finger/toe pad | **YES** "Seek medical care within 24 hours" |
| • Signs of infection: increased pain, swelling, redness, warmth, red streaks, or drainage | |
| • Difficulty moving joint nearest the injury | **NO** Go to D |
| • Fingers and toes numb compared with other fingers and toes | |
| • Blood under nail with increased pain or pressure | |

F

## D. Are any of the following present?

- Pain or swelling without injury
- Inability to remove rings following Home Care Instructions
- Moderate swelling
- Slow-healing wound and diabetic
- Nails discolored and thickened

**YES** "Call back or call PCP for appointment if no improvement"
and
Follow **Home Care Instructions**

**NO** Follow **Home Care Instructions**

## Home Care Instructions
## Finger and Toe Problems

- Ice intermittently (in 20-minute intervals) and elevate the digit for 24 to 48 hours after an injury. Place a small cloth between the ice and the skin.
- Remove rings immediately after the injury, before swelling occurs. Use soap, lotion, petroleum jelly (Vaseline), or another lubricant.
- Immobilize the injured digit by taping it to the next digit.
- Take your usual pain medication (aspirin, acetaminophen, ibuprofen). Do not give aspirin to a child. Avoid aspirin-like products if age <20 years. Avoid acetaminophen if liver disease is present. Avoid ibuprofen if kidney disease or stomach problems exist or in the case of pregnancy. Follow the directions on the label. Use the dosing device that comes with the medication, a measuring device, or a medication syringe from the pharmacy. Household teaspoons often do not give the correct amount of medication.
- For swelling or pain with no known injury, or if signs of infection are present, elevate the digit and apply warm soaks to the area for 20 minutes, 4 times a day.
- Watch for signs of infection as the nail heals. Soak digit in warm water several times a day to combat soreness and to promote healing.

### Additional Instructions

_____

_____

_____

### Report the Following Problems to Your PCP/Clinic/ED

- Signs of infection: increased pain, swelling, redness, warmth, red streaks, fever, or drainage
- Severe pain and swelling that is unresponsive to ice and elevation measures
- Inability to remove rings, and digit is beginning to turn pale, white, or blue
- Severe pain and inability to perform procedure to release blood from under nail
- No improvement in pain, swelling, or ability to use the digit in 48 hours after home care measures
- Problem persists with treatment of >1 week

### Seek Emergency Care Immediately If the Following Occurs

- Fingers or toes become cold or blue compared with other fingers or toes

If the caller agrees with the advice given, document the call and encourage the caller to call back or see PCP if the problem worsens. If the caller does not agree with the advice given, reevaluate and advise the caller to follow up with PCP, Clinic, or ED.

F

# Food Allergy, Known or Suspected

 **Key Questions** Name, Age, Onset, Cause if Known, Allergies, Medications, History

 **Other Protocols to Consider** Allergic Reaction (13); Diarrhea (143); Food Poisoning, Suspected (194); Hives (258); Itching (282); Rash (366); Vomiting (492).

> *Nurse Alert:* Use this protocol only if previously diagnosed with a food allergy or prior reaction to a food substance. If prescribed Epi-Pen for known food allergy, instruct caller to use Epi-Pen as directed by PCP.

*Reminder:* Document caller response to advice, home care instructions, and when to call back.

| ASSESSMENT | ACTION |
|---|---|
| **A. Are any of the following present shortly after eating?** | |
| • Difficulty breathing <br> • Confusion <br> • Difficulty swallowing <br> • Fainting <br> • Severe dizziness | **YES** "Call ambulance" <br> or <br> "Seek emergency care now" <br><br> **NO** Go to B |
| **B. Is the following present within 30 minutes after eating?** | |
| • Swelling of lips, tongue, or mouth | **YES** "Seek medical care now" <br> **NO** Go to C |
| **C. Are any of the following present after eating?** | |
| • Generalized hives or itching <br> • Sore throat <br> • Postnasal drip and throat clearing <br> • Congestion, sneezing, or runny nose <br> • Fatigue <br> • Headache <br> • Persistent diarrhea or vomiting | **YES** "Call back or call PCP for appointment if no improvement" <br> and <br> Follow **Home Care Instructions** <br><br> **NO** Follow **Home Care Instructions** |

## Home Care Instructions
## Food Allergy

- If Epi-Pen used as directed by provider, seek emergency care immediately as symptoms may return once medication has worn off.
- Try to identify the food causing the problem and avoid it. Eggs and milk are the most common food allergies in infants. Peanuts, eggs, chocolate, cow's milk products, soybeans, tree nuts, wheat, fish, and shellfish are the most common causes of food allergies.
- Eliminate the suspected food from the diet for 2 weeks and note whether symptoms disappear. If so, avoid that food in the future. If not, observe for relationship between other foods and symptoms (hives, swelling in mouth, diarrhea).
- Try baking soda baths, Caladryl lotion, or calamine for itching, or take an antihistamine (Benadryl) chewable tablet or liquid (follow instructions on the label). Use the dosing device that comes with the medication, a measuring device, or a medication syringe from the pharmacy. Household teaspoons often do not give the correct amount of medication.

## Additional Instructions

_____

_____

_____

### Report the Following Problems to Your PCP/Clinic/ED

- No improvement in symptoms or condition worsens
- Desire to add suspected food back to diet

### Seek Emergency Care Immediately If Any of the Following Occur

- Fainting
- Difficulty breathing
- Confusion
- Difficulty swallowing
- Severe dizziness

**F**

If the caller agrees with the advice given, document the call and encourage the caller to call back or see PCP if the problem worsens. If the caller does not agree with the advice given, reevaluate and advise the caller to follow up with PCP, Clinic, or ED.

# Food Poisoning, Suspected

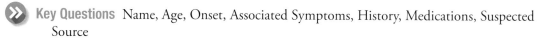 **Key Questions**  Name, Age, Onset, Associated Symptoms, History, Medications, Suspected
Source

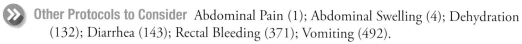 **Other Protocols to Consider**  Abdominal Pain (1); Abdominal Swelling (4); Dehydration
(132); Diarrhea (143); Rectal Bleeding (371); Vomiting (492).

> ***Nurse Alert:***  If caller suspects food poisoning after eating at a restaurant, encourage caller to notify
> the restaurant. Other patrons may have had the same problem. Early notification helps the restaurant to
> track the source and correct the problem.

***Reminder:***  Document caller response to advice, home care instructions, and when to call back.

| ASSESSMENT | ACTION |
|---|---|

**A. Sick 6 to 48 hours after eating canned, smoked, or vacuum-packed foods and are any of the
following present?**

- Altered mental status
- Difficulty breathing or swallowing, or blurred vision
- Vomiting blood
- Bloody stool

 **YES**  "Seek emergency care now"

 **NO**  Go to B

## B. Are any of the following present?

- Pain is severe, worsens, or lasts >4 hours
- Nausea and vomiting >12 hours and unresponsive to home treatment or OTC medications
- Diarrhea >48 hours and unresponsive to home treatment or OTC medications
- Bloody diarrhea
- Signs of dehydration:
  - decreased urine
  - sunken eyes or fontanelle
  - loose dry skin
  - excessive thirst, dry mouth
  - crying without tears
- Dizziness upon standing
- Rash
- Fever

**YES** "Seek medical care within 2 to 4 hours"

**NO** Go to C

## C. Are any of the following present?

- Nausea, vomiting, diarrhea, abdominal pain occurred after eating unrefrigerated meat, poultry, fish, mayonnaise, or egg products
- Others eating the same meal also are ill

**YES** "Call back or call PCP for appointment if no improvement"

**NO** Follow **Home Care Instructions**

F

## Home Care Instructions
## Food Poisoning, Suspected

- Drink small sips of clear fluids (apple juice, tea, broth, sports drinks, clear soda pop, ginger ale) frequently (every 5 to 10 minutes) until nausea and vomiting subside. Increase amount as tolerated during the first 24 hours after vomiting subsides.
- Avoid milk products when experiencing diarrhea.
- Avoid spicy foods, alcohol, dairy products, and coffee for 48 hours after vomiting and diarrhea have subsided.
- Avoid aspirin.
- Prevention:
  - Avoid meats, dressings, sauces, and mayonnaise-based preparations that have been at room temperature for >2 hours. Maintain a food temperature of <40°F (4.4°C) or >140°F (60°C).
  - Do not eat the contents of cans or jars with bulging lids.
  - Defrost meats in the refrigerator or microwave, rather than at room temperature.
  - Wash hands, cutting boards, and countertops frequently, especially after handling raw chicken or eggs.
  - If the food smells unusual or foul, do not eat it.

## Additional Instructions

_____

_____

_____

### Report the Following Problems to Your PCP/Clinic/ED

- Condition persists >48 hours or worsens
- Blood in the stool or vomit (not streaks or flecks)
- Temperature >101°F (38.3°C)

### Seek Emergency Care Immediately If Any of the Following Occur

- Blurred vision
- Difficulty breathing
- Difficulty swallowing
- Decreased level of consciousness
- Signs of dehydration

If the caller agrees with the advice given, document the call and encourage the caller to call back or see PCP if the problem worsens. If the caller does not agree with the advice given, reevaluate and advise the caller to follow up with PCP, Clinic, or ED.

# Foot Problems

**Key Questions**  Name, Age, Onset, Cause, Allergies, History of Diabetes or Vascular Disease, Medications, History

**Other Protocols to Consider**  Ankle Injury (16); Extremity Injury (163); Finger and Toe Problems (183); Joint Pain/Swelling (287).

*Reminder:*  Document caller response to advice, home care instructions, and when to call back.

| ASSESSMENT | ACTION |
|---|---|
| **A. In addition to pain after an injury, fall, or sudden movement, are any of the following present?** | |
| • Deformity <br> • Foot cold or blue compared with other foot | **YES** "Seek emergency care now" <br> **NO** Go to B |
| **B. Are any of the following present?** | |
| • Inability to walk or move foot <br> • Fever and painful, red, swollen toe joints <br> • Diabetic and open or infected wound unresponsive to home care measures | **YES** "Seek medical care within 2 to 4 hours" <br> **NO** Go to C |
| **C. Are any of the following present?** | |
| • Nonhealing wound >1 week <br> • Persistent swelling >1 week <br> • Toe joint swollen, painful, red, and warm and there is no known injury <br> • Red, swollen, painful area on sole of foot | **YES** "Seek medical care within 24 hours" <br> **NO** Go to D |

F

## D. Are any of the following present?

- Pain after walking or running
- Painful, warm, swollen area around toenail
- Injured toe swollen and bruised
- Both feet ache after prolonged walking or standing
- Persistent itching
- Soft, red, peeling skin between toes or on soles of feet
- Excessive sweating or foul odor
- Painful flat hard lump of tough skin on sole of foot
- Lumps of hard skin over toes and sides of feet
- Soles of feet ache upon rising in the morning
- Heel pain
- Cracked dry skin

**YES** "Call back or call PCP for appointment if no improvement"
and
Follow **Home Care Instructions**

**NO** Follow **Home Care Instructions**

## Home Care Instructions
## Foot Problems

- For signs of infection (pain, swelling, redness, red streaks, drainage, or warmth), apply moist hot packs or soaks to area for 20 minutes, 4 to 6 times a day.
- After an injury, elevate foot and apply ice packs to area for 20 minutes, 4 to 6 times a day. Wrap with elastic bandage to keep swelling down for the first 24 to 48 hours. Never apply ice directly to the skin. Place a washcloth between the ice pack and the skin.
- Tape an injured toe to the next toe to provide support and promote healing for 7 to 10 days.
- Apply sponge rings around painful hard lumps to reduce the pressure of a shoe against the area.
- Wear comfortable-fitting shoes.
- Apply OTC remedies (DuoFilm, DuoPlant, Wart-Off) to warts on bottom of feet at night. Follow instructions on the label. Be careful to avoid applying treatment to surrounding sensitive skin.
- For peeling irritated skin, wash and dry frequently. Wear cotton or other natural fiber socks and shoes with porous soles or open-toed shoes. Apply OTC antifungal cream, spray, or powder to the affected area.
- Trim toenails straight across, but do not cut them too short.
- Apply moisturizing hand or body cream (Alpha-Keri, Curel, Vaseline Intensive Care) to dry, cracked skin twice a day. Follow instructions on the label. Avoid going barefoot.
- Rest and elevate feet for discomfort and swelling. Soak aching feet in tub or basin of warm water and Epsom salt.
- Reduce weight-bearing activities until free of pain.
- Apply ice for heel pain for 20 minutes, 4 times a day and after weight-bearing activity.
- For persistent pain on sole and/or heel, perform foot exercises upon arising and throughout the day. In a sitting position, use the affected foot to create each letter in the alphabet.
- Take usual pain medication (acetaminophen or ibuprofen). Do not give aspirin to a child. Avoid aspirin-like products if age <20 years. Avoid acetaminophen if liver disease is present. Avoid ibuprofen if kidney disease or stomach problems exist or in the case of pregnancy. Follow the directions on the label. Use the dosing device that comes with the medication, a measuring device, or a medication syringe from the pharmacy. Household teaspoons often do not give the correct amount of medication.

**Additional Instructions**

### Report the Following Problems to Your PCP/Clinic/ED

- Persistent pain, swelling, or sores
- No improvement with home care measures or condition worsens
- Inability to walk or move foot

### Seek Emergency Care Immediately If the Following Occurs

- Foot turns cold or blue compared with other foot

If the caller agrees with the advice given, document the call and encourage the caller to call back or see PCP if the problem worsens. If the caller does not agree with the advice given, reevaluate and advise the caller to follow up with PCP, Clinic, or ED.

# Foreign Body, Eye

 **Key Questions** Name, Age, Onset, Cause, Medications, History

 **Other Protocols to Consider** Eye Injury (166); Eye Problems (169); Vision Problems (489).

*Reminder:* Document caller response to advice, home care instructions, and when to call back.

| ASSESSMENT | ACTION |
|---|---|
| **A. Are any of the following present?** | |
| • Object is embedded in the eyeball<br>• Severe pain after irrigating chemical substance from eye<br>• Sudden change in vision<br>• Bulging eyeball<br>• Blood in the colored part of the eye<br>• Clear jelly-like discharge from injured eye<br>• Severe pain after foreign body removed<br>• Unequal pupil size | **YES** "Seek emergency care now"<br><br>**NO** Go to B |
| **B. Are any of the following present?** | |
| • Foreign object is over the colored part of the eye<br>• Swelling, pain, or tearing >30 minutes<br>• Injury caused by hot water, chemical, or foreign body, and pain persists after home care treatment<br>• Unable to remove free-floating foreign body | **YES** "Seek medical care within 2 to 4 hours" and Follow **Home Care Instructions**<br><br>**NO** Go to C |
| **C. Are any of the following present?** | |
| • Discomfort or irritation persists 24 hours after the injury or removal of a foreign body<br>• Signs of infection develop after an injury: pain, swelling, redness, drainage, or fever<br>• Unable to remove contact lens | **YES** "Seek medical care within 24 hours"<br><br>**NO** "Call back or call PCP for appointment if no improvement" and Follow **Home Care Instructions** |

201

## Home Care Instructions
## Foreign Body, Eye

- Chemicals in the eye: Immediately flush eye with cold running water for 20 to 30 minutes. Tilt head under running water with the injured eye down. While holding eyelids apart, allow water to run across the inner eye to the outer part of the eye.
- Do not try to remove
  - foreign body embedded in the eye
  - metal chip
  - foreign body over the colored part of the eye
- Foreign body removal (lint, specks of dirt, eyelashes):
  - Pull down the lower lid and remove the particle with the corner of a moistened handkerchief, tissue, or cotton-tipped swab.
  - Pull down the upper lid over the lower lid and hold in place for a moment. Release and look to see if object is visible; if so, remove it.
- Do not rub eye.
- Apply ice pack or cool compresses to reduce discomfort.
- Take your usual pain medication (acetaminophen or ibuprofen). Do not give aspirin to a child. Avoid aspirin-like products if age <20 years. Avoid acetaminophen if liver disease is present. Avoid ibuprofen if kidney disease or stomach problems exist or in the case of pregnancy. Follow the directions on the label. Use the dosing device that comes with the medication, a measuring device, or a medication syringe from the pharmacy. Household teaspoons often do not give the correct amount of medication.

## Additional Instructions

## Report the Following Problems to Your PCP/Clinic/ED

- Increased pain, swelling, drainage, or fever
- Changes in vision
- No improvement in pain after 48 hours
- Unable to remove free-floating foreign body

If the caller agrees with the advice given, document the call and encourage the caller to call back or see PCP if the problem worsens. If the caller does not agree with the advice given, reevaluate and advise the caller to follow up with PCP, Clinic, or ED.

# Foreign Body, Inhaled

 **Key Questions** Name, Age, Onset, Object Inhaled, History, Medications

 **Other Protocols to Consider** Breathing Problems (68); Cough (121); Foreign Body, Swallowing of (214); Piercing Problems (338).

*Reminder:* Document caller response to advice, home care instructions, and when to call back.

| ASSESSMENT | ACTION |
|---|---|

### A. Are any of the following present?

- Choking and unable to speak, cough, or breathe
- Unconscious person who is not breathing

**YES** "Call ambulance and begin rescue breathing"

**NO** Go to B

### B. Are any of the following present?

- Difficulty breathing
- Lips or face turning blue
- Inability to cry or speak
- Suicide attempt
- Aspirated foreign body into the lungs and difficulty breathing

**YES** "Call ambulance"

**NO** Go to C

### C. Are any of the following present?

- Persistent coughing or wheezing >30 minutes after clearing an inhaled foreign body
- Coughing up blood or severe pain after dislodging foreign body from the throat
- Unable to remove foreign object from throat but no other symptoms
- Feeling of suffocation
- Drooling
- Speaking in short words
- Unable to swallow saliva or fluids

**YES** "Seek emergency care now"

**NO** Go to D

F

## D.  Are any of the following present?

- Fever
- Speaking in partial sentences
- Intermittent cough or wheezing after inhaling a foreign object, aerosol, or smoke

**YES**  Seek medical attention within 2 to 4 hours"

**NO**  Go to E

## E.  Are any of the following present?

- Able to speak and cough
- No difficulty breathing
- Frequent episodes of choking on saliva, foods, or fluids
- Speaking in full sentences

**YES**  "Call back or call PCP for appointment if no improvement"
and
Follow **Home Care Instructions**

**NO**  Follow **Home Care Instructions**

## Home Care Instructions
## Foreign Body, Inhaled

- For frequent choking, eat slowly, taking smaller bites.
- If there is a sensation that a fish bone is stuck in the throat, try washing down the bone with bread and milk.

### Additional Instructions

_____

_____

_____

### Report the Following Problems to Your PCP/Clinic/ED

- Fish or chicken bone in throat and persistent scratchy throat >2 hours
- Coughing up blood
- Signs of infection: persistent sore throat, fever, or drainage
- Difficulty swallowing
- No improvement or condition worsens

### Seek Emergency Care Immediately If Any of the Following Occur

- Difficulty breathing, shortness of breath, or wheezing
- Unable to swallow saliva or fluids
- Feeling of suffocation

F

If the caller agrees with the advice given, document the call and encourage the caller to call back or see PCP if the problem worsens. If the caller does not agree with the advice given, reevaluate and advise the caller to follow up with PCP, Clinic, or ED.

# Foreign Body, Nose

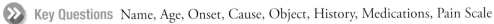 **Key Questions**  Name, Age, Onset, Cause, Object, History, Medications, Pain Scale

**Other Protocols to Consider**  Piercing Problems (338); Congestion (110); Nosebleed (319); Nose Injury (322).

***Reminder:***  Document caller response to advice, home care instructions, and when to call back.

| ASSESSMENT | ACTION |
|---|---|

### A. Are any of the following present?

- Sharp object embedded in nose
- Profuse bleeding
- Irritating or adhesive substance in nose
- Severe nasal pain
- Age younger than 18 months
- Foreign body may be a small disk battery

**YES** "Seek medical care within 2 hours"

**NO** Go to B

### B. Body art or piercing present, and are any of the following present?

- Skin red and warm, and fever or headache
- Vomiting and abdominal pain

**YES** "Seek medical care within 4 to 8 hours"

**NO** Go to C

### C. Are any of the following present?

- Unable to remove foreign object after several tries
- Swelling and tenderness
- Foul-smelling green or yellow nasal drainage from one nostril

**YES** "Seek medical care within 24 hours"

**NO** Go to D

## D. Is the following present?

- Foreign substance or object in nose removed and no other symptoms

**YES**   "Call back or call PCP for appointment if no improvement" and Follow **Home Care Instructions**

**NO**   Follow **Home Care Instructions**

F

## Home Care Instructions
## Foreign Body, Nose

- Apply saline drops or a nasal decongestant in the affected nostril.
- Pinch the unaffected nostril and exhale through the affected nostril.
- If the object is visible, do not attempt removal if unable to hold the head absolutely still. If there is resistance or a chance of pushing the object in farther, stop and seek medical care.

**Additional Instructions**

_____

_____

_____

### Report the Following Problems to Your PCP/Clinic/ED

- Unable to remove foreign object after several tries
- Swelling and tenderness persist or worsen
- Foul-smelling green or yellow nasal drainage from one nostril
- Fever, headache, and/or stiff neck

If the caller agrees with the advice given, document the call and encourage the caller to call back or see PCP if the problem worsens. If the caller does not agree with the advice given, reevaluate and advise the caller to follow up with PCP, Clinic, or ED.

# Foreign Body, Rectum

**Key Questions** Name, Age, Onset, Object, Allergies, Medications, History, Pain Scale

**Other Protocols to Consider** Child Abuse (94); Constipation (114); Rectal Bleeding (371); Rectal Problems (374); Sexual Assault (400).

*Reminder:* Document caller response to advice, home care instructions, and when to call back.

| ASSESSMENT | ACTION |
|---|---|

### A. Are any of the following present?

- Sharp object in rectum
- Profuse bleeding
- Severe pain
- Victim of sexual assault
- Traumatic injury
- High fever, chills, nausea, or vomiting

**YES** "Seek medical care now"

**NO** Go to B

### B. Are any of the following present?

- Unable to remove foreign object after several tries
- Swelling and tenderness
- Foul-smelling drainage
- Rectal bleeding
- Abdominal or shoulder pain

**YES** "Seek medical care within 2 to 4 hours"

**NO** Go to C

### C. Are any of the following present?

- Sensation of rectal fullness
- Rectal pain
- Retained condom
- Unable to pass stool

**YES** "Seek medical care within 24 hours"

**NO** "Call back or call PCP for appointment if no improvement"
and
Follow **Home Care Instructions**

**F**

## Home Care Instructions
## Foreign Body, Rectum

- Do not try to remove sharp object or object that has broken inside rectum.
- Take your usual pain medication (acetaminophen or ibuprofen). Do not give aspirin to a child. Avoid aspirin-like products if age <20 years. Avoid acetaminophen if liver disease is present. Avoid ibuprofen if kidney disease or stomach problems exist or in the case of pregnancy. Follow the directions on the label. Use the dosing device that comes with the medication, a measuring device, or a medication syringe from the pharmacy. Household teaspoons often do not give the correct amount of medication.
- Watch for signs of infection: increased pain, discharge, fever, or swelling.

## Additional Instructions

_____

_____

_____

### Report the Following Problems to Your PCP/Clinic/ED
- Unable to remove foreign object after several tries
- Swelling and tenderness persist or worsen
- Foul-smelling drainage or fever
- Rectal bleeding
- Unable to pass stool
- High fever, chills, nausea, or vomiting

### Seek Emergency Care Immediately If Any of the Following Occur
- Profuse bleeding
- Severe pain

If the caller agrees with the advice given, document the call and encourage the caller to call back or see PCP if the problem worsens. If the caller does not agree with the advice given, reevaluate and advise the caller to follow up with PCP, Clinic, or ED.

# Foreign Body, Skin

>> **Key Questions**  Name, Age, Onset, Object, Allergies, Medications, History

>> **Other Protocols to Consider**  Bites, Tick (57); Piercing Problems (338); Extremity
     Injury (163); Laceration (290); Puncture Wound (362); Tattoo Problems (456).

*Reminder:*  Document caller response to advice, home care instructions, and when to call back.

| ASSESSMENT | ACTION |
|---|---|

### A. Are any of the following present?

- Unable to remove embedded fishhook
- Foreign body embedded in joint space
- Deep foreign body
- Unable to remove foreign substance
- Foreign substance is adhered to the skin
- Unable to remove pierced earring back that is embedded in earlobe or other embedded body piercing or foreign object
- Signs of infection: increased redness, pain, swelling, warmth, drainage, or red streaks
- Super glue in eye
- Severe pain

**YES** "Seek emergency care within 2 to 4 hours"
and
Follow **Home Care Instructions**

**NO** Go to B

### B. Are any of the following present?

- Unable to remove large splinter
- Embedded glass, plastic, or metal object
- Tetanus immunization >5 years ago
- Tick head embedded in skin and unable to remove

**YES** "Seek medical care within 24 hours"

**NO** Go to C

F

## C. Are any of the following present?

- Unable to remove small splinter
- Persistent sensation of a foreign body under the skin

**YES**  "Call back or call PCP for appointment if no improvement"
and
Follow **Home Care Instructions**

**NO**  Follow **Home Care Instructions**

## Home Care Instructions
## Foreign Body, Skin

- Fishhook removal techniques:
  - Push barb through the skin, cut off the barb with wire cutters, and then back it out the way it entered.
  - Push barb in and down slightly to disengage the barb from the skin and pull it out of the skin.
  - Loop fishline through the bend in the fishhook. Push barb in and hold down slightly to disengage barb from skin. Jerk the fishline quickly to remove the hook.
- Remove splinter or object with tweezers or a needle sterilized with a match flame or rubbing alcohol.
- Do not soak splinter area in water or solution, which will cause the wood to swell, thus hindering removal.
- Apply hot packs or soaks 4 to 6 times a day if there are signs of infection and to aid in the removal of a foreign body.
- Apply antibiotic (Neosporin) ointment and a bandage over difficult-to-remove splinters. They often will dislodge in a couple of days.
- After removal, wash the area well with soap and water.
- Techniques for removing tar or superglue:
  - Apply petroleum jelly, Neosporin, mayonnaise, mineral oil, or nail polish remover to the involved area (except near the eyes).
  - Do not force open skin or eyelids.
  - Superglue eventually will flake.
  - If eye is glued shut, apply Neosporin and hot compresses.
  - Tar may leave a stain on the skin.
  - Reduce heat from tar by cooling the area with water or wet towels.

**F**

## Additional Instructions

_____

_____

_____

### Report the Following Problems to Your PCP/Clinic/ED
- Unable to remove foreign body after 48 hours
- Signs of infection: increased redness, pain, swelling, warmth, drainage, or red streaks
- Severe pain

If the caller agrees with the advice given, document the call and encourage the caller to call back or see PCP if the problem worsens. If the caller does not agree with the advice given, reevaluate and advise the caller to follow up with PCP, Clinic, or ED.

# Foreign Body, Swallowing of

 **Key Questions**  Name, Age, Onset, Object, Medications, History, Pain Scale

 **Other Protocols to Consider**  Abdominal Pain (1); Constipation (114); Diarrhea (143);
Piercing Problems (338); Rectal Bleeding (371); Rectal Problems (374);
Vomiting (492).

*Reminder:*  Document caller response to advice, home care instructions, and when to call back.

| ASSESSMENT | ACTION |
|---|---|
| **A. Are any of the following present?**<br><br>• Excessive saliva, drooling, or gagging<br>• Difficulty swallowing<br>• Coughing, choking, or breathing difficulties<br>• Suicide attempt<br>• Object was a battery, magnet, or sharp object | **YES** "Call ambulance"<br>or<br>"Seek emergency care now"<br><br>**NO** Go to B |
| **B. Are any of the following present?**<br><br>• Pain or discomfort in throat or chest<br>• Abdominal pain<br>• Vomiting | **YES** "Seek medical care within 2 to 4 hours"<br><br>**NO** Go to C |
| **C. Are any of the following present?**<br><br>• Metal object<br>• Object size larger than a nickel | **YES** "Seek medical care within 24 hours"<br><br>**NO** Go to D |
| **D. Are any of the following present?**<br><br>• Wood or plastic object<br>• Dull glass object (piece of a jar or cup)<br>• Object size smaller than a penny<br>• Known substance swallowed but no symptoms | **YES** "Call back or call PCP for appointment if no improvement"<br>and<br>Follow **Home Care Instructions**<br><br>**NO** Follow **Home Care Instructions** |

## Home Care Instructions
## Foreign Body, Swallowing of

- If no symptoms, try a sip of fluid. If no difficulty, try swallowing bread or soft food.
- A dull glass object, such as a piece of a jar, cup, or ring, should pass with stools without difficulty in 3 to 4 days.
- Do not give laxatives. Increase fiber (fruit, vegetables, whole grains) in the diet to help stimulate natural elimination.
- Check stools for swallowed object.

## Additional Instructions

_____

_____

_____

### Report the Following Problems to Your PCP/Clinic/ED

- Intermittent choking or gagging
- Abdominal pain
- No evidence of object in stools within 7 days
- Vomiting
- Chest pain
- Fever

### Seek Emergency Care Immediately If the Following Occurs

- Drooling, gagging, choking, or difficulty breathing or swallowing

**F**

If the caller agrees with the advice given, document the call and encourage the caller to call back or see PCP if the problem worsens. If the caller does not agree with the advice given, reevaluate and advise the caller to follow up with PCP, Clinic, or ED.

# Foreign Body, Vagina

 **Key Questions**  Name, Age, Onset, Object, Allergies, Medications, History, Pain Scale

 **Other Protocols to Consider**  Piercing Problems (338); Sexual Assault (400); Vaginal Bleeding (484); Vaginal Discharge/Pain/Itching (486).

*Reminder:*  Document caller response to advice, home care instructions, and when to call back.

| ASSESSMENT | ACTION |
|---|---|
| **A. Are any of the following present?** | |
| • Sharp object embedded in vagina<br>• Profuse bleeding<br>• Severe pain<br>• Sexual assault<br>• Rapid onset: rash, fever, peeling hands or feet, general ill feeling, vomiting, or diarrhea | **YES** "Seek emergency care now"<br><br>**NO** Go to B |
| **B. Are any of the following present?** | |
| • Unable to remove foreign object after several tries<br>• Swelling and tenderness<br>• Foul-smelling discharge<br>• Tampon left in vagina >24 hours and cannot be removed<br>• Unable to remove contraceptive or pleasure device | **YES** "Seek medical care within 24 hours"<br><br>**NO** "Call back or call PCP for appointment if no improvement"<br>and<br>Follow **Home Care Instructions** |

# Home Care Instructions
## Foreign Body, Vagina

- Do not try to remove sharp object or object that has broken inside vagina.
- Take your usual pain medication (acetaminophen, ibuprofen). Do not give aspirin to a child. Avoid aspirin-like products if age <20 years. Avoid acetaminophen if liver disease is present. Avoid ibuprofen if kidney disease or stomach problems exist or in the case of pregnancy. Follow the directions on the label. Use the dosing device that comes with the medication, a measuring device, or a medication syringe from the pharmacy. Household teaspoons often do not give the correct amount of medication.
- Watch for signs of infection: increased pain, discharge, fever, or swelling.

## Additional Instructions

_____

_____

_____

### Report the Following Problems to Your PCP/Clinic/ED
- Unable to remove foreign object after several tries
- Swelling and tenderness persist or worsen
- Foul-smelling drainage or fever
- Rash, fever, peeling hands or feet, general ill feeling, vomiting, or diarrhea

### Seek Emergency Care Immediately If Any of the Following Occur
- Profuse bleeding
- Severe pain

If the caller agrees with the advice given, document the call and encourage the caller to call back or see PCP if the problem worsens. If the caller does not agree with the advice given, reevaluate and advise the caller to follow up with PCP, Clinic, or ED.

# Frostbite

**Key Questions** Name, Age, Onset, Exposure to Freezing Conditions, Allergies, Medication, History

**Other Protocols to Consider** Cold Exposure Problems (100).

> *Nurse Alert:* Use this protocol only if exposed to freezing temperatures and skin symptoms (e.g., hard, cold, waxy, white or blue blotchy appearance, numbness, tingling, pain, or blisters) are present. Tissue damage may not be evident until after reperfusion, and the extent of damage may evolve over weeks to months. Feet, hands, earlobes, nose, cheeks, and chin are the most frequently affected areas of the body.

*Reminder:* Document caller response to advice, home care instructions, and when to call back.

| ASSESSMENT | ACTION |
|---|---|
| **A. Is the following present?** | |
| • Hard, cold, white, or blue blotchy skin (third-degree frostbite) | **YES** "Seek emergency care now" <br> **NO** Go to B |
| **B. Are any of the following present?** | |
| • Symptoms of hypothermia: confusion, drowsiness, rigid muscles, or irrational behavior | **YES** "Go to Cold Exposure Problems protocol (100)" <br> **NO** Go to C |
| **C. Are any of the following present?** | |
| • Frozen area with blistering or peeling skin (second-degree frostbite) <br> • Blisters develop with rewarming or color and sensation do not return with 1 hour of rewarming. <br> • Signs of infection: increased redness, swelling, pain, drainage, red streaks, warmth, or fever | **YES** "Seek medical care within 2 to 4 hours" <br> **NO** Go to D |

## D.  Is the following present?

- Frozen numb area without blistering (first-degree frostbite)

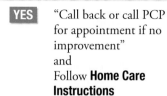 "Call back or call PCP for appointment if no improvement" and Follow **Home Care Instructions**

**NO**  Follow **Home Care Instructions**

F

## Home Care Instructions
## Frostbite

- Remain inside a warm shelter, away from the wind and cold.
- Protect frozen areas from continued exposure.
- Do not thaw or warm the area if there is a possibility it will refreeze; seek medical care immediately.
- Soak cold part in warm water (101°F to 108°F or 38.3°C to 42.2°C) or apply warm compresses to area for 10 to 30 minutes. Skin will thaw, and temperature will return to normal after 1 to 1½ hours.
- Do not use direct heat to rewarm. Avoid using a radiator, campfire, hair dryer, or heating pad to rewarm as they may cause burns.
- Apply firm pressure to the area, but do not rub or massage frozen skin.
- Avoid walking on frostbitten feet, if possible.
- Keep the frostbitten area warm and elevated. Wrap the affected parts in blankets or soft material to prevent bruising.
- Blisters may develop as skin warms. Do not break open the blisters.
- Skin may become red and painful, itch, or tingle. Take usual pain medication (aspirin, acetaminophen, or ibuprofen) as tolerated for discomfort. Do not give aspirin to a child. Avoid aspirin-like products if age <20 years. Avoid acetaminophen if liver disease is present. Avoid ibuprofen if kidney disease or stomach problems exist or in the case of pregnancy. Follow the directions on the label. Use the dosing device that comes with the medication, a measuring device, or a medication syringe from the pharmacy. Household teaspoons often do not give the correct amount of medication.
- Remove wet clothing.

## Additional Instructions

_____

_____

_____

## Report the Following Problems to Your PCP/Clinic/ED

- Persistent hard, white, blue, or numb skin
- Swelling, blistering, or signs of infection
- If blistering occurs, may need an updated tetanus immunization

If the caller agrees with the advice given, document the call and encourage the caller to call back or see PCP if the problem worsens. If the caller does not agree with the advice given, reevaluate and advise the caller to follow up with PCP, Clinic, or ED.

# Gas/Belching

 **Key Questions**  Name, Age, Onset, Cause, Allergies, Medications, History

 **Other Protocols to Consider**  Abdominal Pain (1); Abdominal Swelling (4);
Chest Pain (85); Constipation (114); Heartburn (245); Indigestion (273).

*Reminder:*  Document caller response to advice, home care instructions, and when to call back.

| ASSESSMENT | ACTION |
|---|---|
| **A. Is the following present?** | |
| • Chest, jaw, or neck pain or discomfort | **YES** Go to Chest Pain protocol (85) |
| | **NO** Go to B |
| **B. Are any of the following present?** | |
| • Severe abdominal pain <br> • Shortness of breath <br> • Excessive sweating <br> • Palpitations <br> • Severe nausea and/or vomiting | **YES** "Seek medical care within 2 hours" |
| | **NO** Go to C |
| **C. Are any of the following present?** | |
| • Persistent abdominal discomfort after belching <br> • Pain radiates to back | **YES** "Seek medical care within 24 hours" |
| | **NO** Go to D |
| **D. Are any of the following present?** | |
| • Intermittent abdominal discomfort or swelling <br> • Burping, belching, or hiccups after meals <br> • Belching or heartburn between meals | **YES** "Call back or call PCP for appointment if no improvement" <br> and <br> Follow **Home Care Instructions** |
| | **NO** Follow **Home Care Instructions** |

G

## Home Care Instructions
## Gas/Belching

- Avoid gas-forming foods (parsnips, beans, corn, cabbage, onions, fried food).
- Avoid overindulgence in sweet desserts, fatty foods, and other foods that are known to cause gas.
- Avoid eating too fast or too much.
- Avoid excessive gum chewing.
- Stop smoking if possible or reduce smoking at mealtime.
- Drink an adequate amount of fluids each day.
- Try to reduce stress or excitement, especially at mealtime.
- Sip flat, clear carbonated beverage or peppermint tea to help break up gas.
- Take your usual antacids (Di-Gel, Mylanta-II, Mylicon) to help relieve gas. Follow instructions on the label. Ask pharmacist for other product suggestions. Use the dosing device that comes with the medication, a measuring device, or a medication syringe from the pharmacy. Household teaspoons often do not give the correct amount of medication.

## Additional Instructions

_____

_____

_____

## Report the Following Problems to Your PCP/Clinic/ED

- Symptoms persist or worsen after home care measures
- Severe pain
- Shortness of breath
- Excessive sweating
- Palpitations
- Nausea and vomiting

## Seek Emergency Care Immediately If Any of the Following Occur

- Chest, neck, or jaw pain or discomfort develops
- Light-headedness

If the caller agrees with the advice given, document the call and encourage the caller to call back or see PCP if the problem worsens. If the caller does not agree with the advice given, reevaluate and advise the caller to follow up with PCP, Clinic, or ED.

# Gas/Flatulence

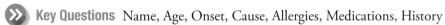

**Key Questions**  Name, Age, Onset, Cause, Allergies, Medications, History

**Other Protocols to Consider**  Abdominal Pain (1); Abdominal Swelling (4); Chest Pain (85); Constipation (114); Indigestion (273).

*Reminder:*  Document caller response to advice, home care instructions, and when to call back.

| ASSESSMENT | | ACTION |
|---|---|---|

### A. Is severe abdominal pain present?

| | YES | Go to Abdominal Pain |
|---|---|---|
| | NO | Go to B |

### B. Is the following present?

- Black tarry stool

| | YES | "Seek emergency care now" |
|---|---|---|
| | NO | Go to C |

### C. Is the following present?

- Severe nausea and vomiting

| | YES | "Seek medical care within 2 to 4 hours" |
|---|---|---|
| | NO | Go to D |

### D. Are any of the following present?

- Persistent abdominal discomfort after passing gas
- Blood in stool
- Pain radiates to back

| | YES | "Seek medical care within 24 hours" |
|---|---|---|
| | NO | Go to E |

G

## E. Are any of the following present?

- Intermittent abdominal discomfort or swelling
- Excessive flatulence
- Pale, bulky, foul-smelling stools
- Recent ingestion of high-fiber or gas-producing foods, such as beans or beer

**YES** "Call back or call PCP for appointment if no improvement" and
Follow **Home Care Instructions**

**NO** Follow **Home Care Instructions**

## Home Care Instructions
## Gas/Flatulence

- Avoid gas-forming foods (parsnips, beans, corn, cabbage, onions, fried food).
- Avoid overindulgence in sweet desserts, fatty foods, and other foods that are known to cause gas.
- Avoid eating too fast or too much.
- Avoid laxatives.
- Drink an adequate amount of fluids each day.
- Maintain regular bowel habits.
- Exercise regularly.
- Try to reduce stress or excitement, especially at mealtime.
- Sip flat, clear carbonated beverage or peppermint tea to help break up gas.
- If lactose intolerant and unable to avoid dairy foods, ask pharmacist for OTC product suggestions.
- As an alternative, try sugar-coated fennel seeds after a meal or sip tea brewed with fennel seeds to break up and disperse gas in the intestinal tract.

## Additional Instructions

_____

_____

_____

### Report the Following Problems to Your PCP/Clinic/ED

- Symptoms persist or worsen after home care measures
- Nausea/vomiting

### Seek Emergency Care Immediately If Any of the Following Occur

- Large amount of blood in stool
- Black tarry stools
- Light-headedness

G

If the caller agrees with the advice given, document the call and encourage the caller to call back or see PCP if the problem worsens. If the caller does not agree with the advice given, reevaluate and advise the caller to follow up with PCP, Clinic, or ED.

# Genital Lesions

 **Key Questions** Name, Age, Onset, Allergies, Medications, History, Pain Scale

 **Other Protocols to Consider** Lice (296); Penis Problems (331); Piercing Problems (338); Scrotal Problems (390); Sexually Transmitted Infection (STI) (403); Skin Lesions: Lumps, Bumps, and Sores (414); Tattoo Problems (456); Vaginal Discharge/Pain/Itching (486).

*Reminder:* Document caller response to advice, home care instructions, and when to call back.

| ASSESSMENT | ACTION |
|---|---|
| **A. Are any of the following present?** | |
| • Severe pain<br>• Signs of infection: increased pain, redness, swelling, drainage, warmth, fever<br>• Age <1 month and small blisters on genitals | **YES** "Seek medical care within 4 to 12 hours"<br><br>**NO** Go to B |
| **B. Are any of the following present?** | |
| • Open sores<br>• New onset of scattered clustered blisters<br>• Fever and general ill feeling<br>• Swollen glands in groin area<br>• Vaginal or penile discharge or bleeding<br>• Severe itching or burning<br>• Sores elsewhere on the body<br>• Pelvic pain<br>• Foreign body<br>• Painful lump at vaginal opening<br>• No improvement >3 days of home treatment for yeast infection | **YES** "Seek medical care within 24 hours"<br><br>**NO** Go to C |

## C.  Are any of the following present?

- Diagnosed herpes, genital warts, or exposure to an STI and requests treatment
- Difficulty passing urine; painful urination or bowel movements
- Painless rash or hard bumps in genital or rectal area >24 hours

   "Seek medical care within 48 hours"

**NO**  Go to D

## D.  Are any of the following present?

- Itchy red rash
- History of recent strenuous activity and sweating
- Pink, scaly, itchy rash on inner thighs, groin, or scrotum
- Raised red, tender, or white or hard bumps
- Painless rash or growths <24 hours

**YES**  "Call back or call PCP for appointment if no improvement"
and
Follow **Home Care Instructions**

**NO**  Follow **Home Care Instructions**

G

## Home Care Instructions
## Genital Lesions

- Soak in a warm bath.
- Avoid bubble bath, harsh or perfumed soaps, scented toilet paper, or hygiene products.
- Avoid sexual activity until symptoms subside.
- Keep area clean and dry.
- Wear cotton underwear and loose garments. Avoid restrictive clothing.
- Try OTC cream (Lotrimin) for itchy rash. Follow instructions on the label.
- If lice are suspected by the presence of small insects or eggs on pubic hairs, see Lice protocol.
- If caller suspects an STI, refer to local public health department or clinic.

## Referral Telephone Numbers

_____

_____

_____

## Additional Instructions

_____

_____

_____

## Report the Following Problems to Your PCP/Clinic/ED

- Signs of infection: pain, redness, swelling, drainage, warmth, red streaks, or swollen glands in the groin
- No improvement after 2 days or condition worsens
- Increased pain or swelling
- Discharge or fever develops
- Suspected exposure to an STI
- Severe pain
- Age <1 month and small blisters on genitals

If the caller agrees with the advice given, document the call and encourage the caller to call back or see PCP if the problem worsens. If the caller does not agree with the advice given, reevaluate and advise the caller to follow up with PCP, Clinic, or ED.

# Glands, Swollen or Tender

**»» Key Questions** Name, Age, Onset, Allergies, Medications, History, Location

**»» Other Protocols to Consider** Mumps (305); Rubella (German Measles) (382); Rubeola (Measles) (385); Skin Lesions: Lumps, Bumps, and Sores (414).

*Reminder:* Document caller response to advice, home care instructions, and when to call back.

| ASSESSMENT | ACTION |
|---|---|

### A. Are any of the following present?

- Swollen node >2 inches across
- Red streaks near the swollen node
- Warmth or redness over the node
- Severe pain
- Node interferes with swallowing, or moving the neck
- Drainage from the node
- Neonate <4 weeks of age

**YES** "Seek medical care within 2 to 4 hours"

**NO** Go to B

### B. Are any of the following present?

- Swollen node 1 to 2 inches across
- Persistent fever unresponsive to fever-reducing measures
- Swollen nodes in groin or posterior cervical or axillary area
- Signs of infection in area near or distal to swollen nodes
- Persistent rash, itching, or swelling in other parts of the body
- Persistent fatigue
- Night sweats
- Node is tender to touch

**YES** "Seek medical care within 24 hours"

**NO** Go to C

G

## C. Are any of the following present?

- History of intermittent nodal swelling
- Nodal swelling in the neck with fever, sore throat, or congestion
- History of allergies
- Swelling and tenderness in underarm area before menstruation

**YES** "Call back or call PCP for appointment if no improvement"
and
Follow **Home Care Instructions**

**NO** Follow **Home Care Instructions**

# Home Care Instructions
## Glands, Swollen or Tender

- Do not squeeze swollen nodes.
- Take your usual pain medication (aspirin, acetaminophen, ibuprofen) as tolerated for discomfort or fever. Do not give aspirin to a child. Avoid aspirin-like products if age <20 years. Avoid acetaminophen if liver disease is present. Avoid ibuprofen if kidney disease or stomach problems exist or in the case of pregnancy. Follow the directions on the label. Use the dosing device that comes with the medication, a measuring device, or a medication syringe from the pharmacy. Household teaspoons often do not give the correct amount of medication.
- Watch for signs of infection.

## Additional Instructions

_____

_____

_____

### Report the Following Problems to Your PCP/Clinic/ED

- Node interferes with breathing, swallowing, or moving the neck
- Persistent underarm swelling or tenderness after menstruation
- Persistent nodal swelling
- Signs of infection: Increased redness, pain, swelling, warmth, red streaks, drainage

If the caller agrees with the advice given, document the call and encourage the caller to call back or see PCP if the problem worsens. If the caller does not agree with the advice given, reevaluate and advise the caller to follow up with PCP, Clinic, or ED.

G

# Hair Loss

 **Key Questions**  Name, Age, Onset, Location, Allergies, Medications, History

 **Other Protocols to Consider**  Fatigue (181); Lice (296); Rash (366); Skin Lesions: Lumps, Bumps, and Sores (414).

***Reminder:*** Document caller response to advice, home care instructions, and when to call back.

| ASSESSMENT | ACTION |
|---|---|
| **A. Are any of the following present?** | |
| • New onset of hair loss and fever >101°F (38.3°C) that is unresponsive to fever-reducing measures | **YES** "Seek medical care within 24 hours" |
| • Signs of infection in hair-loss areas | **NO** Go to B |
| **B. Are any of the following present?** | |
| • Persistent severe fatigue | **YES** "Seek medical care within 48 hours" |
| • Sudden onset after taking a new medication | |
| • History of hypothyroidism | **NO** Go to C |
| • Circular raised, rough pink patch on scalp with a clear center, ½ to 1 inch and itchy | |

## C. Are any of the following present?

- Increased stress level
- Persistent hair loss >2 weeks
- Scaly, itchy, red bald spots
- Recent pregnancy
- Family history of hair loss
- Poor dietary habits
- History of chemotherapy, major surgery, or infection
- History of recent severe diet and weight loss
- Increased use of vitamin A, aspirin, or heparin
- Prolonged use of hair treatments or appliances
- Persistent dandruff or head lice
- History of tight braiding, use of curling iron or hot rollers, or use of chemicals (dye, bleach, or permanent wave application)
- Gradual hair loss over months/years
- Using hormonal contraception

 **YES**    "Call back or call PCP for appointment if no improvement"
and
Follow **Home Care Instructions**

Follow **Home Care Instructions**

H

# Home Care Instructions
## Hair Loss

- Be reassured that hair usually grows back after sudden hair loss.
- Avoid use of rubber bands, barrettes, braids, or other styles that apply tension on the hair.
- Avoid tugging on hair. Use a cream rinse or detangler to reduce snarls when combing wet hair.
- If hair is severely damaged from chemicals or hairdressing techniques, consider a change in style.
- Eat a well-balanced diet and take diet supplements as directed. OTC Biotin is a supplement that helps to improve nail and hair growth. Check for pediatric doses with a pharmacist.
- Watch for patterns of continued hair loss.
- Talk with your hairdresser for recommendations of hair growth stimulation products.
- If there is sudden hair loss after medications or stressful event (usually 1 to 2 months after the event), minimize hair handling. Provide reassurance that hair often grows back 3 to 6 months after the event.

## Additional Instructions

_____

_____

_____

## Report the Following Problems to Your PCP/Clinic/ED

- Persistent hair loss
- New onset of hair loss and fever >101°F (38.3°C)
- Persistent severe fatigue
- Signs of infection in hair-loss areas

If the caller agrees with the advice given, document the call and encourage the caller to call back or see PCP if the problem worsens. If the caller does not agree with the advice given, reevaluate and advise the caller to follow up with PCP, Clinic, or ED.

# Hay Fever Problems

» **Key Questions**  Name, Age, Onset, Cause, History of Known Allergies, Medications, History. If no history of hay fever, see most severe symptom protocol

» **Other Protocols to Consider**  Breathing Problems (68); Common Cold Symptoms (103); Congestion (110); Cough (121); Earache, Drainage (150); Sinus Problems (411); Sore Throat (420); Wheezing (503).

> *Nurse Alert:* Use this protocol only if previously diagnosed with hay fever.

*Reminder:*  Document caller response to advice, home care instructions, and when to call back.

| ASSESSMENT | ACTION |
|---|---|
| **A. Is there difficulty breathing for reasons other than nasal congestion?** | |
| | **YES** Go to Breathing Problems protocol (68) |
| | **NO** Go to B |
| **B. Is chest pain present?** | |
| | **YES** Go to Chest Pain protocol (85) |
| | **NO** Go to C |
| **C. Are any of the following present?** | |
| • Wheezing and age <4 years<br>• Persistent wheezing that is unresponsive to home care measures | **YES** Go to Wheezing protocol (503) |
| | **NO** Go to D |

H

**D. In addition to clear nasal discharge, sniffing, or sneezing, are any of the following present?**

- Fever
- Headache and muscle aches
- Green, brown, or yellow nasal discharge or sputum for >24 hours
- Ear pain or drainage
- Persistent uncontrollable coughing

  "Seek medical care within 24 hours"

**NO** Go to E

**E. Are any of the following present?**

- Symptoms persist, even when triggers are avoided
- Symptoms interfere with sleep or daily activities
- Intermittent coughing
- Nasal itching
- Red, itchy, or watery eyes
- Sore throat
- Clear nasal drainage

**YES** "Call back or call PCP for appointment if no improvement"
and
Follow **Home Care Instructions**

**NO** Follow **Home Care Instructions**

## Home Care Instructions
## Hay Fever Problems

- Take OTC or prescription antihistamines of choice. Check with pharmacist for correct doses. Do not give aspirin to a child. Avoid aspirin-like products if age <20 years. Avoid acetaminophen if liver disease is present. Avoid ibuprofen if kidney disease or stomach problems exist or in the case of pregnancy. Follow the directions on the label. Use the dosing device that comes with the medication, a measuring device, or a medication syringe from the pharmacy. Household teaspoons often do not give the correct amount of medication.
- Avoid use of nasal sprays unless prescribed by PCP. If sprays are used, do not use >5 days.
- Shower and wash hair at night and after having exposure to pollen, dust, or known irritants.
- When pollen count is high, particularly in the morning, stay indoors with the doors and windows closed.
- For itchy eyes, apply cold compresses to the eyelids.
- Avoid pollen and other irritants that worsen the problem.

## Additional Instructions

_____

_____

_____

### Report the Following Problems to Your PCP/Clinic/ED

- Persistent nasal discharge, sneezing, or sniffing that is unresponsive to medication
- Fever
- Sinus pressure or pain
- Green, brown, or yellow nasal discharge or sputum
- Earache
- Uncontrolled coughing
- Symptoms interfere with daily activity
- Persistent wheezing or coughing that is unresponsive to home care measures

### Seek Emergency Care Immediately If Any of the Following Occur

- Chest pain
- Difficulty breathing for reasons other than nasal congestion

If the caller agrees with the advice given, document the call and encourage the caller to call back or see PCP if the problem worsens. If the caller does not agree with the advice given, reevaluate and advise the caller to follow up with PCP, Clinic, or ED.

# Headache

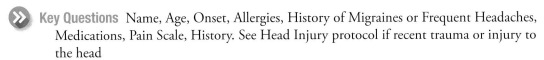

**» Key Questions**  Name, Age, Onset, Allergies, History of Migraines or Frequent Headaches, Medications, Pain Scale, History. See Head Injury protocol if recent trauma or injury to the head

**» Other Protocols to Consider**  Alcohol Problems (9); Congestion (110); Head Injury (242); Neck Pain (309); Neurologic Symptoms (312); Sinus Problems (411); Toothache (465); Vision Problems (489).

> *Nurse Alert:* There are many conditions that cause headaches; some can be potentially life-threatening. Err on the side of caution when triaging callers with a headache.
>
> • Be on the alert for signs of meningitis: headache, stiff neck, fever, petechial rash, vomiting, irritability, altered mental status.

*Reminder:*  Document caller response to advice, home care instructions, and when to call back.

| ASSESSMENT | ACTION |
|---|---|
| **A. Are any of the following present?** | |
| • Sudden severe pain or "worst headache ever" <br> • Sudden onset of weakness, unsteady gait, numbness, and/or tingling on one side of the body <br> • Confusion, difficulty in arousing, acting differently <br> • Sudden onset of difficulty speaking or slurred speech <br> • Stiff neck and fever (pain bending head forward) <br> • Blurred or double vision <br> • Purple or blood-colored flat spots or dots on skin <br> • Child with diabetes and blood glucose is high | **YES** "Call ambulance" <br> or <br> "Seek emergency care now" <br><br> **NO** Go to B |

### B. Are any of the following present?

- Persistent vomiting
- History of high blood pressure and light-headedness
- Fever >103°F (39.4°C) and unresponsive to fever-reducing measures
- Eye pain with redness and decreased vision
- Recent tick bite, headache, rash, and flu-like symptoms
- New onset of severe persistent pain
- Change in ability to walk

**YES** "Seek medical care within 2 hours"

**NO** Go to C

### C. Are any of the following present?

- Persistent migraine unresponsive to usual migraine treatment
- Migraine intensity or character different from past migraines
- Persistent headache >12 hours and no other symptoms
- Pain interferes with activity

**YES** "Seek medical care within 24 hours"

**NO** Go to D

### D. Are any of the following present?

- Congestion
- Fever and sore throat
- Muscles and joints ache
- Recent stressful event
- History of allergies
- Dull and constant pain with tender and tight neck muscles
- Severe dieting and weight loss
- Dental problems

**YES** "Call back or call PCP for appointment if no improvement" and Follow **Home Care Instructions**

**NO** Follow **Home Care Instructions**

H

## Home Care Instructions
## Headache

- Apply cool compresses or ice pack to forehead every 2 hours.
- Rest in a quiet darkened room.
- Take usual pain medication (aspirin, acetaminophen, ibuprofen). Do not give aspirin to a child. Avoid aspirin-like products if age <20 years. Avoid acetaminophen if liver disease is present. Avoid ibuprofen if kidney disease or stomach problems exist or in the case of pregnancy. Follow the directions on the label. Use the dosing device that comes with the medication, a measuring device, or a medication syringe from the pharmacy. Household teaspoons often do not give the correct amount of medication.
- Reduce fever with usual fever-reducing measures.
- For known migraine:
  - take medication as directed by PCP
  - rest with head elevated
  - apply heat to back of neck
  - apply cool compresses to forehead
- If nasal congestion is present, breathe steam for 10 to 20 minutes, 4 times a day or use a vaporizer.
- Keep a migraine journal and take it to next appointment. Try to identify triggers.

### Additional Instructions

_____

_____

_____

### Report the Following Problems to Your PCP/Clinic/ED

- Headache persists >24 hours
- No improvement or pain worsens
- Fever is present
- Thick green or yellow nasal discharge
- High blood glucose if you have diabetes
- Persistent vomiting

### Seek Emergency Care Immediately If Any of the Following Occur

- Sudden onset of weakness, numbness, or tingling on one side of the body
- Fever, stiff neck
- Confusion, severe drowsiness, or difficulty speaking
- Purple or blood-colored flat spots or dots appear on skin
- Change in ability to walk

If the caller agrees with the advice given, document the call and encourage the caller to call back or see PCP if the problem worsens. If the caller does not agree with the advice given, reevaluate and advise the caller to follow up with PCP, Clinic, or ED.

# Head Injury

>> **Key Questions**  Name, Age, Onset, Cause, Allergies, Mechanism of Injury, Medications, Associated Symptoms, History

>> **Other Protocols to Consider**  Back/Neck Injury (31); Confusion (107); Headache (238); Vomiting (492).

> **Nurse Alert:**
> - A neck injury should always be considered whenever there is a head injury. Assess for weakness, incoordination, numbness, neck pain.
> - Altered mental status may be one of the first signs of a head injury after trauma, particularly in a child.

**Reminder:**  Document caller response to advice, home care instructions, and when to call back.

| ASSESSMENT | ACTION |
|---|---|

**A. After a blow or injury to the head, are any of the following present?**

- Difficulty moving arms or legs, weakness, incoordination, or slurred speech
- Severe neck pain

**YES**  "Call ambulance and do not attempt to move the person"

**NO**  Go to B

**B. Are any of the following present?**

- Abnormal breathing or difficulty in breathing
- Altered mental status, difficulty in arousing, confusion, agitation
- Uncontrolled bleeding
- Seizure activity
- Preverbal children do not recognize parents or caregiver
- Persistent visual disturbance
- Persistent vomiting
- Persistent headache
- Numbness or tingling in arm or leg

**YES**  "Call ambulance"
or
"Seek emergency care now"

**NO**  Go to C

## C. Are any of the following present?

- Persistent blood or fluid draining from the nose or ears
- Gaping, split, jagged, or deep wound
- Laceration
- Bruising behind the ears or under the eyes
- Persistent bleeding >10 minutes
- History of loss of consciousness
- Change in behavior since the injury
- Fall >2 feet in a child <1 year old
- Child <1 year old with a soft spongy swollen area over the skull for >12 hours

**YES**    "Seek medical care within 2 hours"

**NO**    Go to D

## D  Are any of the following present?

- Swollen area (goose egg) on the forehead or scalp
- Intermittent headache not responsive to pain medication

**YES**    "Call back or call PCP for appointment if no improvement"
and
Follow **Home Care Instructions**

**NO**    Follow **Home Care Instructions**

H

## Home Care Instructions
## Head Injury

- Apply ice packs or cold compresses to area for 20 minutes every 2 hours to reduce swelling and discomfort. Place a cloth barrier between the ice and the skin.
- Allow a child to sleep after an injury. Awaken every 2 hours for 24 hours to determine level of alertness and responsiveness.
- Avoid heavy activity during first 24 hours after the injury. Rest in a quiet area with head slightly elevated.
- Take acetaminophen for discomfort. Do not give aspirin to a child. Avoid aspirin-like products if age <20 years. Avoid acetaminophen if liver disease is present. Avoid ibuprofen if kidney disease or stomach problems exist or in the case of pregnancy. Follow the directions on the label. Use the dosing device that comes with the medication, a measuring device, or a medication syringe from the pharmacy. Household teaspoons often do not give the correct amount of medication.
- Avoid aspirin and ibuprofen.
- Avoid heavy meals.

## Additional Instructions

_____

_____

_____

### Report the Following Problems to Your PCP/Clinic/ED
- No improvement or condition worsens
- Persistent headache
- Persistent swelling >24 hours after ice pack application
- Blood or clear drainage from nose or ears

### Seek Emergency Care Immediately If Any of the Following Occur
- Confusion, disorientation, agitation, or change in vision
- Altered mental status or difficulty arousing
- Numbness, tingling, or weakness in an arm or leg
- Persistent vomiting, severe headache, speech problems, seizures, or lethargy
- Child does not recognize parents or caregiver
- Persistent numbness and tingling

If the caller agrees with the advice given, document the call and encourage the caller to call back or see PCP if the problem worsens. If the caller does not agree with the advice given, reevaluate and advise the caller to follow up with PCP, Clinic, or ED.

# Heartburn

⟫ **Key Questions**  Name, Age, Onset, Cause, Allergies, Medications, History, Associated Symptoms, Pain Scale

⟫ **Other Protocols to Consider**  Abdominal Pain (1); Chest Pain (85); Gas/Belching (221); Indigestion (273); Vomiting, (492); Swallowing Difficulty (442).

> *Nurse Alert:* Heartburn can mimic chest pain. There are many conditions that cause chest pain; some can be potentially life-threatening. Err on the side of caution when triaging callers with chest pain.

*Reminder:*  Document caller response to advice, home care instructions, and when to call back.

| ASSESSMENT | ACTION |
|---|---|
| **A. In addition to a burning or heavy sensation, are any of the following present?** | |
| • Shortness of breath<br>• Cool, moist skin<br>• Pain in the neck, jaw, shoulders, back, or arms<br>• Blue or gray face, lips, earlobes, or fingernails<br>• Fainting<br>• Vomiting blood or dark coffee-grounds–like emesis | **YES** "Call ambulance"<br><br>**NO** Go to B |
| **B. Are any of the following present?** | |
| • History of diabetes or cardiac disease<br>• Dizziness or light-headedness | **YES** "Seek medical care within 2 to 4 hours"<br><br>**NO** Go to C |
| **C. Are any of the following present?** | |
| • Discomfort persists after taking antacids<br>• Condition worsening, requiring more frequent use of antacids<br>• Difficult or painful swallowing<br>• Sensation that pill is stuck in esophagus | **YES** "Seek medical care within 24 hours"<br><br>**NO** Go to D |

H

## D. Are any of the following present?

- Pain increased with use of medications
- Increased pain bending over, exercising, or lying down soon after eating
- Nausea or vomiting
- Pregnancy
- Frequent belching
- Burping stomach contents into mouth
- Obesity
- Heavy tobacco or alcohol use
- Increased stress

**YES**   "Call back or call PCP for appointment if no improvement" and Follow **Home Care Instructions**

**NO**   Follow **Home Care Instructions**

### Home Care Instructions
### Heartburn

- Try OTC antacids (Maalox, Mylanta, Riopan, Tums) and follow directions on bottle. Try OTC Pepcid AC, Tagamet HB, Zantac, or Prilosec. Discuss pediatric dosage with pharmacist. Consult with PCP if taking other prescription medications. Liquids provide faster relief than tablets. Do not give Pepto-Bismol to a child. Ask pharmacist for additional product suggestions. Use the dosing device that comes with the medication, a measuring device, or a medication syringe from the pharmacy. Household teaspoons often do not give the correct amount of medication.
- Avoid eating or drinking 2 to 3 hours before going to bed.
- Do not lie down, bend over, or exercise soon after eating.
- Elevate head of bed 4 to 6 inches using blocks or bricks, or lie on left side to help speed stomach emptying and reduce reflux.
- Eat small meals, but eat them more than 3 times a day.
- Avoid spicy foods, alcohol, coffee, smoking, chocolate, citrus fruits, tomatoes, vinegar, fatty foods, or any other food or drink that triggers heartburn.
- If aspirin or ibuprofen worsens the problem, try acetaminophen. Do not give aspirin to a child. Avoid aspirin-like products if age <20 years. Avoid acetaminophen if liver disease is present. Avoid ibuprofen if kidney disease or stomach problems exist or in the case of pregnancy. Follow the directions on the label.
- Avoid tight-fitting clothing, with a tight-fitting waistband.

**Additional Instructions**

H

### Report the Following Problems to Your PCP/Clinic/ED

- Discomfort occurs after taking prescribed medication
- No improvement in 3 days or condition worsens
- No relief from antacids or other OTC drugs (such as Pepcid AC or Zantac)
- Frequent use of antacids
- Difficult or painful swallowing

### Call Ambulance If Any of the Following Occur

- Shortness of breath
- Dizziness
- Cool, moist skin
- Pain or discomfort in neck, jaw, shoulders, back, or arms
- Blue or gray face or lips
- Fainting
- Vomiting blood or dark coffee-grounds–like emesis

If the caller agrees with the advice given, document the call and encourage the caller to call back or see PCP if the problem worsens. If the caller does not agree with the advice given, reevaluate and advise the caller to follow up with PCP, Clinic, or ED.

# Heart Rate Problems

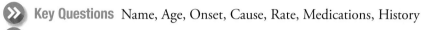 **Key Questions** Name, Age, Onset, Cause, Rate, Medications, History

**Other Protocols to Consider** Alcohol Problems (9); Anxiety (18); Breathing Problems (68); Chest Pain (85); Dizziness (147); Fatigue (181); Headache (238); Weakness (496).

*Reminder:* Document caller response to advice, home care instructions, and when to call back.

| ASSESSMENT | ACTION |
|---|---|

### A. Is heart rate >150 bpm and are any of the following present?

- Chest, neck, jaw, or arm pain or discomfort
- Difficulty breathing
- Skin cool and moist or hot and dry
- Face or lips blue, gray, or very pale
- Fainting

**YES** "Call ambulance"

**NO** Go to B

### B. Are any of the following present?

- Persistent rapid heart rate of >150 bpm for >30 minutes
- Light-headedness, faintness, or dizziness
- Persistent rapid heart rate and history of thyroid disease or heart disease
- Slow heart rate and extreme fatigue or frequent episodes of a slow heart rate
  - Persistent slow heart rate and pauses of >3 seconds (count 1,001, 1,002, 1,003)

**YES** "Seek medical care now"

**NO** Go to C

### C. Are any of the following present?

- Frequent episodes of a rapid heart rate
- Persistent slow heart rate and history of heart disease, general ill feeling, or frequent falls
- Recent history of persistent vomiting or diarrhea

**YES** "Seek medical care within 24 hours"

**NO** Go to D

H

## D. Are any of the following present?

- History of prior treatment for rapid heart rate
- Recent ingestion of diuretics, diet pills, decongestants, cold remedies, β-blockers, thyroid medication, a new medication, or recreational drugs
- History of bronchodilator use and new prescription or increase in dose
- Excessive use of caffeine, tobacco, alcohol, or herbal stimulants
- Difficulty sleeping or persistent fatigue
- Increase in stress
- Exercise <30 minutes before onset of symptoms
- Frequent skipped beats
- Unexplained weight gain, fatigue, and feeling cold
- Fever

**YES**  "Call back or call PCP for appointment if no improvement" and Follow **Home Care Instructions**

**NO**  Follow **Home Care Instructions**

## Home Care Instructions
## Heart Rate Problems

- To slow down heart rate:
  - take a deep breath; hold and pinch nostrils closed. Gently try to exhale through the nose
  - take a deep breath and bear down as if having a bowel movement
  - try to blow up a balloon
  - take a cold shower and let cold water splash on the face and head
  - try to remain calm
  - rest and relax
  - try to identify the trigger and discuss it with PCP if problem persists
  - avoid medications that seem to worsen the problem
  - avoid caffeine and alcohol

## Additional Instructions

_____

_____

_____

### Report the Following Problems to Your PCP/Clinic/ED
- Problem persists or worsens
- Light-headedness or faintness

### Seek Emergency Care Immediately If Any of the Following Occur
- Chest, neck, jaw, or arm pain
- Difficulty breathing
- Cool and moist skin
- Face or lips blue, gray, or very pale
- Fainting
- Loss of consciousness or altered mental status

If the caller agrees with the advice given, document the call and encourage the caller to call back or see PCP if the problem worsens. If the caller does not agree with the advice given, reevaluate and advise the caller to follow up with PCP, Clinic, or ED.

H

# Heat Exposure Problems

 **Key Questions**  Name, Age, Onset, Cause, Temperature, Medications, History

 **Other Protocols to Consider**  Dehydration (132); Dizziness (147); Fainting (178); Fever (184); Muscle Cramps (307); Sunburn (439); Sweating, Excessive (446); Weakness (496).

*Nurse Alert:*

- Hyperthermia may result from prolonged exposure to high temperatures or humidity, excessive exercise, infection, drug use such as amphetamines

*Reminder:*  Document caller response to advice, home care instructions, and when to call back.

| ASSESSMENT | ACTION |
|---|---|

**A. After prolonged exposure to heat or strenuous exercise, are any of the following present?**

- Temperature >102°F (38.9°C), skin is hot and dry, and any of the following:
  - flushed skin
  - no sweating
- Sudden dizziness, headache, weakness, faintness, or loss of consciousness
- Confusion, delirium, or disorientation
- Visual disturbances
- Seizures
- Rapid heart rate
- Rapid breathing
- Age <10 years
- Low or normal temperature, skin cool and moist, and mental confusion or unconsciousness

 **YES** "Call ambulance"
or
"Seek emergency care now"
and
Follow **Emergency Home Care Instructions** while waiting for help to arrive

 **NO** Go to B

**B. After prolonged exposure to heat or strenuous exercise, are any of the following present?**

- Profuse sweating
- Dizziness, weakness, or faintness
- Severe muscle cramps or incoordination
- Slow heart rate
- Dark yellow or orange urine
- Vomiting and inability to tolerate fluids

 **YES** "Follow **Home Care Instructions**, but if no immediate improvement, seek emergency care now"

 **NO** Go to C

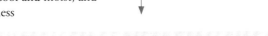

**C. After prolonged exposure to heat or strenuous exercise, are any of the following present?**

- Temperature >100.5°F (38.1°C) and age <3 months, or child is diabetic, bedridden, or has weakened immune system
- Signs of dehydration

 "Seek medical care within 2 to 4 hours"

**NO** Go to D

**D. After prolonged exposure to heat or strenuous exercise, are any of the following present?**

- Fatigue
- Mild muscle cramps
- Flushed skin
- Slight nausea or dizziness
- Feeling hot

 "Call back or call PCP if no improvement"
and
Follow **Home Care Instructions**

**NO** **Home Care Instructions**

H

## Home Care Instructions
## Heat Exposure Problems

### Emergency Home Care Instructions
- Help the victim to lie down in a cool, shady area and loosen clothing or remove clothes.
- Keep the victim cool while awaiting medical assistance. Apply cool towels and use a fan to help cool the victim. Do not put ice directly on the skin. Do not allow the victim to shiver, as it increases body heat. Sponge the victim with tepid water. Do not use an alcohol rub.
- Elevate legs higher than the heart.
- If alert, give the victim cold liquids (water, sports beverages, soft drinks, fruit juices) to drink. Do not drink beverages with alcohol or caffeine. Drinking too fast can cause nausea. Drink one cup every 15 minutes as tolerated and no nausea.

### Moderate or Mild Heat Exposure Instructions
- Use a spray bottle or mister with lukewarm water and spray exposed skin to help cool through evaporation.
- If age <13 years, give Pedialyte or Ricelyte to rehydrate.
- Mix ¼ tsp salt in 1 quart of water. Give ½ cup every 15 minutes for 1½ hours. Do not allow person to consume salt tablets. If thirst persists, give plain water.
- If no nausea, try salty snack foods such as pretzels, potato chips, etc.
- Do not give aspirin or acetaminophen for elevated temperature.
- Apply cool towels and use a fan to help cool down. Do not put ice directly on the skin. Do not allow the person to shiver, as it increases body heat.
- Take a cool shower or bath to reduce body temperature quickly.

## Additional Instructions

_____

_____

_____

### Report the Following Problem to Your PCP/Clinic/ED
- No improvement after following Home Care Instructions

### Seek Emergency Care Immediately If Any of the Following Occur
- Decreasing alertness
- Seizures
- Muscle cramps or incoordination
- Persistent unusually slow heart rate
- Persistent vomiting and inability to tolerate fluids

If the caller agrees with the advice given, document the call and encourage the caller to call back or see PCP if the problem worsens. If the caller does not agree with the advice given, reevaluate and advise the caller to follow up with PCP, Clinic, or ED.

H

# Hiccups

 **Key Questions**  Name, Age, Onset, Allergies, Medications, History

 **Other Protocols to Consider**  Chest Pain (85); Swallowing Difficulty (442).

*Reminder:* Document caller response to advice, home care instructions, and when to call back.

| ASSESSMENT | ACTION |
|---|---|

### A. Are any of the following present?

- Confusion, lethargy
- Difficulty breathing
- Fainting
- Chest, neck, jaw, or arm pain or pressure

**YES** "Call ambulance" or "Seek emergency care now"

**NO** Go to B

### B. Are any of the following present?

- Persistent pain
- Constant hiccups >8 hours

**YES** "Seek medical care within 2 to 4 hours"

**NO** Go to C

### C. Are any of the following present?

- Persistent vomiting
- Pain in shoulder, abdomen, or back

**YES** "Seek medical care within 24 hours"

**NO** Go to D

### D. Are any of the following present?

- Sudden onset after taking a new medication
- Interferes with sleep
- Anxiety or irritability
- Intermittent episodes
- Increased alcohol use
- Mild discomfort
- Recent ingestion of hot or irritating food or drink
- History of cancer

**YES** "Call back or call PCP for appointment if no improvement" and Follow **Home Care Instructions**

**NO** Follow **Home Care Instructions**

## Home Care Instructions
# Hiccups

- Take a deep breath and hold for 15 to 30 seconds.
- Breathe into a paper bag for 1 minute.
- Sip ice water.
- Pull on tongue.
- Apply gentle pressure to closed eyelids.
- Grasp upper lip between teeth and right side of nose and apply gentle pressure.
- Stroke back of tongue.
- Take your usual antacid (Maalox, Mylanta) as directed on container. Ask pharmacist for pediatric dosage. Use the dosing device that comes with the medication, a measuring device, or a medication syringe from the pharmacy. Household teaspoons often do not give the correct amount of medication.
- Divert attention through distraction.

## Additional Instructions

_____

_____

_____

### Report the Following Problem to Your PCP/Clinic/ED
- Persistent or worsening condition

### Seek Emergency Care Immediately If Any of the Following Occur
- Chest, neck, jaw, or arm pain or pressure
- Difficulty breathing
- Confusion or lethargy
- Fainting

If the caller agrees with the advice given, document the call and encourage the caller to call back or see PCP if the problem worsens. If the caller does not agree with the advice given, reevaluate and advise the caller to follow up with PCP, Clinic, or ED.

H

# Hives

>> **Key Questions** Name, Age, Onset, Suspected Cause, Red Raised Itchy Patches on Skin, Allergies, Medications, History, Associated Symptoms

>> **Other Protocols to Consider** Allergic Reaction (13); Bee Stings (42); Bites, Insect (49); Breathing Problems (68); Immunization Reactions (267); Itching (282); Rash (366); Skin Lesions: Lumps, Bumps, and Sores (414); Wheezing (503).

> *Nurse Alert:* A sudden onset of hives can precede an anaphylactic reaction, a severe life-threatening allergic reaction, and can occur within seconds to an hour after exposure to the offending substance such as food, medication, a bee sting, etc. An anaphylactic reaction involves the respiratory, cardiovascular, and central nervous systems. Sudden onset of symptoms may include difficulty breathing; feeling faint; swelling of the tongue, throat, or lips; hives; wheezing or coughing; or a feeling of impending doom. The sooner symptoms occur after exposure to the antigen, the more severe the anaphylaxis.

*Reminder:* Document caller response to advice, home care instructions, and when to call back.

| ASSESSMENT | ACTION |
|---|---|
| **A. Hives, and are any of the following present?** | |
| • Difficulty breathing, chest tightness, or wheezing <br> • Difficulty swallowing or swelling of tongue or back of throat <br> • Confusion, agitation, or decreasing level of consciousness <br> • Fainting <br> • History of bee sting(s) and bee sting allergy <br> • Previous severe allergic reaction to same allergen | **YES** "Call ambulance" <br> **NO** Go to B |
| **B. Are any of the following present?** | |
| • Faintness or dizziness <br> • Severe abdominal pain <br> • Nausea or vomiting <br> • Rapid onset of cough <br> • Sudden onset of hoarseness | **YES** "Seek emergency care now" <br> **NO** Go to C |

## C. Are any of the following present?

- Rapid progression of red, raised, itchy rash on several areas of the body
- Swelling in face or limbs
- Hives after 2 days of antihistamine therapy

**YES** "Seek medical care within 2 to 4 hours"

**NO** Go to D

## D. Are any of the following present?

- Diarrhea or fever
- Joint swelling or pain
- Exposure to plants in the woods (such as poison ivy, poison oak, or poison sumac) that required steroid therapy in the past

**YES** "Seek medical care within 24 hours"

**NO** Go to E

## E. Are any of the following present?

- New medication
- New foods in diet
- New soaps, shampoos, laundry detergent, clothing, cosmetics, toothpaste, or other toiletries
- Recent new contact with plants or animals or new insect bites
- Intermittent hives
- Hives >7 days and interfering with activity

**YES** "Call back or call PCP for appointment if no improvement"
and
Follow **Home Care Instructions**

**NO** Follow **Home Care Instructions**

H

## Home Care Instructions
## Hives

- For widespread hives, take an OTC antihistamine (e.g., Benadryl, Claritin, Alavert) until hives have disappeared. Follow instructions on the label. Do not drive or engage in activities that require concentration. Ask pharmacist for pediatric dosage and other product suggestions. Use the dosing device that comes with the medication, a measuring device, or a medication syringe from the pharmacy. Household teaspoons often do not give the correct amount of medication.
- If medications are suspected as the cause of the reaction, discontinue use and contact PCP.
- Cool baths of plain water, baking soda and water, or oatmeal powder and water may help to relieve itching and discomfort.
- Apply Caladryl or calamine lotion to help control itching and dry lesions. Follow instructions on the label. Limit use of Caladryl on small children because it may cause sedation.
- Avoid the sun. Seek cool areas and take cool showers to help relieve discomfort.

## Additional Instructions

_____

_____

_____

### Report the Following Problems to Your PCP/Clinic/ED

- Persistent hives >7 days
- Persistent itching >24 hours after taking antihistamines

### Seek Emergency Care Immediately If Any of the Following Occur

- Difficulty breathing, chest tightness, or wheezing
- Difficulty swallowing, or swelling of tongue or back of throat
- Confusion, agitation, or decreasing level of consciousness
- Fainting
- Swelling of lips or mouth

If the caller agrees with the advice given, document the call and encourage the caller to call back or see PCP if the problem worsens. If the caller does not agree with the advice given, reevaluate and advise the caller to follow up with PCP, Clinic, or ED.

# Hoarseness

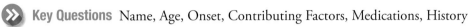

**Key Questions**  Name, Age, Onset, Contributing Factors, Medications, History

**Other Protocols to Consider**  Allergic Reaction (13); Breathing Problems (68); Cough (121); Croup (125); Hay Fever Problems (235); Hives (258); Foreign Body, Inhaled (203); Sore Throat (420).

*Reminder:*  Document caller response to advice, home care instructions, and when to call back.

| ASSESSMENT | ACTION |
|---|---|
| **A. Sudden onset of hoarseness, and are any of the following present?** | |
| • Sore throat, drooling, and difficulty breathing <br> • Sensation of swelling tongue or throat <br> • Recent trauma to neck <br> • Speaking in short three-word sentences | **YES** "Seek emergency care now" <br><br> **NO** Go to B |
| **B. Are any of the following present?** | |
| • Sudden onset of swelling in face <br> • Speaking in partial sentences | **YES** "Seek medical care within 2 to 4 hours" <br><br> **NO** Go to C |
| **C. Are any of the following present?** | |
| • High fever and feels or looks ill <br> • Persistent hoarseness >1 week <br> • History of tobacco use, recent weight loss, and decreased appetite <br> • Dry skin or hair, increased sensitivity to cold, increased fatigue, or unexplained weight gain | **YES** "Seek medical care within 24 hours" <br><br> **NO** Go to D |

H

## D. Are any of the following present?

- Recent sore throat, cough, cold, or fever
- Recently used voice more than usual (yelling, cheering, singing)
- Speaking in complete sentences

**YES** "Call back or call PCP for appointment if no improvement"
and
Follow **Home Care Instructions**

**NO** Follow **Home Care Instructions**

## Home Care Instructions
## Hoarseness

- Avoid tobacco or alcohol.
- Rest voice as much as possible.
- Drink plenty of fluids.
- Take your usual pain medication (aspirin, acetaminophen, ibuprofen) as tolerated for discomfort or fever. Do not give aspirin to a child. Avoid aspirin-like products if age <20 years. Avoid acetaminophen if liver disease is present. Avoid ibuprofen if kidney disease or stomach problems exist or in the case of pregnancy. Follow the directions on the label. Use the dosing device that comes with the medication, a measuring device, or a medication syringe from the pharmacy. Household teaspoons often do not give the correct amount of medication.
- Use honey or throat lozenges for throat discomfort or cough.

**Additional Instructions**

_____

_____

_____

### Report the Following Problems to Your PCP/Clinic/ED
- Condition persists >1 week or worsens
- High fever and appears ill

### Seek Emergency Care Immediately If Any of the Following Occur
- Sore throat, drooling, and difficulty breathing
- Sensation of swelling tongue or throat
- Speaking in short three-word sentences

If the caller agrees with the advice given, document the call and encourage the caller to call back or see PCP if the problem worsens. If the caller does not agree with the advice given, reevaluate and advise the caller to follow up with PCP, Clinic, or ED.

H

# Immunization, Tetanus

 **Key Questions**  Name, Age, Onset, Cause of Injury, Tetanus Immunization Status, Allergies, Medications, History

 **Other Protocols to Consider**  Allergic Reaction (13); Fever (184); Immunization Reactions (267); Laceration (290); Puncture Wound (362).

> *Nurse Alert:* Use this protocol if concerns about a recent tetanus immunization reaction or questions about immunization status and recent injury.

*Reminder:*  Document caller response to advice, home care instructions, and when to call back.

| ASSESSMENT | ACTION |
|---|---|
| **A. After tetanus immunization, are any of the following present?** | |
| • Difficulty breathing, speaking, or swallowing<br>• Sudden swelling in back of throat or tongue<br>• Chest pain<br>• Fainting<br>• Confusion, agitation, or decreased level of consciousness<br>• Palpitations | **YES** "Call ambulance"<br>or<br>"Seek emergency care now"<br><br>**NO** Go to B |
| **B. After tetanus immunization, are any of the following present?** | |
| • Rash or flushing<br>• Generalized hives | **YES** "Seek medical care within 2 to 4 hours"<br><br>**NO** Go to C |
| **C. Sustained injury within 48 hours, and are any of the following present?** | |
| • No prior tetanus immunization<br>• >5 years since last tetanus immunization<br>• Fewer than four tetanus immunizations since birth<br>• Fever, pain, redness, swelling at injection site >48 hours after injection | **YES** "Seek medical care within 24 hours"<br><br>**NO** Go to D |

## D. Are any of the following present?

- Fever, pain, redness, swelling at tetanus injection site <48 hours after injection

**YES** "Call back or call PCP for appointment if no improvement" and Follow **Home Care Instructions**

**NO** Follow **Home Care Instructions**

## Home Care Instructions
## Immunization, Tetanus

- Apply ice pack to injection site for 20 minutes every 2 hours throughout a 24-hour period to help reduce swelling and discomfort. Place a cloth barrier between ice and skin.
- Take your usual pain medication (aspirin, acetaminophen, ibuprofen) if needed for fever or discomfort. Do not give aspirin to a child. Avoid aspirin-like products if age <20 years. Avoid acetaminophen if liver disease is present. Avoid ibuprofen if kidney disease or stomach problems exist or in the case of pregnancy. Follow the directions on the label.
- Record date of booster. A booster provides protection for 5 years.
- Tetanus immunization should be given within 72 hours of injury.
- Monitor injection site for signs of infection.
- Provide reassurance; pain and swelling are normal reactions for first 48 hours.

## Additional Instructions

_____

_____

_____

## Report the Following Problems to Your PCP/Clinic/ED

- Child cries >3 hours after injection
- Redness, swelling, pain, or fever occurs >48 hours after injection

## Seek Emergency Care Immediately If Any of the Following Occur

- Difficulty breathing, speaking, or swallowing
- Sudden swelling in back of throat or tongue
- Chest pain or fainting
- Palpitations
- Confusion, agitation, or decreased level of consciousness

If the caller agrees with the advice given, document the call and encourage the caller to call back or see PCP if the problem worsens. If the caller does not agree with the advice given, reevaluate and advise the caller to follow up with PCP, Clinic, or ED.

# Immunization Reactions

>> **Key Questions**  Name, Age, Onset, Cause, Allergies, Medications, History, Date and Type of Immunization

>> **Other Protocols to Consider**  Allergic Reaction (13); Fever (184); Immunization, Tetanus (264).

> *Nurse Alert:*  Use this protocol if concerns about a recent immunization and possible reaction or questions about immunization reactions. Serious reactions are rare but do occur.
>
> - Minor reaction: pain or swelling at the site of injection (usually within 2 days); fever, headache, or muscle aches (usually occur within 7 days).
> - Severe reaction: anaphylaxis; difficulty breathing; feeling faint; swelling of the tongue, throat, or lips; hives; wheezing or coughing; or a feeling of impending doom (can occur within seconds to an hour after exposure). The sooner the symptoms occur after exposure to the antigen, the more severe the anaphylaxis.
> - VAERS—Vaccine Adverse Event Reporting System is a national program for monitoring vaccine safety. Call for reporting forms: 1-800-822-7967, or locate on the Internet at http://www.vaers.hhs.gov
> - National Vaccine Injury Compensation Program provides compensation to individuals whose injuries may have been caused by certain vaccines. Call 1-800-338-2382.
> - National Immunization Hotline provides vaccine information. Call 1-800-232-2522.
> - Vaccine website information: www.cdc.gov/vaccines

*Reminder:*  Document caller response to advice, home care instructions, and when to call back.

| ASSESSMENT | ACTION |
|---|---|

### A. After an immunization, are any of the following present?

- Difficulty breathing or speaking
- Sudden swelling in back of throat
- Chest pain or fainting
- Palpitations
- Confusion, agitation, or decreased level of consciousness

**YES**  "Call ambulance"
or
"Seek emergency care now"

**NO**  Go to B

I

## B. Are any of the following present?

- Rash or flushing
- Hives
- Temperature >105°F (40.6°C) or temperature >100.4°F (38.0°C) rectally in child <12 weeks of age
- High-pitched, unfamiliar cry for >1 hour

**YES** "Seek medical care within 2 to 4 hours"

**NO** Go to C

## C. Are any of the following present?

- Persistent fever and rash >24 hours 7 to 10 days after measles immunization
- Child cries constantly >3 hours after immunization
- Increasing redness, swelling, pain at the injection site, or fever >48 hours after immunization

**YES** "Seek medical care within 24 hours"

**NO** Go to D

## D. Are any of the following present?

- Fever, pain, redness, or swelling at tetanus injection site
- Swollen glands in neck after MMR immunization
- Rash or swollen glands 7 to 14 days after MMR immunization and painful joints 2 to 4 weeks afterward

**YES** "Call back or call PCP for appointment if no improvement"
and
Follow **Home Care Instructions**

**NO** Follow **Home Care Instructions**

## Home Care Instructions
## Immunization Reactions

- Take usual pain medication (aspirin, acetaminophen, ibuprofen) for fever. Infants less than 8 weeks of age should not be given an antipyretic for fever without first consulting their health care provider. Do not give aspirin to a child. Avoid aspirin-like products if age <20 years. Avoid acetaminophen if liver disease is present. Avoid ibuprofen if kidney disease or stomach problems exist or in the case of pregnancy. Follow the directions on the label. Use the dosing device that comes with the medication, a measuring device, or a medication syringe from the pharmacy. Household teaspoons often do not give the correct amount of medication.
- Women should avoid pregnancy for 4 weeks after rubella immunization.
- Discuss with your PCP the safety of immunizations if the child is ill or taking immune suppressors or cortisone.
- Expect side effects to include fever, fussiness, and redness at injection site.

## Additional Instructions

_____

_____

_____

### Report the Following Problems to Your PCP/Clinic/ED

- Persistent fever and rash >3 days after measles immunization
- Child has a high-pitched cry for >1 hour or cries constantly >3 hours after immunization
- Temperature >105°F (40.5°C) or >100.4°F in infants <12 weeks of age
- Redness, swelling, pain, fever >48 hours

### Seek Emergency Care Immediately If Any of the Following Occur

- Difficulty breathing or speaking
- Sudden swelling in back of throat
- Chest pain or fainting
- Confusion, agitation, or decreased level of consciousness

If the caller agrees with the advice given, document the call and encourage the caller to call back or see PCP if the problem worsens. If the caller does not agree with the advice given, reevaluate and advise the caller to follow up with PCP, Clinic, or ED.

# Impetigo

**Key Questions**  Name, Age, Onset, Known Diagnosis or Exposure to Impetigo, Sores with Honey-Colored Crusts, Medications, History

**Other Protocols to Consider**  Rash (366); Skin Lesions (414).

*Reminder:*  Document caller response to advice, home care instructions, and when to call back.

| ASSESSMENT | ACTION |
|---|---|
| **A. Are any of the following present?** | |
| • Red or cola-colored urine<br>• Bright red and tender face<br>• Flank pain<br>• Very rapid spread<br>• Abdominal swelling | **YES** "Seek emergency care now"<br><br>**NO** Go to B |
| **B. Are any of the following present?** | |
| • Blister or sore >1 inch across<br>• Red streak extends from sore<br>• History of diabetes, steroid therapy, cancer, HIV, or other immunosuppression | **YES** "Seek medical care within 2 to 4 hours"<br><br>**NO** Go to C |
| **C. Are any of the following present?** | |
| • Child younger than 1 year old<br>• Two or more household members have sores<br>• More than two sores<br>• Sores in nostril, ear canal, or around mouth<br>• Swollen nodes in area near sores<br>• Temperature >100°F (37.8°C) or sore throat<br>• Sores increase in number >2 days of treatment<br>• Red, yellow, brown, green, or white drainage from sore | **YES** "Seek medical care within 24 hours"<br><br>**NO** Go to D |

## D. Are any of the following present?

- Sore <1 inch across
- Small red bump changed to a cloudy blister or pimple and then a sore with a yellow-brown scab

**YES**    "Call back or call PCP for appointment if no improvement"
and
Follow **Home Care Instructions**

**NO**    Follow **Home Care Instructions**

I

## Home Care Instructions
## Impetigo

- To remove scabs, apply a cloth soaked in a solution of antibacterial soap and water to the scab. Rub scab gently; do not scrub.
- Wash sores with antibacterial soap.
- Apply antibiotic (Mycitracin, Neosporin, Polysporin) ointment 3 times a day after sores are washed. Follow instructions on the label.
- Avoid touching, scratching, or picking at sores to help prevent spreading and infection.
- Wash hands after touching sores.
- Keep fingernails short, and wash hands frequently with antibacterial soap.
- Do not share towels with other family members. Impetigo is highly contagious and can spread easily to other household members.
- Keep child out of school until he/she has taken antibiotics for >24 hours; for mild infections, wash well with soap and water and cover the scabs with antibiotic ointment and a bandage before sending the child to school or day care.

## Additional Instructions

_____

_____

_____

If the caller agrees with the advice given, document the call and encourage the caller to call back or see PCP if the problem worsens. If the caller does not agree with the advice given, reevaluate and advise the caller to follow up with PCP, Clinic, or ED.

# Indigestion

>> **Key Questions** Name, Age, Onset, Symptoms Usually Occur Soon After Eating, Allergies, Medications, History

>> **Other Protocols to Consider** Abdominal Pain (1); Abdominal Swelling (4); Chest Pain (85); Diarrhea (143); Gas/Belching (221); Gas/Flatulence (223); Heartburn (245); Rectal Bleeding (371); Vomiting (492); Swallowing Difficulty (442).

> **Nurse Alert:** Indigestion and heartburn can mimic chest pain. There are many conditions that cause chest pain; some can be potentially life-threatening. Err on the side of caution when triaging callers with symptoms like chest pain.

**Reminder:** Document caller response to advice, home care instructions, and when to call back.

| ASSESSMENT | ACTION |
|---|---|

### A. Is there a burning or heavy sensation in the chest, and are any of the following present?

- Shortness of breath
- Cool moist skin
- Pain in the neck, jaw, shoulders, back, or arms
- Blue or gray face, lips, earlobes, or fingernails
- History of cardiac disease or diabetes
- Pain occurs with exertion
- Feeling of impending doom
- Chest pain and palpitations

 **YES** "Call ambulance"

 **NO** Go to B

### B. Are any of the following present?

- Belching blood
- Vomiting blood or dark coffee-grounds–like emesis
- Black tarry stool
- Severe abdominal pain

 **YES** "Seek emergency care now"

 **NO** Go to C

## C. Are any of the following present?

- Discomfort persists after taking medication
- Condition worsening, requires more frequent use of medication
- Frequent vomiting, weight loss, or decreased appetite
- Difficult or painful swallowing

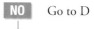 "Seek medical care within 24 hours"

 Go to D

## D. Are any of the following present?

- Pain increased with use of ibuprofen, or steroids
- Increased pain when bending, exercising, or lying down soon after eating
- Frequent belching or gas
- Acid taste in mouth
- Bloated or full feeling
- Itching
- Recent increase in stress
- Symptoms appear soon after eating or drinking
- Mild nausea or diarrhea after eating
- Previously diagnosed with reflux esophagitis
- Recently started new medication

**YES** "Call back or call PCP for appointment if no improvement"
and
Follow **Home Care Instructions**

**NO** Follow **Home Care Instructions**

# Home Care Instructions
# Indigestion

- Try OTC medications (Maalox, Mylanta, Riopan, Tums, Pepcid, Prilosec) and follow instructions on the label. Liquids often provide faster relief than tablets. Consult with PCP if taking other prescription medications. Use the dosing device that comes with the medication, a measuring device, or a medication syringe from the pharmacy. Household teaspoons often do not give the correct amount of medication.
- Do not give Pepto-Bismol that contains bismuth subsalicylate to a child. Use children's Pepto-Bismol that contains calcium carbonate.
- Avoid eating 2 to 3 hours before bed.
- Do not lie down for 2 to 3 hours after eating or bend over or exercise soon after eating.
- Elevate head of bed 4 to 6 inches using blocks or bricks.
- Eat small, frequent meals.
- Avoid spicy foods, alcohol, coffee, smoking, chocolate, citrus fruits, tomatoes, vinegar, fatty foods, and carbonated beverages.
- If ibuprofen worsens the problem, try acetaminophen. Do not give aspirin to a child. Avoid aspirin-like products if age <20 years. Avoid acetaminophen if liver disease is present. Avoid ibuprofen if kidney disease or stomach problems exist or in the case of pregnancy. Follow the directions on the label.
- Avoid tight-fitting clothing, such as belts, pants, or skirts with a tight waistband.
- Take time to eat and drink, thoroughly chewing food.
- Avoid chewing gum or other activities that result in swallowing air.
- Avoid foods and drinks known to cause stomach upset and heartburn. Try taking OTC medications (Pepcid AC, Pepto-Bismol, or Prilosec) before eating foods causing symptoms. Follow instructions on the label.
- Try Gas-X for belching and follow instructions on the label.
- Sip a tonic made of 4 ounces ginger ale, 1 tsp grated ginger root, 1 tsp honey to soothe an upset stomach. Do not give honey to children less than 1 year of age.
- Avoid straining during bowel movements, urinating, and lifting.

## Additional Instructions

_____

_____

_____

## Report the Following Problems to Your PCP/Clinic/ED

- Persistent discomfort unresponsive to home care measures after >3 days or condition worsens
- No relief from antacids
- Difficult or painful swallowing

If the caller agrees with the advice given, document the call and encourage the caller to call back or see PCP if the problem worsens. If the caller does not agree with the advice given, reevaluate and advise the caller to follow up with PCP, Clinic, or ED.

# Influenza

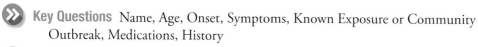

>> **Key Questions**  Name, Age, Onset, Symptoms, Known Exposure or Community Outbreak, Medications, History

>> **Other Protocols to Consider**  Common Cold Symptoms (103); Congestion (110); Cough (121); Fever (192); Headache (238); Swine Flu (H1N1 Virus) Exposure (452); Sore Throat (420); West Nile Virus (499).

> *Nurse Alert:*  Use this protocol if exposure to influenza is known or suspected, there is a community outbreak, or previously diagnosed with influenza.

*Reminder:*  Document caller response to advice, home care instructions, and when to call back.

| ASSESSMENT | ACTION |
|---|---|
| **A. Are any of the following present?**<br><br>• Altered mental status<br>• Difficulty breathing for reasons other than congestion<br>• Fever >104.9°F (40.5°C)<br>• Flat purple or dark red spots on face or trunk and stiff or painful neck<br>• Severe headache<br>• Skin or lips turning blue<br>• New onset of drooling or unable to swallow | **YES** "Seek emergency care now"<br><br>**NO** Go to B |
| **B. Are any of the following present?**<br><br>• Stiff or painful neck<br>• Fever >103.1°F (39.5°C) or >100.4°F (38.0 C) in infant <12 weeks of age<br>• Fever, and child appears very ill, lethargic, or very irritable<br>• Signs of dehydration<br>• Age <6 weeks | **YES** "Seek medical care immediately"<br><br>**NO** Go to C |

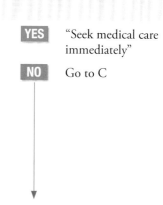

## C. Are any of the following present?

- Known exposure and any of the following: fatigue, fever <103.1°F (39.5°C), dry cough, sore throat, GI symptoms, runny nose or congestion, muscle aches
- History of immunosuppression, 6 weeks to 23 months of age, pregnancy, sickle cell disease, asthma

**YES** "Seek medical care within 24 hours"

**NO** Go to D

## D. Are any of the following present?

- Mild symptoms
- No symptoms but parent or person concerned

**YES** "Call back or call PCP for appointment if no improvement"
and
Follow **Home Care Instructions**

**NO** Follow **Home Care Instructions**

## Home Care Instructions
## Influenza

- Wash hands frequently with soap and water or alcohol-based hand rubs.
- Reinforce that influenza is highly contagious. Maintain good respiratory etiquette; cover mouth and nose with a tissue when coughing or sneezing.
- Avoid contact with sick individuals.
- If sick, avoid contact with other people. Stay home from school or work at least 24 hours after fever is gone.
- Get plenty of rest and drink plenty of fluids.
- Do not give aspirin to a child. Avoid aspirin-like products if age <20 years. Avoid acetaminophen if liver disease is present. Avoid ibuprofen if kidney disease or stomach problems exist or in the case of pregnancy. Follow the directions on the label.
- Give antivirals such as Tamiflu within 48 hours of symptom onset.

## Additional Instructions

_____

_____

_____

## Report the Following Problems to Your PCP/Clinic/ED

- Stiff or painful neck
- Fever >103.1°F (39.5°C) or >100.4°F in infant <12 weeks of age
- Fever, and child appears very ill, lethargic, or very irritable
- Signs of dehydration

## Seek Emergency Care If Any of the Following Occur

- Altered mental status
- Difficulty breathing
- Fever >104.9°F (40.5°C)
- Flat purple or dark red spots on face or trunk and stiff or painful neck
- Severe headache
- Skin or lips turning blue
- New onset of drooling or unable to swallow

If the caller agrees with the advice given, document the call and encourage the caller to call back or see PCP if the problem worsens. If the caller does not agree with the advice given, reevaluate and advise the caller to follow up with PCP, Clinic, or ED.

# Insomnia

 **Key Questions**  Name, Age, Onset, Cause, Allergies, Medications, History

 **Other Protocols to Consider**  Alcohol Problems (9); Anxiety (18); Depression (135); Heartburn (245); Substance Abuse, Use, or Exposure (434); Suicide Attempt, Threat (437).

*Reminder:*  Document caller response to advice, home care instructions, and when to call back.

| ASSESSMENT | | ACTION |
|---|---|---|
| **A. Is the following present?** | | |
| • Suicidal ideation | **YES** | "Seek emergency care now" |
| | **NO** | Go to B |
| **B. Are any of the following present?** | | |
| • Persistent pain, itching, coughing, or fever that interferes with sleep and is unresponsive to home care measures | **YES** | "Seek medical care within 24 hours" |
| • Persistent depression, anxiety, or stress | **NO** | Go to C |
| **C. Are any of the following present?** | | |
| • Persistent difficulty sleeping >7 days | **YES** | "Call back or call PCP for appointment if no improvement" and Follow **Home Care Instructions** |
| • Consistently unable to sleep >2 to 3 hours | | |
| • Requesting medication for sleep | | |
| • Urinary or bowel problems that frequently interrupt sleep | | |
| • Problem interferes with work, school, or other daily activity | | |
| • Ingestion of caffeine products | **NO** | Follow **Home Care Instructions** |
| • Intermittent episodes lasting 3 to 5 days | | |
| • Recent withdrawal from drugs or alcohol | | |
| • Prescribed sleep medication ineffective | | |
| • Taking a new medication | | |
| • Ingestion of OTC products | | |
| • Feeling overwhelmed | | |

I

## Home Care Instructions
## Insomnia

- Increase daily exercise. Avoid strenuous exercise 2 to 3 hours before bedtime. Do gentle stretching exercises for 10 minutes before retiring.
- Read or listen to soothing music at bedtime. Avoid using e-readers or other electronic products with brightly lit screens.
- Avoid caffeine and other stimulants 11 hours before bedtime.
- Take a warm bath or shower 2 hours before retiring.
- Drink warm milk before bed.
- Try relaxation techniques, such as deep breathing exercises or visualizing flower-filled meadows.
- Identify stress factors and try to reduce them. If awakening prompts worry about things to be done, devise a plan of action, list the items, and try to go back to sleep.
- Avoid eating 3 hours before bedtime. Sip 1 tbsp of apple cider vinegar diluted with water or juice 30 minutes after dinner to help speed gastric flow through the stomach and reduce gastric reflux.
- If difficulty sleeping is due to gastric reflux, sleep lying on the left side as tolerated to help speed stomach emptying and prevent reflux into the esophagus.
- If stress, anxiety, or depression interferes with sleep, seek help from a local counseling center or mental health services.
- Consider taking Benadryl or melatonin on a short-term basis. Follow the instructions on the label and consult pharmacist for pediatric dosing.
- Plug in a red, blue, or green nightlight to avoid turning on bright lights to use the restroom at night.
- Keep the bedroom dark, cool, and quiet. Use a fan or other appliance to block noise.
- Wear loose-fitting nightclothes.
- Call back immediately if feeling overwhelmed.

## Additional Instructions

_____

_____

_____

### Report the Following Problems to Your PCP/Clinic/ED

- No improvement with home care measures or problem worsens
- Problem interferes with work, school, or other daily activity
- Feeling overwhelmed

### Seek Emergency Care Immediately If the Following Occurs

- Suicidal ideation

If the caller agrees with the advice given, document the call and encourage the caller to call back or see PCP if the problem worsens. If the caller does not agree with the advice given, reevaluate and advise the caller to follow up with PCP, Clinic, or ED.

# Itching

 **Key Questions**  Name, Age, Onset, Medications, History, Associated Symptoms

 **Other Protocols to Consider**  Allergic Reaction (13); Bedbug Exposure or Concerns (37); Chickenpox (91); Penis Problems (331); Lice (296); Pinworms (345); Rash (366); Rubella (German Measles) (382); Rubeola (Measles) (385); Vaginal Discharge/Pain/ Itching (486); Wound Healing and Infection (509).

***Reminder:*** Document caller response to advice, home care instructions, and when to call back.

| ASSESSMENT | ACTION |
|---|---|

### A. Are any of the following present?

- Severe itching in several areas of the body, generalized hives, difficulty breathing, or swelling in the face, mouth, or throat
- Used Epi-Pen as directed by PCP

**YES** "Seek emergency care now"

**NO** Go to B

### B. Are any of the following present?

- Generalized itching, or yellow skin and eyes
- Itching rash started after taking a new medication
- Intense itching, particularly at night; red dots in folds of skin; and other household members have similar symptoms
- Persistent itching interferes with activity
- Itching scalp and bald spots
- Persistent itchy rash and recent exposure to poison oak or ivy and unresponsive to home care measures

**YES** "Seek medical care within 24 hours"

**NO** Go to C

## C.  Are any of the following present?

- Multiple insect bites
- Itching around anus, vagina, or genitals
- Itching scalp or pubic area, and white round spots along hair shaft will not detach
- Itching hands that are frequently exposed to moisture or chemicals
- Itching after wearing new clothing
- New-onset itchy rash and recent exposure to poison oak or ivy

**YES**  "Call back or call PCP for appointment if no improvement"
and
Follow **Home Care Instructions**

**NO**  Follow **Home Care Instructions**

I

## Home Care Instructions
## Itching

- Apply cool compress to affected area. Soak cloth in ice water.
- Soak in baking soda or oatmeal bath or Aveeno Bath, make an oatmeal sponge using a cotton cloth and cooked oatmeal, or apply baking soda paste mixed with white vinegar.
- Apply Caladryl lotion or Domeboro solution to insect bites and poison oak or ivy rashes. Follow instructions on the label.
- Itching around the anus may be caused by hemorrhoids or pinworms. See Hemorrhoids or Pinworms protocol, as appropriate.
- Apply OTC NIX Creme Rinse or Rid treatments for lice. Follow instructions on the label. See Lice protocol.
- If sensitivity to clothing exists, wash clothes before wearing and rinse twice. Wear cotton clothing. Avoid wool and synthetic clothing next to skin.
- Take OTC antihistamines (Benadryl, Chlor-Trimeton) for severe, persistent itching. Follow instructions on the label and consult pharmacist for pediatric dosing. Use the dosing device that comes with the medication, a measuring device, or a medication syringe from the pharmacy. Household teaspoons often do not give the correct amount of medication.
- Wrap a young child's hands or place in gloves to prevent scratching at night. Keep nails short.
- Apply OTC hydrocortisone creams to rash for short periods of time. Do not use longer than 3 days.
- Apply moisturizing cream (Curel, Vaseline Intensive Care) to dry, itching skin. Follow instructions on the label.
- For itching feet, wash frequently and dry well. Expose to air as much as possible. Wear cotton, rather than synthetic, socks.

## Additional Instructions

_____

_____

_____

### Report the Following Problems to Your PCP/Clinic/ED

- No improvement or condition worsens after >3 days of home care measures
- Other household members have the same symptoms

### Seek Emergency Care Immediately If the Following Occur

- Severe itching over several areas of the body, generalized hives, swelling in the face or throat, and difficulty breathing

If the caller agrees with the advice given, document the call and encourage the caller to call back or see PCP if the problem worsens. If the caller does not agree with the advice given, reevaluate and advise the caller to follow up with PCP, Clinic, or ED.

# Jaundice

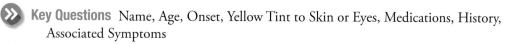

>> **Key Questions** Name, Age, Onset, Yellow Tint to Skin or Eyes, Medications, History, Associated Symptoms

>> **Other Protocols to Consider** Abdominal Pain (1); Abdominal Swelling (4); Itching (282); Newborn Problems (315); Stools, Abnormal (429).

*Reminder:* Document caller response to advice, home care instructions, and when to call back.

| ASSESSMENT | ACTION |
|---|---|

### A. Are any of the following present?

- Yellow-tinted skin in newborn within first 24 hours of life
- Yellow tint involves arms or legs
- Rectal temperature >100.4°F (38°C) or <96.8°F (36°C); in a newborn, seek medical care immediately
- Newborn with yellow tint below waistline
- Unable to awaken infant for two feedings in a row (4 to 6 hours)
- Newborn >2 days old and no wet diapers for >8 hours

**YES** "Seek medical care within 2 to 4 hours"

**NO** Go to B

### B. Are any of the following present?

- Dark urine
- Yellow skin
- White, yellow, or clay-colored stools
- Fatigue
- Headache
- Nausea, vomiting, or loss of appetite
- Abdominal pain
- Newborn >7 days of age and new onset of yellow skin
- Newborn 2 to 4 days old and no stool for >24 hours
- Wet diapers <6 per day or <3 per day if breast-feeding and less than 5 days old
- Newborn and yellow skin persists >14 days of age

**YES** "Seek medical care within 24 hours"

**NO** "Call back or call PCP for appointment if no improvement"
and
Follow **Home Care Instructions**

## Home Care Instructions
# Jaundice

### Newborn
- If newborn is breast-fed, feed every 1½ to 2½ hours (8 or more times in 24 hours).
- If newborn is bottle-fed, feed every 2 to 3 hours during the day.
- Place newborn near a window during sleep periods, with the skin exposed during the day to absorb the sun's rays.
- If supplement is offered, use formula or breast milk. Do not use water.
- Remember that jaundice occurs in many newborns and usually peaks at 3 to 5 days and disappears in 1 to 2 weeks. Newborns excrete bilirubin through stool. (The more they feed, the more stool they excrete.)
- Tips for awakening a sleepy newborn:
  - Unwrap blankets and undress the newborn.
  - Change the diaper.
  - Massage the newborn's legs, back, and arms.
  - Give the newborn a back rub by walking fingers down the spine.
  - Perform "sit-ups" by holding the newborn away from you and gently lifting the newborn toward your face.
- If newborn has not eaten in 6 hours, feed pumped breast milk or formula.

## Additional Instructions

_____

_____

_____

## Report the Following Problems to Your PCP/Clinic/ED
- Persistent yellowing of the skin with or without symptoms
- Unable to awaken newborn for feeding

If the caller agrees with the advice given, document the call and encourage the caller to call back or see PCP if the problem worsens. If the caller does not agree with the advice given, reevaluate and advise the caller to follow up with PCP, Clinic, or ED.

# Joint Pain/Swelling/Injury

>> **Key Questions**  Name, Age, Onset, Cause, Allergies, Medications, History, Pain Scale

>> **Other Protocols to Consider**  Ankle Injury (16); Extremity Injury (163); Leg Pain/Swelling (293); Pregnancy Problems (358); Sickle Cell Disease Problems (408).

*Reminder:*  Document caller response to advice, home care instructions, and when to call back.

| ASSESSMENT | ACTION |
|---|---|

### A. Are any of the following present?

- New onset and unable to walk or bear weight
- Dislocation or deformity
- Fingers or toes of affected part are cold or blue

**YES** "Seek emergency care now"

**NO** Go to B

### B. Are any of the following present?

- Swelling and pain in thigh or calf
- New onset and hesitant to walk or bear weight
- Joint, calf, or thigh painful, swollen, warm, or red with no known injury
- Purple rash on the arms and/or legs
- Swelling in one extremity and a recent long trip, pregnant, history of cancer, prolonged bed rest, or history of blood clots in legs

**YES** "Seek medical care within 2 to 4 hours"

**NO** Go to C

## C. Are any of the following present?

- Pregnant and recent onset of symptoms
- Pain persists or worsens with:
  - walking or standing
  - rest
  - raising the leg
  - flexing the foot
  - using hand, arm, or shoulder
- History of heart, liver, kidney disease, immunosuppression, diabetes or recent illness, such as sore throat or skin infection
- New prescription medication
- Skin over joint red or shiny
- Pain in knee or hip and limping
- Joint pain and two of the following: headache, sore throat, cough
- Child not using arm or hand
- Fever
- Recent weight gain of >10 pounds

**YES**  "Seek medical care within 24 hours"

**NO**  Go to D

## D. Are any of the following present?

- Pregnancy
- Pain in other joints
- General ill feeling
- Sudden onset with no known injury
- Mild swelling
- Chronic pain unrelieved with home care measures

**YES**  "Call back or call PCP for appointment if no improvement"
and
Follow **Home Care Instructions**

**NO**  Follow **Home Care Instructions**

# Home Care Instructions
## Joint Pain/Swelling

- Elevate the affected limb higher than the heart. Place pillows under the calves to elevate swollen ankles.
- For ankle swelling, reduce salt in diet.
- Apply heat to area (if no known injury): use caution when applying heat and diabetic. Do not fall asleep on a heating pad.
- Do not massage painful thighs or calves.
- Take your usual pain medication (acetaminophen, ibuprofen). Do not give aspirin to a child. Avoid aspirin-like products if age <20 years. Avoid acetaminophen if liver disease is present. Avoid ibuprofen if kidney disease or stomach problems exist or in the case of pregnancy. Follow the directions on the label. Use the dosing device that comes with the medication, a measuring device, or a medicine syringe from the pharmacy. Household teaspoons often do not give the correct amount of medication.
- Rest.
- For known injury, apply ice pack to joint for 20 to 30 minutes every 2 hours for first 24 to 48 hours. Do not apply ice directly on skin; place a washcloth or other cloth barrier between ice and skin.

## Additional Instructions

_____

_____

_____

### Report the Following Problems to Your PCP/Clinic/ED
- No improvement or condition worsens
- Increased pain
- Decreased mobility
- Fever

### Seek Emergency Care Immediately If Any of the Following Occur
- Fingers or toes of affected part are cold or blue

If the caller agrees with the advice given, document the call and encourage the caller to call back or see PCP if the problem worsens. If the caller does not agree with the advice given, reevaluate and advise the caller to follow up with PCP, Clinic, or ED.

# Laceration

**Key Questions**  Name, Age, Onset, Cause, Allergies, Pain Scale, Medications, Tetanus Immunization Status, Location (If caused by a bite, see Bites, Animal/Human (46), Marine Animal (53), and Snake (55).)

**Other Protocols to Consider**  Foreign Body, Skin (211); Immunization, Tetanus (264); Piercing Problems (338); Puncture Wound (362); Wound Care: Suture or Staples (506); Wound Healing and Infection (509).

*Reminder:* Document caller response to advice, home care instructions, and when to call back.

| ASSESSMENT | ACTION |
|---|---|
| **A. Are any of the following present?** | |
| • Large gaping wound <br> • Partial or complete amputation <br> • Deep wound to the head, back of mouth or throat, chest, neck, genitals, or abdomen <br> • Difficulty breathing <br> • Pulsating or squirting blood <br> • Visible bone in laceration <br> • Penetrating injury (knife, bullet, metal object) <br> • Self-injury suspected | **YES** "Call ambulance" or "Seek emergency care now" and "Do not remove knife or other penetrating cause of injury" <br><br> **NO** Go to B |
| **B. Are any of the following present?** | |
| • Gaping, split, jagged, or deep wound <br> • Newly sutured, stapled, or glued wound now split open <br> • Severe pain <br> • Unable to move or limited movement of injured part <br> • History of diabetes <br> • Persistent bleeding after 10 minutes of direct pressure <br> • Numbness or weakness <br> • Laceration through eyelid, lip border, or eyebrow <br> • High-pressure injection injury <br> • Unable to remove dirt or other foreign material from wound <br> • Taking a steroid or a blood-thinning medication <br> • Signs of infection: increased redness, drainage, fever, increased pain, red streaks, or swelling in a healing wound | **YES** "Seek medical care within 2 to 4 hours" <br><br> **NO** Go to C |

### C.  Are any of the following present?

- Persistent pain unrelieved by home care measures
- Tetanus immunization >5 years ago
- Wound over a joint and difficulty keeping edges of wound together
- Wound not healing well after 7 to 10 days

 **YES**  "Seek medical care within 24 hours"

 **NO**  Go to D

### D.  Are any of the following present?

- Small laceration in the mouth
- Edges of wound stay together and bleeding is controlled
- No history of tetanus immunization or immunization history unknown
- Headache, muscle aches, general ill feeling, or fever
- Parent or caller concerned about scarring

**YES**  "Call back or call PCP for appointment if no improvement" and Follow **Home Care Instructions**

**NO**  Follow **Home Care Instructions**

L

## Home Care Instructions
## Laceration

- Apply direct pressure over the wound with a clean bandage or cloth to control the bleeding.
- Clean the wound with soap and water.
- Pull edges of the wound together and hold in place with a butterfly or sterile strip bandage. Do not overlap skin edges. Leave butterfly or sterile strip in place until it falls off.
- May apply antibiotic ointment 2 to 3 times a day.
- Cover the wound with a clean, dry dressing.
- Check the wound daily for signs of infection. Replace soiled dressings daily or more often, as needed.
- For lacerations in the mouth, suck on an ice cube or flavored ice to reduce swelling and control bleeding.

## Additional Instructions

_____

_____

_____

### Report the Following Problems to Your PCP/Clinic/ED

- Increase in pain, swelling, or bleeding
- Headache, muscle aches, general ill feeling, or fever
- Signs of infection, numbness, or tingling
- Laceration is not healing well after 1 week to 10 days
- Newly sutured, stapled, or glued wound now split open
- Unable to move or limited movement of injured part

### Seek Emergency Care Immediately If Any of the Following Occur

- Difficulty breathing

If the caller agrees with the advice given, document the call and encourage the caller to call back or see PCP if the problem worsens. If the caller does not agree with the advice given, reevaluate and advise the caller to follow up with PCP, Clinic, or ED.

# Leg Pain/Swelling

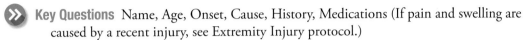 **Key Questions**  Name, Age, Onset, Cause, History, Medications (If pain and swelling are caused by a recent injury, see Extremity Injury protocol.)

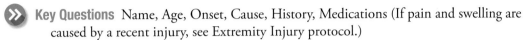 **Other Protocols to Consider**  Ankle Injury (16); Extremity Injury (163); Muscle Cramps (307); Pregnancy Problems (358); Tattoo Problems (456).

*Reminder:*  Document caller response to advice, home care instructions, and when to call back.

| ASSESSMENT | ACTION |
|---|---|

**A. In addition to leg swelling, are any of the following present?**

- Chest pain
- Severe shortness of breath
- Sudden onset and cold or blue foot or toe(s)
- Sudden onset and no pulse in foot of affected leg and numbness or tingling
- Unable to walk

**YES**  "Call ambulance"
or
"Seek emergency care now"

**NO**  Go to B

**B. Are any of the following present?**

- Severe swelling and/or pain in thigh, calf, ankle, or toes
- Child is reluctant to use or move the leg
- Fever
- Area over the ankle, calf, or thigh is warm to touch; red streaks extending from area
- Sudden swelling in one leg or ankle
- Signs of infection and immunosuppressed
- Persistent pain or swelling and recent trauma to leg

**YES**  "Seek medical care within 2 to 4 hours"

**NO**  Go to C

L

## C. Are any of the following present?

- Pain persists or worsens with
  - walking or standing
  - rest
  - raising the leg
  - flexing the foot
- New prescription medication
- Swelling increases at night
- Pregnancy and recent onset of symptoms
- No improvement with home care
- Recent weight gain of >10 pounds
- History of blood clots, cancer, diabetes, cardiac disease, immunosuppression, liver or kidney disease
- Signs of infection, swelling, pain, warmth, drainage, red streaks
- Fever
- Limping and pain in knee or hip
- Increased pain with movement or weight bearing and interferes with activity

**YES**  "Seek medical care within 24 hours"

**NO**  Go to D

## D. Are any of the following present?

- Pain in other joints
- General ill feeling
- Pain over the shin bone in the lower leg after exercising
- Persistent pain but does not interfere with activity
- Muscle cramps that awaken during sleep

**YES**  "Call back or call PCP for appointment if no improvement"
and
Follow **Home Care Instructions**

**NO**  Follow **Home Care Instructions**

## Home Care Instructions
## Leg Pain/Swelling

- Elevate legs on pillows so that the feet are higher than the heart. Do not place anything under the knees. Place pillows under the calves.
- Reduce salt in the diet.
- Rest and decrease activity.
- Apply heat to the area. If shins become painful after exercising, apply ice. Do not apply ice directly to the skin. Use a washcloth or other cloth barrier between ice and the skin.
- Do not massage area.
- Avoid sitting or standing for long periods of time, but if such activity is unavoidable, move toes and calf muscles frequently.
- Try usual medication for discomfort. Do not give aspirin to a child. Avoid aspirin-like products if age <20 years. Avoid acetaminophen if liver disease is present. Avoid ibuprofen if kidney disease or stomach problems exist or in the case of pregnancy. Follow the directions on the label. Use the dosing device that comes with the medication, a measuring device, or a medicine syringe from the pharmacy. Household teaspoons often do not give the correct amount of medication.

## Additional Instructions

_____

_____

_____

### Report the Following Problems to Your PCP/Clinic/ED

- No improvement or condition worsens
- Increased pain
- Decreased mobility
- Fever

### Seek Emergency Care Immediately If Any of the Following Occur

- Chest pain
- Severe shortness of breath
- Cold or blue foot or toe(s)
- No pulse in foot of affected leg

If the caller agrees with the advice given, document the call and encourage the caller to call back or see PCP if the problem worsens. If the caller does not agree with the advice given, reevaluate and advise the caller to follow up with PCP, Clinic, or ED.

# Lice

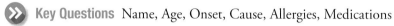 **Key Questions**  Name, Age, Onset, Cause, Allergies, Medications

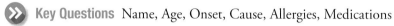 **Other Protocols to Consider**  Bedbug Exposure or Concerns (37); Itching (282); Rash (366); Skin Lesions: Lumps, Bumps, and Sores (414).

> *Nurse Alert:* Use this protocol if undergoing treatment for lice, history of lice (small gray or brown bugs), and lice or nits (white eggs) are present and attached to the hair shaft on the scalp, groin, underarm, or eyelashes.
>
> ● If symptoms of an allergic reaction develop after using a lice treatment medication (rash, swelling of the lips, tongue, or throat or difficulty breathing), go to the Allergic Reaction protocol (13).

*Reminder:*  Document caller response to advice, home care instructions, and when to call back.

| ASSESSMENT | ACTION |
|---|---|
| **A. Lice present and are any of the following present?** | |
| ● Persistent rash and itch that interfere with sleep<br>● Rash persists after 1 week of treatment<br>● Sores spread or show signs of infection<br>● New eggs appear after treatment<br>● Rash clears, then returns<br>● Local skin reaction to OTC or prescribed treatment medication<br>● Pregnancy<br>● Fever, malaise, or enlarged nodes | **YES** "Seek medical care within 24 to 48 hours" See Allergic Reaction protocol (13) if suspected allergic reaction to medication<br><br>**NO** Go to B |
| **B. No lice seen and are any of the following present?** | |
| ● Undergoing treatment for lice and has questions regarding medication or preventing the spread to others<br>● Known exposure to someone with lice or suspicion of infestation | **YES** "Call back or call PCP for appointment if no improvement" and Follow **Home Care Instructions**<br><br>**NO** Follow **Home Care Instructions** |

## Home Care Instructions
# Lice

- Search for lice when hair is wet and comb through small sections at a time with a fine comb, louse comb, or flea comb used on cats and dogs. Repeat every 2 to 3 days for 2 weeks.
- Check the scalps and bodies of other household members for rash or itching. If present, treat with antilice shampoo.
- If lice are found, apply antilice product (prescribed or OTC—Rid, Nix, or Pronto shampoos) to dry hair for 10 minutes and follow instructions on the label. Do not use Rid on children who are allergic to ragweed. Do not use Nix on children with asthma. Be sure to read the label for warnings and contraindications. Retreat in 7 to 10 days. Ask pharmacist for additional product suggestions.
- Rinse over a sink with cool water (Nix kills eggs).
- Use a fine-toothed comb to remove eggs from the shaft of the hairs. Scotch tape applied to the shaft of the hair is also effective in removing nits.
- To remove eggs on eyelashes, apply petrolatum to lashes twice a day for 8 days.
- Soak brushes and combs in antilice shampoo for 1 hour.
- Wash clothing and linens in hot water. Wash clothing inside out to destroy lice or eggs hiding in the seams. Dry on high heat (if possible) and iron seams. Place clothing and items that cannot be washed in a plastic bag for 3 days.
- Clean furniture, carpets, and mattresses. Vacuum and immediately throw away the vacuum bag.
- Avoid sharing personal items, such as combs, brushes, hats, or towels.
- Lice are highly contagious. Avoid head-to-head contact.
- Blow dry hair every day to help remove and prevent lice infestation.
- If lice are resistant to antilice medications, apply real mayonnaise or olive oil liberally to the hair and cover the hair with a shower cap for at least 3 hours. The mayonnaise or olive oil will help to smother the lice.
- A child can return to school after one application of antilice shampoo.

## Additional Instructions

_____

_____

_____

## Report the Following Problems to Your PCP/Clinic/ED

- The rash, lice, or nits disappear, then return
- Signs of infection: redness, pain, drainage, or fever
- Questions concerning the medication for the ill, infants, children, or pregnant women
- Mild allergic reaction to the medication
- Rash itching >1 week after treatment

## Seek Emergency Care Immediately If the Following Occur

- Severe allergic reaction to medication

If the caller agrees with the advice given, document the call, and encourage the caller to call back or see PCP if the problem worsens. If the caller does not agree with the advice given, reevaluate and advise the caller to follow up with PCP, Clinic, or ED.

# Menstrual Problems

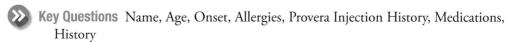

>> **Key Questions**  Name, Age, Onset, Allergies, Provera Injection History, Medications, History

>> **Other Protocols to Consider**  Abdominal Pain (1); Sexually Transmitted Infection (STI) (403); Vaginal Bleeding (484); Vaginal Discharge/Pain/Itching (486).

*Reminder:*  Document caller response to advice, home care instructions, and when to call back.

| ASSESSMENT | ACTION |
| --- | --- |

### A. Are any of the following present?

- Persistent severe bleeding that requires use of more than one full-size sanitary pad per hour for 8 hours
- Passage of large blood clots or tissue and different than usual menstrual cycle
- Severe pain and possible pregnancy
- Sexually active and last menstrual period is 6 to 8 weeks ago and abdominal or shoulder pain or vaginal bleeding

**YES**  "Seek emergency care now"

**NO**  Go to B

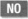

### B. Are any of the following present?

- Unusually severe pain and no possibility of pregnancy
- Unexplained fever (temperature >100°F or 37.8°C) and abdominal pain
- Fainting or dizziness sitting up or standing
- Use of tampons and sudden high fever, sunburn-type rash, general ill feeling, dizziness, vomiting, watery diarrhea, rapid pulse, or headache

**YES**  "Seek medical care within 2 to 4 hours"

**NO**  Go to C

### C. Are any of the following present?

- Cramping interferes with school, work, or daily activity
- Persistent vaginal discharge
- Persistent vaginal bleeding for >10 days or <21 days since last period
- Possible pregnancy and bleeding and no pain

**YES**  "Seek medical care within 24 hours"

**NO**  Go to D

## D. Are any of the following present?

- Persistent pain after bleeding stops
- Late period and history of increased stress, strenuous activity, significant weight loss, recent illness, stopped taking birth control pills
- Light bleeding or mild abdominal discomfort mid-cycle
- Irritability, bloating, headaches, or breast tenderness before period
- Breakthrough bleeding and taking birth control pills or other hormonal contraceptives
- Irregular periods
- Postcoital bleeding

**YES**  "Call back or call PCP for appointment if no improvement"
and
Follow **Home Care Instructions**

**NO**  Follow **Home Care Instructions**

## Home Care Instructions
## Menstrual Problems

- Take usual pain medication (acetaminophen, ibuprofen, naproxen). Avoid ibuprofen if pregnant. Do not give aspirin to a child. Avoid aspirin-like products if age <20 years. Avoid acetaminophen if liver disease is present. Avoid ibuprofen if kidney disease or stomach problems exist. Follow the directions on the label.
- Apply heating pad or hot water bottle to abdomen for 20 to 30 minutes for abdominal discomfort or take a warm bath. Do not fall asleep on a heating pad.
- Change tampons frequently, at least every 4 hours. Use pads at night. Avoid using tampons if skin infection is present and near the genitals.
- If period is >2 weeks late, use home pregnancy kit on first morning urine sample.
- For premenstrual symptoms, decrease salt, caffeine, and sugar in the diet and alcohol and cigarette use before menstruation.
- Increase exercise to help reduce cramping and premenstrual symptoms.

## Additional Instructions

_____

_____

_____

### Report the Following Problems to Your PCP/Clinic/ED
- No improvement in 3 days or condition worsens
- Menstrual cramps interfere with school, work, or daily activity
- Fainting or dizziness sitting up or standing
- Unexplained fever and abdominal pain

### Seek Emergency Care Immediately If Any of the Following Occur
- Persistent severe bleeding requiring use of more than one full-size sanitary pad per hour for 8 hours
- Passage of blood clots or tissue

If the caller agrees with the advice given, document the call and encourage the caller to call back or see PCP if the problem worsens. If the caller does not agree with the advice given, reevaluate and advise the caller to follow up with PCP, Clinic, or ED.

M

# Mouth Problems

 **Key Questions**  Name, Age, Onset, Allergies, Medications, History

 **Other Protocols to Consider**  Piercing Problems (338); Skin Lesions: Lumps, Bumps, and Sores (414); Sore Throat (420); Swallowing Difficulty (442); Toothache (465); Tooth Injury (468).

*Reminder:*  Document caller response to advice, home care instructions, and when to call back.

| ASSESSMENT | ACTION |
|---|---|
| **A. Are any of the following present?** | |
| • Sudden swelling in back of throat or tongue<br>• Jaw feels locked in place, inability to open mouth<br>• Unable to swallow own saliva<br>• New-onset jaw pain and pain radiates to neck and shoulders or arms |  "Seek emergency care now"<br><br> Go to B |
| **B. Are any of the following present?** | |
| • Penetrating injury to mouth with sharp object<br>• Persistent bleeding<br>• Severe pain<br>• Gaping laceration to lip, tongue, or inside mouth<br>• Pain with facial swelling<br>• Sensation of bone or food stuck in throat<br>• Teeth do not align as usual |  "Seek medical care within 2 to 4 hours"<br><br> Go to C |

## C. Are any of the following present?

- Fever and mouth sores
- Blisters in mouth, hands or feet
- White patches on tongue, gums, or inner cheeks
- General ill feeling
- Pain with biting, chewing, or opening mouth
- Persistent mouth pain unresponsive to home care measures
- History of phenytoin (Dilantin) use
- Foul odor despite regular hygiene
- Red, swollen, tender gums with fever
- Difficulty swallowing
- Jaw locks in certain positions and able to adjust and open mouth
- Signs of infection: increased pain, swelling, drainage, red streaks, warmth

**YES** "Seek medical care within 24 hours"

**NO** Go to D

## D. Are any of the following present?

- History of oral herpes, canker sores, recent viral illness, or new medication
- Taking large doses of vitamins
- Red, swollen, tender gums and no fever
- Sore spot on tongue
- Poor eating habits or change in diet
- Recent increase in stress
- Dental caries
- Intermittent swelling over the jaw
- Clicking, snapping or popping sound with jaw movement
- Jaw pain and ear or eye pain

**YES** "Call back or call PCP for appointment if no improvement"
and
Follow **Home Care Instructions**

**NO** Follow **Home Care Instructions**

M

## Home Care Instructions
## Mouth Problems

- Iced fluids may soothe mouth sores but will worsen a toothache.
- Rinse mouth with warm water and ½ tsp salt or baking soda 4 times a day, or rinse with an antiseptic mouthwash.
- Avoid spicy, citrus, or salty foods until sores are healed. A soft diet may be tolerated in children who have mouth sores or difficulty swallowing.
- If chewing increases jaw pain, avoid chewing gum or tough foods and alternate hot and cold packs to jaw 6 times a day.
- Avoid touching sores.
- Brush, floss, and rinse teeth and mouth at least twice daily.
- Take usual pain medication (acetaminophen or ibuprofen) for fever and discomfort. Do not give aspirin to a child. Avoid aspirin-like products if age <20 years. Avoid acetaminophen if liver disease is present. Avoid ibuprofen if kidney disease or stomach problems exist or in the case of pregnancy. Follow the directions on the label. Use the dosing device that comes with the medication, a measuring device, or a medicine syringe from the pharmacy. Household teaspoons often do not give the correct amount of medication.
- Use OTC product containing Orabase to provide protective coating and diminish discomfort. Note: Products such as Orabase contain benzocaine that should not be used in children less than 2 years of age. For children 1 year of age or older, a liquid antacid can be placed on mouth lesions to diminish pain.

## Additional Instructions

_____

_____

_____

## Report the Following Problems to Your PCP/Clinic/ED

- Mouth lesion persists >2 weeks
- Persistent pain or bleeding
- Signs of infection: pain, swelling, drainage, warmth, or fever
- Difficulty swallowing
- No improvement or condition worsens

## Seek Emergency Care Immediately If Any of the Following Occur

- Sudden swelling in back of throat or tongue
- Jaw feels locked in place, inability to open mouth
- Unable to swallow own saliva

If the caller agrees with the advice given, document the call and encourage the caller to call back or see PCP if the problem worsens. If the caller does not agree with the advice given, reevaluate and advise the caller to follow up with PCP, Clinic, or ED.

# Mumps

>> **Key Questions**  Name, Age, Onset, Known or Suspected Mumps, History, Medications

>> **Other Protocols to Consider**  Fever (184); Glands, Swollen or Tender (229);
Neck Pain (309).

> *Nurse Alert:* Use this protocol if diagnosed with mumps or caller has known exposure to mumps, has swollen glands, and has questions about mumps.

*Reminder:*  Document caller response to advice, home care instructions, and when to call back.

| ASSESSMENT | ACTION |
|---|---|

### A. Person has diagnosed mumps and are any of the following present?

- Stiff neck or severe headache
- Repeated vomiting
- Severe abdominal pain
- Confusion
- Decreased level of consciousness
- Difficulty breathing
- Severe dizziness on standing

**YES** "Seek emergency care now"

**NO** Go to B

### B. Are any of the following present?

- Swollen gland >8 days
- Fever >5 days
- Skin red over swollen gland
- Painful testicle
- Severe pain

**YES** "Seek medical care within 24 hours"

**NO** Go to C

### C. Are any of the following present?

- Swollen and tender gland in front of ear and around jaw
- Chewing increases pain
- Fever
- No prior mumps vaccine
- Exposure to mumps 16 to 18 days earlier

**YES** "Call back or call PCP for appointment if no improvement" and Follow **Home Care Instructions**

**NO** Follow **Home Care Instructions**

M

## Home Care Instructions
# Mumps

- Isolate person with mumps until the swelling is gone. Avoid unvaccinated individuals such as children <1 year of age.
- Rest until fever subsides.
- Apply an ice collar or ice pack to swollen glands for discomfort. Do not place ice directly on skin; place a cloth barrier between the ice and the skin.
- Take usual pain medication (acetaminophen, ibuprofen). Do not give aspirin to a child. Avoid aspirin-like products if age <20 years. Avoid acetaminophen if liver disease is present. Avoid ibuprofen if kidney disease or stomach problems exist or in the case of pregnancy. Follow the directions on the label. Use the dosing device that comes with the medication, a measuring device, or a medicine syringe from the pharmacy. Household teaspoons often do not give the correct amount of medication.
- Eat a liquid or soft diet until pain subsides. Avoid sour or citrus foods.
- Avoid mumps exposure to people who are immunosuppressed (including individuals receiving chemotherapy or those with AIDS).

## Additional Instructions

_____

_____

_____

## Report the Following Problems to Your PCP/Clinic/ED
- Swollen gland >8 days
- Fever >5 days
- Skin red over swollen gland
- Painful testicle

## Seek Emergency Care Immediately If Any of the Following Occur
- Stiff neck or severe headache
- Repeated vomiting
- Severe abdominal pain
- Confusion
- Decreased level of consciousness
- Difficulty breathing
- Severe dizziness on standing

If the caller agrees with the advice given, document the call and encourage the caller to call back or see PCP if the problem worsens. If the caller does not agree with the advice given, reevaluate and advise the caller to follow up with PCP, Clinic, or ED.

# Muscle Cramps

 **Key Questions**  Name, Age, Onset, Cause, Allergies, History, Pain Scale, Medications

 **Other Protocols to Consider**  Back Pain (34); Extremity Injury (163); Joint Pain/ Swelling (287); Leg Pain/Swelling (293).

*Reminder:*  Document caller response to advice, home care instructions, and when to call back.

| ASSESSMENT | ACTION |
|---|---|
| **A. Are any of the following present?** | |
| • Cramping following an injury and inability to move or use limb<br>• Tender, swollen calf with no known injury<br>• Extremity pale, blue, or cool compared with other limb, or extremity numb | **YES** "Seek medical care within 2 to 4 hours"<br>**NO** Go to B |
| **B. Are any of the following present?** | |
| • Tender red area on calf with no known injury<br>• Sudden onset after taking new medication<br>• Cramping interferes with activity<br>• Frequent use of diuretics | **YES** "Seek medical care within 24 hours"<br>**NO** Go to C |
| **C. Are any of the following present?** | |
| • Cramping occurs during or several hours after strenuous exercise<br>• Excessive sweating and inadequate fluid replacement<br>• Calf pain frequently occurs with exercise and disappears with rest<br>• Prolonged sitting, standing, or lying in an awkward position<br>• Leg cramps occur at night | **YES** "Call back or call PCP for appointment if no improvement"<br>and<br>Follow **Home Care Instructions**<br>**NO** Follow **Home Care Instructions** |

M

## Home Care Instructions
## Muscle Cramps

- Perform dynamic stretching exercises for 15 to 20 minutes before strenuous exercise.
- After strenuous exercise or excessive sweating, rest in a cool place and replace lost fluid. Drink a mixture of ¼ tsp salt in 1 quart of water, a sports drink, juice, soda, or water.
- Discuss diuretic use with health care provider. When taking OTC diuretics, make sure lost fluid is adequately replaced. Follow instructions on the label.
- Stretch the muscle cramp after prolonged sitting, standing, or lying in an awkward position by extending the leg and pulling the foot back, or stand and press the foot against the floor.
- Apply moist heat for cramping or an ice pack for injury for 20 minutes, 4 to 6 times a day, for the first 24 hours. Do not apply ice directly to the skin. Use a washcloth or other barrier to protect the skin from burning. Do not fall asleep on a heating pad. If diabetic, use caution when applying heat or cold.
- Take your usual pain medication (acetaminophen, ibuprofen). Do not give aspirin to a child. Avoid aspirin-like products if age <20 years. Avoid acetaminophen if liver disease is present. Avoid ibuprofen if kidney disease or stomach problems exist or in the case of pregnancy. Follow the directions on the label. Use the dosing device that comes with the medication, a measuring device, or a medicine syringe from the pharmacy. Household teaspoons often do not give the correct amount of medication.

## Additional Instructions

_____

_____

_____

## Report the Following Problems to Your PCP/Clinic/ED

- Persistent and frequent cramping
- Cramping after taking prescribed medication
- Increased pain, swelling, redness, or inability to use limb
- Persistent discomfort interferes with activity
- Extremity becomes pale, blue, or cool compared with other limb, or extremity numb
- No improvement or condition worsens

If the caller agrees with the advice given, document the call and encourage the caller to call back or see PCP if the problem worsens. If the caller does not agree with the advice given, reevaluate and advise the caller to follow up with PCP, Clinic, or ED.

# Neck Pain

>> **Key Questions**  Name, Age, Onset, Cause, Associated Symptoms, Medications, History, Pain Scale

>> **Other Protocols to Consider**  Back/Neck Injury (31); Chest Pain (85); Glands, Swollen or Tender (229); Mumps (305); Mouth Problems (302); Numbness and Tingling (325).

*Nurse Alert:* There are many conditions that can cause neck pain. When neck pain is associated with several other symptoms, triage with caution and note signs that may be an indication of a more serious condition such as meningitis (pain bending head forward, headache, fever, vomiting, confusion, photophobia) or a heart attack (chest, neck, back or jaw pain, sweating, palpitations, nausea, and/or vomiting).

*Reminder:*  Document caller response to advice, home care instructions, and when to call back.

| ASSESSMENT | ACTION |
|---|---|
| **A. Is neck pain related to an injury?** | |
| | **YES**  Go to Back/Neck Injury protocol (31) |
| | **NO**  Go to B |
| **B. Is chest pain present?** | |
| | **YES**  Go to Chest Pain protocol (85) |
| | **NO**  Go to C |

### C. Sudden onset of pain, and are any of the following present?

- History of a cardiac condition
- Jaw pain
- Sweating, palpitations, nausea, and/or vomiting
- Difficulty breathing
- Pain worsens when head is bent toward chest and any of the following:
  - confusion/drowsiness
  - severe headache
  - light sensitivity
  - fever
  - purple or blood-colored rash
- Numbness, tingling, weakness in both arms or legs
- Changes in bowel or bladder control
- Head involuntarily turns to side

**YES**  "Seek emergency care now"

**NO**  Go to D

### D. Are any of the following present?

- Weakness or numbness in one arm
- Signs of infection: pain, swelling, redness, drainage, warmth, or red streaks
- Fever >103°F (39.4°C)
- Fever >101°F (38.3°C) and history of diabetes, immunosuppressed, or IV drug abuse
- Swollen, painful lymph nodes > 1 inch (2.5 cm)
- Swollen, painful nodes and difficulty swallowing

**YES**  "Seek medical care within 2 to 4 hours"

**NO**  Go to E

### E. Are any of the following present?

- Rash
- Sore throat associated with neck pain
- Pain interferes with sleep or activity
- Swelling on one or both sides of the neck

**YES**  "Seek medical care within 24 hours"

**NO**  Go to F

### F. Are any of the following present?

- Slept in an awkward position
- New exercise or activity
- Recently carried heavy bag, purse, or other object using a shoulder strap
- Pain worsens with lateral movement
- History of prolonged sitting at a computer terminal or work station
- Intermittent pain and history of prior neck problems

**YES**  "Call back or call PCP for an appointment if no improvement"
and
Follow **Home Care Instructions**

**NO**  Follow **Home Care Instructions**

## Home Care Instructions
## Neck Pain

- Apply heat to neck for 20 minutes every 2 hours. Be careful with heat if diabetic. Do not sleep on a heating pad.
- Sleep with a towel folded around neck to lessen neck movement.
- Carry purse or bag under arm, rather than over the shoulder.
- Avoid prolonged sitting. Frequently stretch and move around.
- Exercise regularly to develop strong neck muscles.
- Soak in hot bath or whirlpool.
- Take usual pain medication (acetaminophen, ibuprofen) as directed by your physician. Do not give aspirin to a child. Avoid aspirin-like products if age <20 years. Avoid acetaminophen if liver disease is present. Avoid ibuprofen if kidney disease or stomach problems exist or in the case of pregnancy. Follow the directions on the label. Use the dosing device that comes with the medication, a measuring device, or a medicine syringe from the pharmacy. Household teaspoons often do not give the correct amount of medication.
- Maintain good posture and proper body alignment.

## Additional Instructions

_____

_____

_____

N

### Report the Following Problems to Your PCP/Clinic/ED

- Rash, fever, or increased pain bending neck forward
- No improvement or condition worsens

### Seek Emergency Care Immediately if Any of the Following Occur

- Chest pain
- Difficulty breathing
- Numbness, tingling, or weakness in both arms or legs
- Severe headache and confusion
- Sweating, palpitations, nausea, and/or vomiting
- Swelling to one side of the neck with pain on palpation with or without fever
- Loss of bowel or bladder control
- Pain worsens when head is bent toward chest, confusion/drowsiness, severe headache, light sensitivity, fever, purple- or blood-colored rash

If the caller agrees with the advice given, document the call and encourage the caller to call back or see PCP if the problem worsens. If the caller does not agree with the advice given, reevaluate and advise the caller to follow up with PCP, Clinic, or ED.

# Neurologic Symptoms

 **Key Questions**  Name, Age, Onset, Medications, History

 **Other Protocols to Consider**  Back/Neck Injury (31); Confusion (107); Dizziness (147); Headache (238); Head Injury (242); Numbness and Tingling (325); Vision Problems (489); Weakness (496).

> *Nurse Alert:*
>
> ● Sudden changes in vision, weakness, numbness, speech, or mental status may be signs of a serious neurologic disorder. Prompt treatment may prevent extensive damage to the brain or spinal cord and reduce permanent disability.
>
> ● Ask how current condition is different from normal.

*Reminder:*  Document caller response to advice, home care instructions, and when to call back.

| ASSESSMENT | ACTION |
|---|---|

### A. Did any of the following symptoms suddenly occur?

- Numbness or weakness in face, arm, or leg
- Unexplained dizziness or falls
- Difficulty breathing
- Altered mental status
- Inability to stand, walk, or bear weight
- Difficulty speaking
- Facial drooping on one side
- Difficulty swallowing
- Unable to move a limb
- Visual changes
- Sudden, severe headache
- Recent history of head trauma and elevated blood pressure

**YES** "Call ambulance"
or
"Seek emergency care now"

**NO** Go to B

## B. Are any of the following present?

- Transient focal neurologic deficits that completely resolve within hours
- New and sudden onset of bladder or bowel incontinence
- New onset of back pain and numbness to groin or rectal area
- Unable to urinate and bladder full
- Headache worse than prior headaches
- Low blood glucose and weakness, confusion, dizziness, headache, tremors, or vision problems, and unresponsive to usual home remedies

 **YES**  "Seek medical care immediately"

**NO**  Go to C

## C. Is the following present?

- Tremors and history of heavy alcohol use

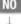 **YES**  "Seek medical care within 24 hours"

**NO**  Go to D

## D. Are any of the following present?

- Poor attention span
- Transient tingling in hands or feet
- New onset of tremors and no history of diabetes, alcohol abuse, or seizures

**YES**  "Call back or call PCP for appointment if no improvement"
and
Follow **Home Care Instructions**

**NO**  Follow **Home Care Instructions**

N

## Home Care Instructions
## Neurologic Symptoms

- Provide reassurance that foot or hand tingling after prolonged sitting or pressure to the area will resolve with movement and stretching.
- Avoid crossing legs at the knees or ankles.
- Avoid smoking.
- Take medications as prescribed.
- Avoid driving or operating machinery when experiencing transient symptoms.

## Additional Instructions

_____

_____

_____

### Report the Following Problems to Your PCP/Clinic/ED

- Weakness or numbness in the face, arms, or legs
- Difficulty understanding
- Persistent vision changes
- Persistent dizziness
- No improvement or condition worsens

### Seek Emergency Care Immediately if Any of the Following Suddenly Occur

- Unexplained dizziness or falls
- Difficulty breathing
- Altered mental status
- Inability to stand, walk, or bear weight
- Difficulty speaking or swallowing
- Facial drooping on one side
- Unable to move a limb
- Severe headache
- Visual changes

If the caller agrees with the advice given, document the call and encourage the caller to call back or see PCP if the problem worsens. If the caller does not agree with the advice given, reevaluate and advise the caller to follow up with PCP, Clinic, or ED.

# Newborn Problems

 **Key Questions**  Name, Age, Onset, Cause, Birth History, Medications

 **Other Protocols to Consider**  Bottle-Feeding Problems (59); Breast-Feeding Problems (63); Circumcision Care (97); Crying, Excessive, in Infants (128); Fever (184); Jaundice (285); Sleep Apnea, Infant (418).

> ***Nurse Alert:*** There are many conditions that affect newborns. When there are multiple associated symptoms, use the protocol that is the primary concern and has the highest probability of a referral to a higher level of care. Ask how the baby's current condition is different from the usual pattern and how the baby is acting at time of call.

***Reminder:***  Document caller response to advice, home care instructions, and when to call back.

| ASSESSMENT | ACTION |
|---|---|
| **A. Are any of the following present?** | |
| • Seizure | **YES**  "Call ambulance" |
| • Unresponsiveness | or |
| • Rectal temperature >100.4°F (38°C) | "Go to Emergency |
| • Temperature <96.8°F (36°C) and unresponsive to warming | Department now" |
| • Bulging soft spot with vomiting, fever, or acting sick | **NO**  Go to B |
| • Fall onto a hard surface with obvious injury | |
| • Nonblanching rash | |
| • Bruising | |

N

## B. Are any of the following present?

- Fall onto a hard surface with no obvious injury
- Refuses to drink >6 hours
- Umbilical cord bleeding >10 minutes of direct pressure
- Red streaks or red area around umbilicus
- Clumps of blisters on one part of body
- Chicken pox, widespread blisters
- Breathing quickly
- Distressed and grunting with breathing
- Difficult to comfort
- Nasal flaring
- Pale or blue skin, lips, or nail beds
- Yellow tint below waistline, arms, or legs
- Yellow skin and <24 hours old

**YES**  "Seek medical care immediately"

**NO**  Go to C

## C. Are any of the following present?

- Bulging soft spot and infant acting normally
- Umbilical cord intermittently bleeding >3 days
- Pimples or blisters near the cord
- Moderate amount of drainage from navel but no fever
- Yellow sticky discharge from eye
- Red eyes or swollen eyelids
- Newborn >7 days of age with yellow skin
- Yellow or green penile discharge after circumcision (no fever)
- No stool >24 hours
- White, yellow, or clay-colored stools

**YES**  "Seek medical care within 24 hours"

**NO**  Go to D

## D. Are any of the following present?

- Intermittent bulging soft spot with no signs or symptoms of illness
- Scant bleeding from umbilical cord
- Pink tissue inside the navel
- Foul odor from cord for >2 days (with no fever or redness)
- Grunting with breathing and no distress

**YES**  "Call back or call PCP for appointment if no improvement"
and
Follow **Home Care Instructions**

**NO**  Follow **Home Care Instructions**

## Home Care Instructions
## Newborn Problems

### Provide Reassurance

- Swollen breasts are normal in the first week of life.
- Red streaks in the white part of the eye are related to the birthing process and will resolve in 2 to 3 weeks.
- Watery eyes are often a result of a blocked tear duct and will resolve within a year. Watch for signs of infection, redness, swelling, and drainage.
- A clear, white, or pink-tinged vaginal discharge is normal and will resolve in 2 to 3 days.
- Swelling in the scrotum will resolve in 6 to 12 months.
- Tips for awakening a sleepy newborn:
  - Unwrap blankets and undress the newborn.
  - Change the diaper.
  - Massage the newborn's legs, back, and arms.
  - Give the newborn a back rub by walking fingers down the spine.
  - Perform "sit-ups" by holding the newborn away from you and gently lifting the newborn toward your face.
- See "Other Protocols to Consider" (viii) for associated symptoms or conditions and additional home care instructions.

### Additional Instructions

N

### Report the Following Problems to Your PCP/Clinic/ED

- Refusal to drink >6 hours
- Umbilical cord bleeding >10 minutes of direct pressure
- Red streaks or red area around umbilicus
- Clumps of blisters on one part of body
- Breathing quickly, grunting when breathing, or nasal flaring
- Difficult to comfort
- Newborn >7 days of age with yellow skin
- Pale or blue skin, lips, or nail beds
- No stool >24 hours or white, yellow, or clay-colored stools
- No improvement or condition worsens
- Newborn looks or acts sick

### Seek Emergency Care Immediately if Any of the Following Occur

- Seizure
- Unresponsiveness
- Temperature >100.4°F (38°C)
- Bulging soft spot with vomiting, fever, or a newborn that acts sick
- Nonblanching rash of dark red or purple spots

If the caller agrees with the advice given, document the call and encourage the caller to call back or see PCP if the problem worsens. If the caller does not agree with the advice given, reevaluate and advise the caller to follow up with PCP, Clinic, or ED.

# Nosebleed

 **Key Questions** Name, Age, Onset, Cause, Medications, History

 **Other Protocols to Consider** Foreign Body, Nose (206); Headache (238); Head Injury (242); Nose Injury (322); Piercing Problems (338).

*Reminder:* Document caller response to advice, home care instructions, and when to call back.

| ASSESSMENT | ACTION |
|---|---|
| **A. Are any of the following present?** | |
| • Unable to stop the bleeding after 30 minutes of constant pressure <br> • Altered mental status <br> • Rapid heart rate, pale skin, or shortness of breath | **YES** "Seek emergency care now" <br> **NO** Go to B |
| **B. Are any of the following present?** | |
| • Difficulty breathing (for reasons other than a stuffy nose) <br> • Light-headedness, dizziness <br> • Nosebleed follows a severe headache <br> • History of high blood pressure or bleeding disorder <br> • Taking blood-thinning medications, aspirin, or nonsteroidal anti-inflammatory drugs and persistent nosebleeds <br> • Foreign body in nose and profuse bleeding <br> • Recent head injury and bloody or fluid nasal drainage | **YES** "Seek medical care within 2 hours" <br> **NO** Go to C |
| **C. Are any of the following present?** | |
| • Recent injury and persistent deformity or obstruction <br> • More than three nosebleeds in the past 48 hours <br> • Recent nasal surgery, bleeding has stopped and restarted <br> • Recent nasal surgery and persistent bleeding | **YES** "Seek medical care within 24 hours" <br> **NO** Go to D |

N

319

## D. Are any of the following present?

- History of allergies or hay fever
- History of frequent controlled nosebleeds
- History of repetitive use of nasal sprays
- Frequent use of cocaine

**YES**  "Call back or call PCP for appointment if no improvement"
and
Follow **Home Care Instructions**

**NO**  Follow **Home Care Instructions**

## Home Care Instructions
## Nosebleed

- In a sitting position, with the head bent forward, firmly pinch the nose closed for 15 minutes with an ice-cold washcloth. Breathe through the mouth.
- If the bleeding stops but then recurs, pinch the nose closed for another 15 minutes.
- Do not blow nose.
- Avoid aspirin and anti-inflammatory products.
- Avoid smoking and strenuous activity for 24 hours after a nosebleed.
- Keep mucous membranes moist. Use saline nasal drops or spray several times a day.
- Avoid hot liquids (such as soup, coffee, or tea).
- Use a humidifier in the bedroom to help keep nasal passages moist.

## Additional Instructions

_____

_____

_____

### Report the Following Problems to Your PCP/Clinic/ED
- Difficulty breathing, light-headedness, or dizziness
- Problem persists or worsens

### Seek Emergency Care Immediately if Any of the Following Occur
- Change in mental status
- Rapid heart rate, pale skin, or shortness of breath
- Bleeding persists after >30 minutes of pressure

If the caller agrees with the advice given, document the call and encourage the caller to call back or see PCP if the problem worsens. If the caller does not agree with the advice given, reevaluate and advise the caller to follow up with PCP, Clinic, or ED.

N

# Nose Injury

**Key Questions**  Name, Age, Onset, Cause, Associated Symptoms, Medications, History, Pain Scale

**Other Protocols to Consider**  Headache (238); Head Injury (242); Laceration (290); Nosebleed (319); Piercing Problems (338).

*Nurse Alert:*

- A neck injury should always be considered whenever there is a blow to the head. Assess for weakness, incoordination, numbness, and neck pain.
- Altered mental status may be one of the first signs of a head injury after trauma to the head.

*Reminder:*  Document caller response to advice, home care instructions, and when to call back.

| ASSESSMENT | ACTION |
|---|---|

### A. Blow to the nose, and are any of the following present?

- Persistent bleeding for >30 minutes
- Signs of head injury:
  - lethargy
  - confusion/combativeness
  - difficulty speaking
  - visual disturbance
  - severe headache
  - coordination problems
  - nausea and/or vomiting
- Sudden onset of neck pain, numbness, tingling, or weakness in arms
- Persistent clear or pink nasal drainage

**YES** "Call ambulance"
or
"Seek emergency care now"

**NO** Go to B

### B. Are any of the following present?

- History of sinus surgery
- Gaping, split or jagged, or deep wound
- Deformity after 72 hours and home care measures

**YES** "Seek medical care within 2 to 4 hours"

**NO** Go to C

## C. Are any of the following present?

- Difficulty breathing through one or both nostrils after swelling has subsided

  **YES** "Seek medical care within 24 hours"

  **NO** Go to D

## D. Are any of the following present?

- Nasal swelling
- Pain
- Controlled nosebleed
- Abrasion or bruising around nose and eyes
- Nose appears deformed 24 to 72 hours after injury

  **YES** "Call back or call PCP for appointment if no improvement" and Follow **Home Care Instructions**

  **NO** Follow **Home Care Instructions**

N

## Home Care Instructions
## Nose Injury

- Apply ice pack to nose for 20 to 30 minutes every 2 hours for the first 48 hours to help reduce swelling and pain. Do not apply ice directly to the skin. Wrap ice in a towel or washcloth.
- To stop a nosebleed, apply continuous pressure to the soft part of the nose for 15 minutes. Sit up and lean forward. Avoid swallowing blood; spit it out. Breathe through mouth.
- If bleeding stops but then recurs, pinch the nose closed for another 15 minutes.
- Expect swelling, bruising, and deformity for the first 48 to 72 hours.

## Additional Instructions

_____

_____

_____

## Report the Following Problems to Your PCP/Clinic/ED

- Deformity lasting >72 hours after swelling subsides
- Difficulty breathing through one or both nostrils
- No improvement or condition worsens

## Seek Emergency Care Immediately if Any of the Following Occur

- Persistent bleeding for >30 minutes
- Signs of head injury:
  - lethargy
  - confusion, combativeness
  - difficulty speaking
  - visual disturbance
  - severe headache
  - coordination problems
  - nausea and/or vomiting
- Sudden onset of neck pain, numbness, tingling, or weakness in arms
- Persistent clear or pink nasal drainage

If the caller agrees with the advice given, document the call and encourage the caller to call back or see PCP if the problem worsens. If the caller does not agree with the advice given, reevaluate and advise the caller to follow up with PCP, Clinic, or ED.

# Numbness and Tingling

>> **Key Questions** Name, Age, Onset, Cause, Location, Associated Symptoms, Medications, History

>> **Other Protocols to Consider** Arm/Hand Problems (24); Back/Neck Injury (31); Back Pain (34); Breathing Problems (68); Chest Pain (85); Headache (238); Head Injury (242); Neurologic Symptoms (312); Weakness (496).

> ### Nurse Alert:
> - Sudden changes in vision, weakness, numbness, speech, or mental status may be signs of a serious neurologic disorder. Prompt treatment may prevent extensive damage to the brain or spinal cord and reduce permanent disability.
> - Ask how current condition is different from normal.

**Reminder:** Document caller response to advice, home care instructions, and when to call back.

| ASSESSMENT | ACTION |
|---|---|
| **A. Are any of the following present?** | |
| • Confusion <br> • Change in mental status | **YES** Go to Confusion Protocol (107) |
| | **NO** Go to B |
| **B. Is the following present?** | |
| • Severe headache | **YES** Go to Headache protocol (238) |
| | **NO** Go to C |

N

### C. Are any of the following present?

- One side of the body affected
- Sudden weakness in arms and/or legs
- Difficulty speaking, slurred speech
- Blurred vision
- Loss of bladder or bowel control
- Fingers or toes are cold or blue compared with other fingers or toes
- Headache prior to onset of symptoms
- Chest pain

**YES**  "Call ambulance"
or
"Seek emergency care now"

**NO**  Go to D

### D. Are any of the following present?

- History of recent heavy lifting or strenuous exercise
- Area painful, swollen, and/or warm
- Severe pain

**YES**  "Seek medical care within 2 to 4 hours"

**NO**  Go to E

### E. Are any of the following present?

- Numbness, tingling, and/or a sharp pain in the hand or arm at night
- History of recent illness or surgery
- Gradual onset
- Stiff or painful neck and no known injury
- Diagnosed carpal tunnel and worsening symptoms
- Pregnant

**YES**  "Seek medical care within 24 hours"

**NO**  Go to F

### F. Are any of the following present?

- Symptoms followed prolonged sitting or lying in one position
- Rapid breathing, dizziness, and hands, face, or lips affected

**YES**  "Call back or call PCP for appointment if no improvement"
and
Follow **Home Care Instructions**

**NO**  Follow **Home Care Instructions**

## Home Care Instructions
## Numbness and Tingling

- Avoid sitting in one position for long periods of time.
- Periodically tighten and release muscles in affected area to stimulate circulation.
- Protect numb area from injury.
- Avoid repetitive motions; take breaks and do stretching exercises.
- Apply heat or cold to stiff neck.
- To slow rapid breathing and control numbness and tingling,
  - Sit down and focus on slowing breathing, one breath every 5 seconds.
  - Cover mouth and nose with a paper bag and breathe in and out 10 times.
  - If no improvement, continue breathing in the bag for 1 minute.
  - Breathe without the bag for a few minutes.
  - Repeat breathing with and without the bag until condition improves.

## Additional Instructions

_____

_____

_____

### Report the Following Problems to Your PCP/Clinic/ED
- No improvement in 20 to 30 minutes or condition worsens
- Symptoms interfere with daily activities

### Seek Emergency Care Immediately if Any of the Following Occur
- Change in mental status
- Sudden weakness in arms or legs
- Difficulty speaking or slurred speech
- Loss of bowel or bladder control
- Chest pain
- Vision changes
- Fingers or toes are blue

If the caller agrees with the advice given, document the call and encourage the caller to call back or see PCP if the problem worsens. If the caller does not agree with the advice given, reevaluate and advise the caller to follow up with PCP, Clinic, or ED.

# Overdose

**Key Questions** Name, Age, Onset, Name of Medication(s) or Substance(s), Amount, History, Medications

**Other Protocols to Consider** Depression (135); Diarrhea (143); Poisoning, Suspected (347); Substance Abuse, Use, or Exposure (434); Suicide Attempt, Threat (437); Vomiting (492).

*Reminder:* Document caller response to advice, home care instructions, and when to call back.

| ASSESSMENT | ACTION |
|---|---|

**A. Suspected overdose, and are any of the following present?**

- Severe difficulty breathing or respiratory rate <10 breaths per minute
- Chest pain
- Suicide attempt
- Seizure activity
- Combined alcohol and drug overdose
- Intoxication in a victim younger than 17 years of age
- Cocaine/crack use and chest pain
- Change in mental status

**YES** "Call ambulance"

**NO** Go to B

**B. Possible drug ingestion, and are any of the following present?**

- Wheezing or shortness of breath
- Severe abdominal pain

**YES** "Seek emergency care now" and Follow **Home Care Instructions**

**NO** Go to C

### C. Possible ingestion, no symptoms, and are any of the following present?

- Nausea, vomiting, or diarrhea
- Ingestion of aspirin, acetaminophen, or other medication, hallucinogen, or unknown mushroom
- Victim is a child in the presence of open spilled containers, such as pill bottles, or has substance on face, skin, or clothes
- Smell of suspected ingested product on breath or clothes

**YES** "Call Poison Control Center" (Telephone number: 1-800-222-1222)
and
Follow **Home Care Instructions**

**NO** "Call back or call PCP for appointment if no improvement"
and
Follow **Home Care Instructions**

## Home Care Instructions
## Overdose

- Follow instructions as directed by the Poison Control Center (Telephone number: 1-800-222-1222). Provide the center with the following information:
  - Identify the substance ingested. Read the exact name from the label on the container, including the strength, or describe the markings on the pill or capsule.
  - Describe how much was ingested or is missing from the container.
  - Indicate time the substance was ingested.
- Read the instructions on the container for accidental ingestion.
- Take the container or mushroom with you to the hospital.
- If the Poison Control Center's telephone number is not readily available, call an ambulance.
- Do not induce vomiting if the person has an altered level of consciousness or has difficulty swallowing. Do not induce vomiting until directed to do so by the Poison Control Center. Do not induce vomiting if acid, alkalis, or petroleum products were ingested, including battery, sulfuric, or hydrochloric acid; bleach; Drano; drain or oven cleaners; gasoline; furniture polish; kerosene; or lighter fluid. Neutralize with milk, water, or milk of magnesia.
- All overdoses should be evaluated by a physician unless told by the Poison Control Center that the ingestion is nothing to be concerned about.
- Do not try to arouse an overdose victim by placing him/her in the shower or forcing coffee.
- Do not give anything to eat or drink unless instructed to do so by the Poison Control Center, or as instructed above when the Poison Control Center is unavailable.

## Additional Instructions

_____

_____

_____

## Report the Following Problems to Your PCP/Clinic/ED

- Persistent problems or illness after initial treatment
- Suicide attempt or threat
- Unsure whether or not a substance was ingested and nausea or vomiting occurs

If the caller agrees with the advice given, document the call and encourage the caller to call back or see PCP if the problem worsens. If the caller does not agree with the advice given, reevaluate and advise the caller to follow up with PCP, Clinic, or ED.

# Penis Problems

>> **Key Questions**  Name, Age, Onset, Cause, Medications, History

>> **Other Protocols to Consider**  Circumcision Care (97); Genital Lesions (226); Piercing Problems (338); Scrotal Problems (390); Sexually Transmitted Infection (STI) (403); Skin Lesions: Lumps, Bumps and Sores (414); Tattoo Problems (456); Urination, Difficult (473).

*Reminder:*  Document caller response to advice, home care instructions, and when to call back.

| ASSESSMENT | ACTION |
|---|---|
| **A. Are any of the following present?** | |
| • Persistent painful erection after application of ice pack for 30 minutes <br> • Severe pain or swelling <br> • Trauma to penis and deformity or bleeding <br> • Foreign body in penis | **YES** "Seek emergency care now" <br> **NO** Go to B |
| **B. Are any of the following present?** | |
| • Unable to pull foreskin back over head of penis <br> • Unable to urinate <br> • Pain with urination <br> • Flank pain <br> • Pain in groin after urinating and temperature 100°F (37.8°C) <br> • Pain or swelling in scrotum or testicle(s) | **YES** "Seek medical care within 2 to 4 hours" <br> **NO** Go to C |
| **C. Are any of the following present?** | |
| • Persistent swelling, hard lump, or sore on penis <br> • Known or suspected exposure to an STI <br> • Painful rash or sores <br> • Penile discharge >24 hours <br> • Redness or swelling at tip of penis <br> • Blood in urine <br> • Blood in semen <br> • Rash with blisters on penis <br> • Swollen foreskin | **YES** "Seek medical care within 24 hours" <br> **NO** Go to D |

P

## D. Are any of the following present?

- Pain during or after intercourse
- Difficulty having or maintaining an erection and history of diabetes or taking antidepressants, antianxiety medications, blood pressure medications, or diuretics
- Premature ejaculation
- Loss of sexual interest
- Penis caught in zipper
- Swelling and small cut on infant penis
- Painless rash or growth >24 hours

**YES** "Call back or call PCP for appointment if no improvement" and Follow **Home Care Instructions**

**NO** Follow **Home Care Instructions**

## Home Care Instructions
## Penis Problems

- If pain during intercourse, consider using OTC lubricating jelly (K-Y jelly). Do not use petroleum jelly.
- If tip of penis is painful after intercourse, explore probable causes, such as allergy to contraceptive cream or condom, and change to alternative methods.
- If tip of penis is red from rubbing against a diaper, push penis down when diapering infant.
- If client has sexual dysfunction problems and is taking prescription medications, has diabetes, or has emotional problems, client should discuss with PCP.
- To release penis caught in zipper:
  - cut off the bottom of the zipper and pull the edges back
  - apply petroleum jelly to penis and zipper track and pull zipper in the direction that originally caused the problem
  - if unable to release penis, seek medical care immediately
- Look for hair wrapped around infant's penis and cut to release pressure. Swelling should go down. If unable to remove hair or swelling persists, seek medical care immediately.
- If an STI is suspected, partner also should be treated. Use a condom until both partners have finished taking prescription medication.

**Additional Instructions**

_____

_____

_____

### Report the Following Problems to Your PCP/Clinic/ED

- No improvement or problem worsens after home care measures
- Persistent sexual dysfunction problems

### Seek Emergency Care Immediately If Any of the Following Occur

- Persistent painful erection
- Severe pain or swelling
- Inability to urinate

If the caller agrees with the advice given, document the call and encourage the caller to call back or see PCP if the problem worsens. If the caller does not agree with the advice given, reevaluate and advise the caller to follow up with PCP, Clinic, or ED.

# Pertussis (Whooping Cough)

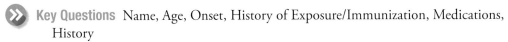 **Key Questions** Name, Age, Onset, History of Exposure/Immunization, Medications, History

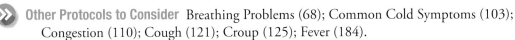 **Other Protocols to Consider** Breathing Problems (68); Common Cold Symptoms (103); Congestion (110); Cough (121); Croup (125); Fever (184).

*Nurse Alert:*

- Use the protocol if previously diagnosed with pertussis, for known or suspected exposure to pertussis, recent local community outbreak of pertussis, and severe cough. Pertussis is highly contagious.

*Reminder:* Document caller response to advice, home care instructions, and when to call back.

| ASSESSMENT | ACTION |
|---|---|

### A. Are any of the following present?

- Altered mental status
- Severe difficulty breathing
- Difficulty breathing and unable to speak
- Seizures

  Apnea
- New onset of drooling
- Unable to swallow
- Nonblanching dark red or purple rash, headache, pain bending head forward, or fever

**YES** "Call ambulance"
or
"Seek emergency care now"

**NO** Go to B

### B. Are any of the following present?

- Skin, lips, or tongue turns blue during coughing spells
- Productive or severe cough
- High fever unresponsive to fever-reducing measures
- Infant unable to feed because of coughing
- Persistent nosebleed
- Fever and signs of dehydration
- Infant, 3 months old or younger (no recent immunization) and temperature >100.4°F (38°C)
- Cough and cold symptoms >1 week and chest pain, weakness, fever

**YES** "Seek medical care immediately"

**NO** Go to C

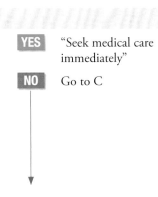

## C. Are any of the following present?

- Family members and classmates exposed to person with known pertussis and request prophylaxis
- Cough lasting more than 2 weeks
- Subconjunctival hemorrhage
- Rectal prolapse or abdominal hernia and persistent coughing
- Fever >72 hours and unresponsive to fever-reducing measures
- Taking antibiotics for pertussis and persistent fever or worsening condition
- Green, brown, or yellow sputum >72 hours
- Coughing up blood

 "Seek medical care within 24 hours"

 Go to D

## D. Is the following present?

- Community epidemic and recent onset of runny nose, cough, watery eyes

**YES** "Call back or call PCP for appointment if no improvement"
and
Follow **Home Care Instructions**

**NO** Follow **Home Care Instructions**

 P

## Home Care Instructions
## Pertussis

- Practice good respiratory hygiene. Cover mouth when coughing or sneezing. Discard tissues in a paper bag. Cough into sleeve to help prevent droplets from contaminating others. Bend elbow and raise upper arm to cover mouth.
- Practice good hand washing to help prevent transmission of the disease. Wash with soap and water or alcohol-based hand rub.
- Take antibiotics as prescribed, and finish the complete course.
- Sip warm liquids to soothe coughing spasms.
- Give small frequent feedings.
- Avoid cough triggers (smoke, pollutants, etc.)
- Give acetaminophen (if infant older than 2 months) or ibuprofen (if infant older than 6 months) for fever and achiness. Do not give aspirin to a child. Avoid aspirin-like products if age <20 years. Avoid acetaminophen if liver disease is present. Avoid ibuprofen if kidney disease or stomach problems exist or in the case of pregnancy. Follow the directions on the label. Use the dosing device that comes with the medication, a measuring device, or a medicine syringe from the pharmacy. Household teaspoons often do not give the correct amount of medication.
- Increase fluid consumption (juices, tea, broths, gelatin).
- Expected course: 1 to 2 weeks of cold symptoms followed by severe coughing spells. Can last up to 6 weeks. Chronic cough can last for 1 to 2 months.
- Once diagnosed, avoid public contact until on antibiotics for at least 3 days. Pertussis is highly contagious.

## Additional Instructions

_____

_____

_____

## Report the Following Problems to Your PCP/Clinic/ED

- No improvement or condition worsens
- Fever >72 hours
- Green, brown, or yellow sputum develops and lasts >72 hours
- Coughing up blood
- Signs of dehydration

## Seek Emergency Care Immediately If Any of the Following Occur

- Breathing worsens
- Skin, lips, or tongue blue or gray
- Chest pain
- New onset of drooling or unable to swallow
- Altered mental status
- Seizures
- Nonblanching dark red or purple rash, headache, pain bending head forward, or fever

If the caller agrees with the advice given, document the call and encourage the caller to call back or see PCP if the problem worsens. If the caller does not agree with the advice given, reevaluate and advise the caller to follow up with PCP, Clinic, or ED.

P

# Piercing Problems

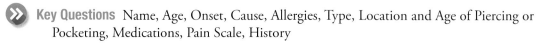 **Key Questions**  Name, Age, Onset, Cause, Allergies, Type, Location and Age of Piercing or Pocketing, Medications, Pain Scale, History

**Other Protocols to Consider**  Ear Injury, Foreign Body (154); Foreign Body, Skin (211); Genital Lesions (226); Penis Problems (331); Lacerations (290); Mouth Problems (302); Skin Lesions: Lumps, Bumps, and Sores (414); Wound Healing and Infection (509).

***Reminder:*** Document caller response to advice, home care instructions, and when to call back.

| ASSESSMENT | ACTION |
|---|---|

### A. Are any of the following present 2 to 4 days after the piercing/pocketing?

- Rapidly increasing pain, swelling, or redness
- Red streaks extending from wound
- White, yellow, or green foul-smelling wound drainage
- Fever
- Enlarged nodes (>1 in diameter) and overlying redness
- Gaping laceration to earlobe, eyelid, eyebrow, tongue, nipple, or genitals
- Unable to remove embedded piercing or other foreign object

**YES** "Seek medical care within 2 to 4 hours"

**NO** Go to B

### B. Are any of the following present?

- Increased pain or swelling
- Increased redness or red streaks extending from inflamed area
- Enlarged nodes (>1 in diameter)
- Thick white, yellow, or green foul-smelling drainage
- Temperature >100.4°F (38°C)
- Chills, feeling of illness, or headache
- No improvement with home care measures
- Warmth over the area
- Darkened hard and painful area around the piercing
- Minor tear from piercing and last tetanus shot >5 years
- No improvement after 3 days of home care

**YES** "Seek medical care within 24 hours"

**NO** Go to C

## C.  Are any of the following present?

- Small blisters, redness, and/or itching around the piercing
- Bleeding, bruising, discoloration, or swelling
- White-yellow crust at jewelry opening
- White thick secretion at opening
- Tongue turns yellow-white

**YES**  "Call back or call PCP for appointment if no improvement"
and
Follow **Home Care Instructions**

**NO**  Follow **Home Care Instructions**

P

## Home Care Instructions
## Piercing Problems

- Apply a cotton ball or gauze pad saturated in salt water solution (¼ tsp in 1 cup water) to pierced area several times a day for at least 1 minute. Rinse with clear water and pat dry with paper products.
- Apply salt water soaks before cleaning the piercing and before activity to prevent the crust from being pulled into the piercing, and remove matter.
- Remember that healing times can vary and that stinging, burning, or aching may persist for several days. Itching usually is a sign of healing.
- Avoid aspirin during the healing period. OTC medication (ibuprofen or acetaminophen) can help to relieve the discomfort and reduce swelling. Do not give aspirin to a child. Avoid aspirin-like products if age <20 years. Avoid acetaminophen if liver disease is present. Avoid ibuprofen if kidney disease or stomach problems exist or in the case of pregnancy. Follow the directions on the label.
- Elevate head of the bed for above-the-neck piercing.
- Do not use alcohol, povidone–iodine (Betadine), peroxide, or other harsh cleaners on piercing. They will cause excessive drying.
- Do not apply ointments to the piercing. They may trap bacteria in the piercing and delay healing.

### Cleaning Body Piercing

- Using recommended cleaning solution, clean the piercing 1 to 2 times a day throughout the healing period, usually 6 to 8 weeks (6 to 12 months for ear cartilage, hand web, navel, and penis or clitoris piercings).
- Wash hands with antibacterial soap. Do not touch the healing piercing unless hands are clean.
- Apply cleaning solution to the piercing and jewelry.
- After the first several cleanings, rotate the jewelry to make sure the solution reaches all areas of the piercing.
- Allow cleaning solution to remain on the piercing for 1 minute.
- Rinse the area under running water and rotate jewelry.
- Pat dry with disposable paper products.

### Oral Piercings

- Rinse the mouth for 30 to 60 seconds with saline solution (¼ tsp salt with 1 cup water) after meals, but no more than 4 to 5 times a day.
- If the tongue begins to turn yellow-white, reduce the number of cleansings per day.
- Use a new, soft-bristle brush to gently clean the mouth and around the piercing.
- Keep the mouth as hygienic as possible throughout the healing period. Remember the piercing is an open wound similar to a cut and should be treated properly to prevent infection.

## Additional Instructions

_____

_____

_____

**Report the Following Problems to Your PCP/Clinic/ED**

- No improvement or condition worsens after home care measures
- Increased pain or swelling
- Increased redness or red streaks extending from inflamed area
- Thick white, yellow, or green foul-smelling drainage
- Temperature >100.4°F (38°C)
- Warmth over the area
- Darkened hard and painful area around the piercing

If the caller agrees with the advice given, document the call and encourage the caller to call back or see PCP if the problem worsens. If the caller does not agree with the advice given, reevaluate and advise the caller to follow up with PCP, Clinic, or ED.

P

# Pinkeye

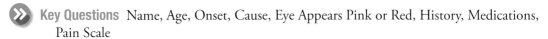

**Key Questions**  Name, Age, Onset, Cause, Eye Appears Pink or Red, History, Medications, Pain Scale

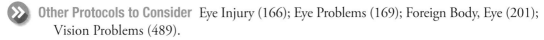

**Other Protocols to Consider**  Eye Injury (166); Eye Problems (169); Foreign Body, Eye (201); Vision Problems (489).

*Nurse Alert:* Use this protocol if previously diagnosed with pinkeye, known or suspected exposure to someone with pinkeye, and eye appears pink or red. Pinkeye is highly contagious.

*Reminder:* Document caller response to advice, home care instructions, and when to call back.

| ASSESSMENT | ACTION |
|---|---|
| **A. Are any of the following present?** | |
| • Injury to the eye<br>• Foreign body in the eye | **YES** Go to Eye Injury protocol (166)<br>or<br>Foreign Body, Eye protocol (201) |
| | **NO** Go to B |
| **B. Are any of the following present?** | |
| • History of glaucoma<br>• Abdominal pain or nausea<br>• Unable to move eye<br>• Partial loss of field of vision<br>• Newborn with a fever >100.4°F (38°C) | **YES** "Seek emergency care now"<br>**NO** Go to C |
| **C. Are any of the following present?** | |
| • Red swollen eyelids<br>• Ulcer or gray-white sore on eyeball<br>• Severe pain<br>• Flashes of light<br>• Age <5 years and severe redness or swelling around eye | **YES** "Seek medical care within 2 to 4 hours"<br>**NO** Go to D |

## D. Are any of the following present?

- Persistent blinking, tearing with pain
- Yellow/green eye discharge
- Eyelids slightly puffy with red rims
- Blurred vision
- Sensitivity to light
- History of previous eye infections
- Eyelids stuck together upon awakening
- Redness >7 days
- Exposure to welders or ultraviolet light
- Earache on same side as pinkeye

**YES**  "Seek medical care within 24 hours"

**NO**  Go to E

## E. Are any of the following present?

- Blood in the white part of the eye with no change in vision
- Cold symptoms: congestion, earache, sore throat, or cough
- Exposure to environmental irritants: smog, smoke, pool water, shampoo, onions, household cleaning products, or jalapeño peppers
- History of hay fever or allergies, and eye itching
- Clear eye discharge

**YES**  "Call back or call PCP for appointment if no improvement"
and
Follow **Home Care Instructions**

**NO**  Follow **Home Care Instructions**

## Home Care Instructions
## Pinkeye

- Rinse eyes frequently with warm water, every 1 to 2 hours when awake. Use a soft warm moist cloth to remove crusting and drainage.
- If exposed to chemical irritants, rinse eyes with warm water for 5 minutes.
- Apply alternating warm and cold compresses to eyes for 10 minutes every 2 hours for 24 hours.
- Do not share towels or linens with other household members.
- To control itching, try Benadryl for 24 to 48 hours. Follow instructions on the label. Use the dosing device that comes with the medication, a measuring device, or a medicine syringe from the pharmacy. Household teaspoons often do not give the correct amount of medication.
- Encourage children to avoid touching eyes and to wash hands frequently.

## Additional Instructions

_____

_____

_____

### Report the Following Problems to Your PCP/Clinic/ED
- Red swollen eyelids
- Ulcer or gray-white sore on eyeball
- Severe pain
- Flashes of light
- Persistent blinking, tearing, or pain
- Persistent eye drainage

### Seek Emergency Care Immediately If Any of the Following Occur
- Unable to move eye
- Abdominal pain or nausea

If the caller agrees with the advice given, document the call and encourage the caller to call back or see PCP if the problem worsens. If the caller does not agree with the advice given, reevaluate and advise the caller to follow up with PCP, Clinic, or ED.

# Pinworms

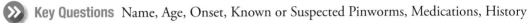

>> **Key Questions**  Name, Age, Onset, Known or Suspected Pinworms, Medications, History

>> **Other Protocols to Consider**  Bedbug Exposure or Concerns (37); Itching (282); Rectal Problems (374).

*Reminder:*  Document caller response to advice, home care instructions, and when to call back.

| ASSESSMENT | ACTION |
|---|---|
| **A. Are any of the following present?** | |
| • Signs of infection (pain, swelling, redness, drainage, warmth, or fever) in rectal area | **YES**  "Seek medical care within 24 hours" |
| • Severe rectal itching worsening at night and early morning | **NO**  Go to B |
| • ¼ to ½ white, thread-like worms in rectal or vaginal area | |
| • Worms visible in stool | |
| **B. Are any of the following present?** | |
| • Mild redness, itching, or tenderness in rectal area | **YES**  "Call back or call PCP for appointment if no improvement" and Follow **Home Care Instructions** |
| • Child has difficulty sleeping, irritability, or vaginal irritation | |
| • Exposed to bedclothes or bed linens of child with pinworms | |
| • Rectal symptoms persist >1 week after treatment | **NO**  Follow **Home Care Instructions** |
| • Family member diagnosed with pinworms and concerned about transmission | |

P

## Home Care Instructions
## Pinworms

- To detect pinworms in a child, shine a light on the child's anus in a darkened room several hours after bedtime. If present, the worms will move back into the anus.
- Trim nails closely and encourage good hand washing.
- Discourage nail biting or thumb sucking.
- Wash linen and underwear in hot soapy water until pinworms are gone.
- Vacuum or mop bedroom daily for 2 weeks after treatment.
- Bathe every morning and clean the affected area. Showers are preferable.
- Wear shorts or panties under pajamas.
- To reduce itching:
  - Apply zinc oxide or 1% hydrocortisone cream ointment to affected area.
  - Take a warm bath with Epsom salts or table salt.
- A prescription medication may be necessary to eliminate the pinworms. Take medication completely and as directed.
- Try OTC pinworm medication (Reese's) and follow instructions on the label.

## Additional Instructions

## Report the Following Problems to Your PCP/Clinic/ED

- Signs of infection: pain, swelling, redness, drainage, or warmth
- Condition persists >3 weeks after treatment

If the caller agrees with the advice given, document the call and encourage the caller to call back or see PCP if the problem worsens. If the caller does not agree with the advice given, reevaluate and advise the caller to follow up with PCP, Clinic, or ED.

# Poisoning, Suspected

 **Key Questions**  Name, Age, Onset, Cause, History, Associated Symptoms, Medications

 **Other Protocols to Consider**  Depression (135); Diarrhea (143); Food Poisoning, Suspected (194); Overdose (328); Substance Abuse, Use, or Exposure (434); Suicide Attempt, Threat (437); Vomiting (492).

> *Nurse Alert:* Use this protocol if known or suspected poisoning. Ask what was swallowed, how much, when, and any associated symptoms. Ask about other children who might have also been exposed who might not readily volunteer the information if they think they might be in trouble.

*Reminder:*  Document caller response to advice, home care instructions, and when to call back.

| ASSESSMENT | ACTION |
|---|---|
| **A. Are any of the following present?** | |
| • Altered mental status, unresponsive<br>• Severe difficulty breathing or respirations <10 breaths per minute<br>• Chest pain<br>• Suicide attempt<br>• Seizure activity<br>• Change in level of consciousness | **YES** "Call ambulance and take container and substance with you to hospital." Instruct to start CPR or rescue breathing if no pulse or respirations<br><br>**NO** Go to B |
| **B. Are any of the following present?** | |
| • Excessive sweating or saliva<br>• Wheezing or shortness of breath<br>• Blue lips, mouth, or nail beds | **YES** "Seek emergency care now and take container and substance with you to hospital."<br><br>**NO** Go to C |

P

## C. Are any of the following present?

- Nausea, vomiting, diarrhea
- Abdominal pain
- Burns on lips, tongue, or skin
- Palpitations
- Headache, irritability, or fever
- History of psychiatric problems

**YES** "Seek medical care now" and Follow **Home Care Instructions**

**NO** Go to D

## D. Are any of the following present and no symptoms?

- Children with open spilled containers, pill bottles, or substance on face, skin, or clothes
- Smell of product on breath or clothes
- Suspected ingestion of aspirin, acetaminophen, or other medication, hallucinogen, or unknown mushroom

**YES** "Call Poison Control" (Telephone number: 1-800-222-1222) and Follow **Home Care Instructions**

**NO** "Call back or call PCP for appointment if no improvement" and Follow **Home Care Instructions**

# Home Care Instructions
## Poisoning, Suspected

- Follow instructions as directed by the Poison Control Center. Provide the Center with the following information:
  - Identify the substance ingested. Read the exact name from the container label.
  - Describe how much was ingested or is missing from the container.
  - Indicate the time the substance was ingested.
- Read the instructions on the container for accidental ingestion.
- Take the container, remaining contents, plant, or mushroom with you to the hospital.
- If the Poison Control Center is not readily available, call an ambulance.
- Do not induce vomiting if the person has an altered level of consciousness or has difficulty swallowing. Do not induce vomiting until directed to do so by the Poison Control Center. Do not induce vomiting if any of the following have been ingested: acid, alkalis, or petroleum products; battery, sulfuric, or hydrochloric acid; bleach; drain or oven cleaners; gasoline; furniture polish; kerosene; or lighter fluid.
- All overdoses should be evaluated by a physician unless the Poison Control Center indicates there is no reason for concern.
- Do not try to arouse the victim by placing in the shower or forcing the ingestion of coffee.
- Do not give anything to eat or drink unless instructed to do so by the Poison Control Center.

## Additional Instructions

_____

_____

_____

### Report the Following Problems to Poison Control
- Persistent problems or illness after initial treatment
- Unsure whether or not substance was ingested and nausea or vomiting occurs

### Seek Emergency Care Immediately If Any of the Following Occur
- Excessive swallowing or saliva
- Wheezing or breathing problems
- Blue lips, mouth, or nail beds

If the caller agrees with the advice given, document the call and encourage the caller to call back or see PCP if the problem worsens. If the caller does not agree with the advice given, reevaluate and advise the caller to follow up with PCP, Clinic, or ED.

P

# Postoperative Problems

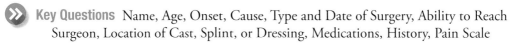

>> **Key Questions**  Name, Age, Onset, Cause, Type and Date of Surgery, Ability to Reach Surgeon, Location of Cast, Splint, or Dressing, Medications, History, Pain Scale

>> **Other Protocols to Consider**  Breathing Problems (68); Cast/Splint Problems (83); Chest Pain (85); Constipation (114); Fever (184); Leg Pain/Swelling (293); Vomiting (492); Swelling (449); Wound Care: Sutures or Staples (506); Wound Healing and Infection (509).

*Reminder:*  Document caller response to advice, home care instructions, and when to call back.

| ASSESSMENT | ACTION |
|---|---|

### A. Are any of the following present?

- Sudden onset of severe pain
- Surgical wound split or gaping and large amount of fluid drainage or material protruding from the wound
- If cast, splint, or orthopedic surgery:
  - fingers or toes cold, blue, or numb
  - severe pain, swelling, or tightness unresponsive to elevation or home care measures
- Chest pain
- Coughing up blood or pink frothy sputum
- Leg swelling and no pulse in foot of affected leg, numbness, or tingling
- Shortness of breath

**YES**  "Call ambulance"
or
"Seek emergency care now"

**NO**  Go to B

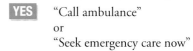

### B. Are any of the following present?

- Surgical wound split or gaping
- Signs of infection (pain, swelling, drainage, warmth, or red streaks extending from the wound)
- Swelling and pain in thigh, calf, ankle, or toes
- Dressing, splint, or cast feels too tight
- Large amount of bleeding from incision and unresponsive to home care measures
- Area over ankle, calf, shin, or thigh is warm to the touch or red
- Sudden swelling in one leg or ankle
- Temperature >100.4°F (38°C)

**YES**  "Seek medical care within 2 to 4 hours hours"

**NO**  Go to C

## C. Are any of the following present?

- History of diabetes, HIV infection, chronic disease, use of steroids, blood thinners, or chemotherapy and wound is not healing well
- Pain gradually worsens
- Pain unrelieved by prescribed medication
- Cracked or unstable cast, splint, or appliance
- Persistent oozing or bleeding at the incision site
- Persistent nausea and vomiting

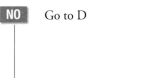

**YES** "Seek medical care within 24 hours"

**NO** Go to D

## D. Are any of the following present?

- Itching around wound edges
- Persistent swelling or tightness within cast or splint but improves with home care measures
- Small amount of bloody drainage on dressing
- Constipation
- Has questions about activity or diet
- Wound vacuum-assisted closure (VAC) device in place and
  - leaking
  - container full
  - turned off for 72 hours

**YES** "Call back or call PCP for appointment if no improvement"
and
Follow **Home Care Instructions**

**NO** Follow **Home Care Instructions**

P

## Home Care Instructions
## Postoperative Problems

- Take pain medications at regular intervals.
- Follow home care plan as directed by health care provider, including antibiotics, wound checks, exercise, diet, bowel care, and elevation.
- Keep wound clean and dry as directed by health care provider.
- Remember that itching along the edges of the wound is a sign of healing.
- If dressing is loose or there is a small amount of drainage, reinforce dressing. Remember that some drainage usually is expected.
- After orthopedic surgery, apply ice pack over the dressing for the first 48 hours.
- If there is a moderate to severe amount of bleeding, reinforce dressing and apply pressure over the wound for 10 minutes. If no improvement, contact PCP.
- Monitor temperature daily.
- Consider alternative methods for pain control: deep breathing, relaxation, ice, heat, elevation, positioning, or distraction.
- For wound VAC problems:
  - If wound VAC is off for 72 hours, replace dressing with wet-to-dry dressing, and contact home health nurse to replace dressing.
  - If VAC is leaking around the tube or at dressing edges, remove VAC dressing and replace it with wet-to-dry dressing, and notify home health nurse.
  - If canister is full, discard it in the garbage and replace it with a new canister.

**Additional Instructions**

_____

_____

_____

**Report the Following Problems to Your PCP/Clinic/ED**

- Pain persists or worsens
- Signs of infection: redness, swelling, pain, foul-smelling drainage, warmth, or red streaks extending from the wound
- Signs of circulation problems; fingers or toes become cold, blue, or numb
- Temperature >100.4°F (38°C)
- Headache, muscle aches, general ill feeling, and fever
- Persistent nausea and vomiting

**Seek Emergency Care Immediately If Any of the Following Occur**

- Sudden onset of severe pain
- Surgical wound split or gaping and large amount of fluid drainage or material protruding from the wound
- If cast, splint, or orthopedic surgery:
  - fingers or toes cold, blue, or numb
  - severe pain, swelling, or tightness unresponsive to elevation or home care measures
- Chest pain
- Coughing up blood or pink frothy sputum
- Leg swelling and no pulse in foot of affected leg, numbness, or tingling
- Shortness of breath

If the caller agrees with the advice given, document the call and encourage the caller to call back or see PCP if the problem worsens. If the caller does not agree with the advice given, reevaluate and advise the caller to follow up with PCP, Clinic, or ED.

P

# Postpartum Problems

 **Key Questions**  Name, Age, Onset, Date of Delivery, Medications, History

 **Other Protocols to Consider**  Abdominal Pain (1); Bottle-Feeding Problems (59); Breast-Feeding Problems (63); Constipation (114); Depression (135); Vaginal Discharge/Pain/Itching (486); Wound Healing and Infection (509).

> *Nurse Alert:* There are many conditions that can occur following a delivery. When there are multiple associated symptoms, focus on the primary concern that has the highest probability of a referral to a higher level of care.

*Reminder:*  Document caller response to advice, home care instructions, and when to call back.

| ASSESSMENT | ACTION |
|---|---|

### A. Are any of the following present?

- Shortness of breath or difficulty breathing
- Vaginal bleeding requiring use of more than one full-size pad per hour and weakness, dizziness
- Altered mental status
- Skin pale, moist, and cool
- Severe lower abdominal pain <48 hours after delivery
- Thoughts of harming infant or self
- Cesarean section and incision is separating

 "Call ambulance"
or
"Seek emergency care now"

 Go to B

## B. Are any of the following present?

- Temperature >100°F (37.8°C) 4 to 10 days after delivery
- Bleeding with fever or abdominal pain
- Increased bleeding and abdominal cramping first week after delivery (saturating one pad with bright red bleeding in <1 hour)
- Abnormal vaginal discharge with bleeding, fever, or pain, or discharge is foul smelling
- Vomiting, diarrhea, fever, or rash
- Calf swelling, pain, or redness
- Clots of blood larger than a lemon
- Headache unrelieved by home care measures
- Muscle aches, fever, and painful red area on breast
- Chills or fever and headache
- Vaginal bleeding requiring use of more than one full-size pad per hour

**YES**   "Seek medical care within 2 to 4 hours"

**NO**   Go to C

## C. Are any of the following present?

- Persistent depression >2 to 3 weeks
- Urgency, frequency, or pain with urination
- Abnormal vaginal discharge without fever
- Increased pain at episiotomy incision site
- Increased pain, swelling, foul-smelling drainage, redness, or warmth at cesarean section incision site

**YES**   "Seek medical care within 24 hours"

**NO**   Go to D

## D. Are any of the following present?

- Engorged, tender, hard breasts
- Cramping
- Constipation
- Stretching or pulling sensation at episiotomy site

**YES**   "Call back or call PCP for appointment if no improvement" and Follow **Home Care Instructions**

**NO**   Follow **Home Care Instructions**

P

## Home Care Instructions
## Postpartum Problems

- Balance activity and rest for first 2 weeks after delivery.
- Can usually return to work after 6-week checkup if cleared by physician (8 weeks for cesarean section).
- Remember that contractions 3 to 4 days after delivery are normal and are stimulated by breast-feeding.
- Bowel movements may not occur 1 to 2 days after delivery. Drink 6 to 8 glasses of water and juices a day and increase intake of fruits, vegetables, and bran. Laxatives (Metamucil) may help. Follow instructions on the label.
- Sit in a warm bath or sitz bath to relieve discomfort.
- Apply dry heat to perineum after bath for 10 minutes. May try exposing perineum a foot away from a 25-W light bulb or using a hair dryer on the low setting.
- After toileting or changing pad, clean area using soap and warm water in a squirt bottle or antiseptic wipes, cleaning from front to back.
- Change pad after toileting.
- Remember that a blood and mucous vaginal discharge may persist for several weeks after delivery, and the discharge increases with activity.
- Vaginal bleeding 4 to 8 weeks after delivery is not a cause for alarm and usually is the return of menstruation.
- Discomfort and dryness during intercourse after delivery can be reduced with use of K-Y Jelly. Avoid intercourse until discharge has stopped and stitches are healed. Discuss contraception options with PCP. If breast-feeding, milk letdown may occur.
- Wear a good supportive bra 24 hours a day for 10 days. If breasts become tender and hard, take a warm bath or apply warm compresses to breasts.
- Remember that depression after delivery is not unusual and should subside. Discuss depression with PCP.

### Cesarean Section Delivery
- Expect vaginal bleeding for as long as 6 weeks.
- Do not insert anything into the vagina for 6 weeks.
- Avoid stairs and lifting anything heavier than 10 lb.
- Do not soak in tub.
- Get plenty of rest.
- Change dressing daily until drainage has stopped.
- Remove sterile strips after 7 to 10 days.

### Postpartum Depression (Blues)
- Get as much rest as possible, nap while infant naps.
- Exercise, such as walking.
- Eat a well-balanced diet.
- Encourage family and friends to help with meal preparation, chores, infant care, and housework.
- Talk about your feelings.

## Additional Instructions

_____

_____

_____

**Report the Following Problems to Your PCP/Clinic/ED**

- No improvement with home care measures or condition worsens
- Fever, abdominal pain, or unusual vaginal discharge
- Signs of infection: increased redness, pain, red streaks from the wound, warmth, foul-smelling or thick green drainage, or fever
- Persistent depression

**Seek Emergency Care Immediately If Any of the Following Occur**

- Shortness of breath or difficulty breathing
- Vaginal bleeding requiring use of more than one full-size pad per hour and weakness or dizziness
- Altered mental status
- Skin pale and moist

If the caller agrees with the advice given, document the call and encourage the caller to call back or see PCP if the problem worsens. If the caller does not agree with the advice given, reevaluate and advise the caller to follow up with PCP, Clinic, or ED.

P

# Pregnancy Problems

>> **Key Questions** Name, Age, Onset, Gestation, Number of Pregnancies, History, Medications

>> **Other Protocols to Consider** Back Pain (34); Constipation (114); Diarrhea (143); Foot Problems (197); Headache (238); Heartburn (245); Swelling (449).

*Nurse Alert:* There are many conditions that can occur during pregnancy. When there are multiple associated symptoms, focus on the primary concern that has the highest probability of a referral to a higher level of care.

*Reminder:* Document caller response to advice, home care instructions, and when to call back.

| ASSESSMENT | ACTION |
|---|---|

### A. Pregnancy of >20 weeks, and are any of the following present?

- Imminent delivery with fetal head crowning
- Severe headache, double or blurred vision, disorientation, dizziness, or irritability
- Previous trauma to mitral valve area, fall, blunt injury to abdomen, etc.
- Passing large clots
- Seizure
- Severe abdominal pain
- Leaking fluid with prolapsed umbilical cord
- Diagnosed preeclampsia with new symptoms

**YES** "Call ambulance"
or
"Seek emergency care now"

**NO** Go to B

### B. Are any of the following present?

- No fetal movement
- Sudden swelling in face, hands, legs, or lower back
- Headache, spots in front of eyes, dizziness, fainting, or vomiting
- Regular contractions or leaking vaginal fluid

**YES** "Seek medical care immediately"

**NO** Go to C

358

## C. Are any of the following present?

- Known hypertension and blood pressure is increasing
- Leg pain, swelling, redness, or warmth that worsens with weight bearing
- Pain, vaginal bleeding, or fever
- Persistent headache unresponsive to pain relievers
- Persistent vomiting of all foods and fluids and/or abdominal pain
- Fewer than 10 fetal movements in 1 hour

 **YES** "Seek medical care within 2 hours"

**NO** Go to D

## D. Are any of the following present?

- Urgent, frequent, or painful urination
- Sudden weight gain >3 pounds per week during the second trimester or >1 lb per week during the third trimester
- Cough with pain, shortness of breath, or yellow, green, or bloody sputum
- Fever >101°F (38.3°C) for >2 days
- Earache or sore throat >2 days
- Generalized rash of unknown cause and itching
- Diarrhea and fever, bloody stools, >10 stools a day, severe abdominal pain, vomiting

**YES** "Seek medical care within 24 hours"

**NO** Go to E

## E. Are any of the following present?

- Nausea and vomiting (morning sickness) during first trimester
- Dizziness, light-headedness, or fainting
- Heartburn
- Hemorrhoids
- Swelling of hands, fingers, feet, or legs
- Aches and pain in back, legs, feet, or groin

**YES** "Call back or call PCP for appointment if no improvement" and Follow **Home Care Instructions**

**NO** Follow **Home Care Instructions**

P

## Home Care Instructions
## Pregnancy Problems

- If diagnosed with preeclampsia or preterm labor, rest while lying on left side.

### Nausea and Vomiting
- Do not eat or drink for 1 hour after last emesis.
- Take small sips of clear fluid for first 12 hours after vomiting.
- Increase fluids as tolerated.
- After 12 hours of no vomiting, try bland foods (crackers, dry toast, bananas).
- Resume normal diet after 12 hours if no emesis.
- Morning sickness:
  - Eat dry bread, cereal, or crackers upon rising in the morning.
  - Get up slowly.
  - Open window for fresh air while sleeping or cooking.
  - Eat several small meals during the day. Avoid fluids with meals.
  - Drink ginger ale or orange or grape juice between meals.
  - Avoid fatty or highly seasoned foods.
  - Avoid lying down immediately after a meal.
  - Eat crackers, cheese, or pretzels if nauseated.

### Light-headedness and Dizziness
- Get up slowly; avoid sudden changes in posture.
- Avoid lying flat on back or standing for prolonged periods of time.
- Avoid hot, stuffy rooms.
- Do not skip meals.

### Heartburn
- Sleep with several pillows or elevate the head of the bed on several blocks.
- Eat frequent small meals.
- Change position frequently.
- Suck on hard candy or sip hot tea.
- Antacids (Maalox, Tums) may help reduce discomfort. Follow instructions on the label.

### Hemorrhoids
- Avoid straining with bowel movements.
- Drink 10 to 12 glasses of water a day.
- Eat lots of fresh fruits, whole grains, and vegetables.
- Take warm baths.
- Use hemorrhoidal creams, suppositories, or medicated pads (Preparation H) as needed for discomfort. Follow instructions on the label.

### Swelling
- Minimize salt in diet.
- Massage feet.

- Elevate legs above the heart.
- Wear supportive hose.
- Avoid tight-fitting clothing or bands around the abdomen.
- Sleep on left side.

### Aches and Pains
- Massage affected areas.
- Apply moist heat to area.
- Lie on affected side and draw leg up to chest.
- Crawl on all fours and rock pelvis forward several times a day.
- Take acetaminophen for discomfort if desired, and follow instructions on the label. Do not take aspirin.

## Additional Instructions

_____

_____

_____

### Report the Following Problems to Your PCP/Clinic/ED
- Conditions persist or worsen after home care measures
- Less than 10 movements <1 hour

### Seek Emergency Care Immediately If Any of the Following Occur
- Imminent delivery
- Severe headache, double or blurred vision, disorientation, dizziness
- Passing large clots
- Severe abdominal pain
- Leaking vaginal fluid with prolapsed umbilical cord
- Sudden swelling in face, hands, legs, or lower back
- Headache, spots in front of eyes
- Regular contractions or leaking vaginal fluid
- No fetal movement

If the caller agrees with the advice given, document the call and encourage the caller to call back or see PCP if the problem worsens. If the caller does not agree with the advice given, reevaluate and advise the caller to follow up with PCP, Clinic, or ED.

P

# Puncture Wound

>> **Key Questions** Name, Age, Onset, Cause, Location, Medications, Tetanus Immunization Status, Pain Scale, History

>> **Other Protocols to Consider** Bites, Animal/Human (46); Bruising (71); Foreign Body, Skin (211); Immunization, Tetanus (264); Laceration (290); Piercing Problems (338); Tattoo Problems (456); Wound Healing and Infection (509).

*Nurse Alert:* Puncture wounds are at high risk for infection when foreign debris and bacteria are pushed deep into the tissue. Puncture wounds to the hand such as a cat bite have the highest rate of infection because of the relatively poor blood supply of many structures in the hand. Local infections and cellulitis are the leading cause of morbidity from bite wounds and can potentially lead to sepsis, particularly in immunocompromised individuals.

*Reminder:* Document caller response to advice, home care instructions, and when to call back.

| ASSESSMENT | ACTION |
|---|---|

**A. Is there a deep wound to the head, chest, neck, scrotum, abdomen, or are any of the following present?**

- Inability to control bleeding with pressure or spurting blood
- Decreased level of consciousness
- No pulse distal to injury
- Difficulty breathing
- Pale skin, sweating, or rapid heartbeat
- Skin cold, blue, and numb distal to the wound
- High-pressure injection injury
- Contaminated needlestick

 "Call ambulance"
or
"Seek emergency care now"
and
Follow **Emergency Instructions**

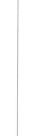 Go to B

### B. Are any of the following present?

- Numbness or tingling
- Difficulty moving affected part
- Puncture wound into a joint
- Visible debris in the wound and unable to remove
- Puncture wound through shoe sole
- Fever, drainage, or red streaks
- Severe pain
- Increasing swelling or bruising around wound and injured person takes blood-thinning medication
- Persistent foreign body sensation
- Foot wound and history of diabetes

**YES** "Seek medical care within 2 to 4 hours"

**NO** Go to C

### C. Are any of the following present?

- Unable to remove large splinter
- History of diabetes
- No tetanus immunization or booster >5 years

**YES** "Seek medical care within 24 hours"

**NO** Go to D

### D. Are any of the following present?

- Persistent pain or swelling >5 days
- Minor puncture wound
- Unable to remove small splinter
- Gradual swelling
- Gradual bruising
- No improvement in pain or swelling >3 days and unresponsive to home care measures

**YES** "Call back or call PCP for appointment if no improvement" and Follow **Home Care Instructions**

**NO** Follow **Home Care Instructions**

## Emergency Instructions
## Puncture Wound

- If bleeding is profuse or spurting, apply pressure with a clean bandage or cloth directly over the wound, and call an ambulance. Do not check to see if the bleeding has stopped. Do not try to remove embedded material from the wound. Seek medical care.

## Home Care Instructions
## Puncture Wound

- Clean well with soap and water.
- Soak the affected area for 10 to 15 minutes several times a day using warm water or Epsom salts in warm water. This will help to prevent infection and promote healing.
- Apply a bandage to the wound for a few days after the injury to help keep the wound clean.
- Watch for signs of infection: increased redness, pain, swelling, drainage, streaks, or fever.
- If no tetanus immunization within 5 years for a dirty or contaminated wound, contact PCP or clinic for tetanus immunization within 24 hours of injury.
- If no tetanus immunization within 5 years, contact PCP or clinic for tetanus immunization within 72 hours of injury.
- Apply antibiotic ointment 2 to 3 times a day. Soak affected area before applying ointment.
- DO NOT soak a splinter area in water or solution, which will cause the wood to swell and hinder removal.

### Additional Instructions

### Report the Following Problems to Your PCP/Clinic/ED

- Signs of infection: increased redness, pain, swelling, drainage, streaks, or fever
- Numbness, tingling, or increased pain
- Wound does not heal within 2 weeks
- Persistent foreign body sensation

### Seek Emergency Care Immediately If Any of the Following Occur

- Difficulty breathing
- Pale skin, sweating, or rapid heartbeat
- Pulses absent distal to wound
- Skin cyanotic distal to wound

If the caller agrees with the advice given, document the call and encourage the caller to call back or see PCP if the problem worsens. If the caller does not agree with the advice given, reevaluate and advise the caller to follow up with PCP, Clinic, or ED.

P

# Rash

>> **Key Questions** Name, Age, Onset, Cause, Location, Medications, History, Immunization Status, Associated Symptoms

>> **Other Protocols to Consider** Allergic Reaction (13); Bedbug Exposure or Concerns (37); Bee Stings (42); Bites, Insect (49); Chickenpox (91); Diaper Rash (141); Heat Exposure Problem (252); Hives (258); Itching (282); Rubella (German Measles) (382); Rubeola (Measles) (385); Scabies (388); Skin Lesions: Lumps, Bumps, and Sores (414); Tattoo Problems (456).

### Nurse Alert:

- There are many conditions that cause a rash. When a rash is associated with several other symptoms, use the protocol that is the primary concern and has the highest probability of a referral to a higher level of care.

*Reminder:* Document caller response to advice, home care instructions, and when to call back.

| ASSESSMENT | ACTION |
|---|---|

### A. Is the following present?

- Sudden onset of severe hives and rash, and difficulty breathing, drooling, chest tightness, or swelling in back of throat or tongue

**YES** "Call ambulance"

**NO** Go to B

## B. Are any of the following present?

- Used Epi-Pen as directed by the PCP
- Purple- or blood-colored flat spots or dots, headache, pain bending head forward, vomiting, or fever
- Unusual drowsiness, refusal to drink, and noisy or fast breathing
- Rash, fever, red tongue, and enlarged lymph nodes
- Sudden onset of illness and rapid progression of widespread redness, scaliness, fever, and enlarged lymph nodes
- Red peeling rash in rectal area
- Rapidly spreading red or purple rash that develops into blisters on mucous membranes (lips, mouth, eyes, genitals)
- Fever, headache, or respiratory infection followed by blistering rash

**YES** "Seek emergency care now"

**NO** Go to C

## C. Are any of the following present?

- Severe facial or eye swelling
- Rash around eyes, vision changes, or weeping lesions
- Open sores with signs of infection: redness, swelling, pain, red streaks, drainage, warmth
- Fever in a menstruating child/adolescent who uses tampons
- Bright-red painful area
- Fever and painful rash
- Red rash peels off in sheets of skin
- Purple- or blood-colored spots or dots
- Age <1 month and grouping of small water blisters
- Rash or flu-like symptoms; fever, chills, sore throat, headache 2 to 4 weeks after a tick bite

**YES** "Seek medical care within 2 to 4 hours"

**NO** Go to D

## D. Is the following present?

- New antibiotic or medication and new onset of rash or hives

**YES** "Call PCP now"

**NO** Go to E

### E. Are any of the following present?

- Persistent rash for >48 hours that is unresponsive to home care measures
- Persistent hives after taking Benadryl for 24 hours
- Extensive rash, cause unknown
- Rash and itching interfere with sleep
- Multiple grouping of painful blisters

**YES**  "Seek medical care within 24 hours"

**NO**  Go to F

### F. Are any of the following present?

- Prolonged exposure to heat
- Rash restricted to diaper and upper leg area
- Exposure to poison oak, ivy, or sumac
- Change in laundry detergent and contact areas affected
- Exposure to chemicals
- Recent immunization
- Other household members have similar rash
- Raised, red, itchy rash followed by blisters
- Small blisters in mouth and on hands and feet
- Blisters form golden crusts
- Scaly or blistery rash on the face or in folds of skin on elbows or knees
- Dull red spots, runny nose, cough, sore throat, fever, red eyes (suspicion of rubella)
- Pink rash, swollen glands at back of the neck, fever, and no prior immunization or history of measles infection
- Circular, raised, rough pink patch with clear center ½ to 1 inch and itchy
- Tick bite and expanding rash

**YES**  "Call back or call PCP for appointment if no improvement"
and
Follow **Home Care Instructions**

**NO**  Follow **Home Care Instructions**

## Home Care Instructions
## Rash

- Try to identify the cause and avoid the irritant.
- Cleanse the area with soap and water to remove the irritant, then use only water to cleanse the area.
- Apply compresses soaked in water and Domeboro.

### To Control Itching
- Take a cool bath with baking soda, Aveeno, or oatmeal (1 cup in a tub of cool water) several times a day, or apply cold packs to localized rashes for 20 minutes every 3 to 4 hours.
- For severe itching, apply 1% hydrocortisone cream and follow the instructions on the label. Refrigerate it for optimal cooling relief. Avoid using it when jock itch, athlete's foot, impetigo, or ringworm is suspected.
- Apply a baking soda paste mixed with white vinegar, or OTC preparations such as calamine lotion or Aveeno, to the affected area.
- Give an antihistamine (Benadryl, Chlor-Trimeton) and follow the instructions on the label.
- Cut the child's fingernails and discourage scratching.
- Cover the infant's hands with socks to discourage scratching.
- Apply wet dressings soaked in Burow's solution, 1 part solution to 10 to 40 parts water. Change frequently, as often as eight times in 2 hours.

### For Possible Allergic Reaction
- If rash is related to a new medication, stop the medication. Call PCP if it is a prescription medication.
- Take antihistamines as directed on the container until rash and itching are gone.
- Watch for signs of worsening reaction (swelling or difficulty swallowing or breathing) and see PCP.

### For Possible Heat Rash
- Apply calamine lotion or hydrocortisone cream.
- Take a cool bath or shower without soap every 2 to 3 hours as needed for relief, and air-dry.
- Apply baby powder to the affected area.

### For Poison Oak, Ivy, or Sumac Exposure
- Wash the exposed area within 1 hour of exposure, if possible.
- Soak the area with cool water or rub it with ice for 20 minutes, as needed.
- Wash all clothes and any animal exposed to the plants.

### For Suspected Measles/Chickenpox/Rubella
- Keep the child home until the rash is gone to avoid exposing others to the disease.
- Avoid spreading infection to others.
- Wash hands well with soap and water after contact with the infected person.
- Keep weeping areas covered when there is the possibility of contact with others.
- Use cotton balls or gauze to apply lotions or ointments to open areas.

## Additional Instructions

### Report the Following Problems to Your PCP/Clinic/ED

- No improvement in 24 to 48 hours with home care measures or condition worsens
- Fever, sore throat, or joint pain
- Signs of infection
- Unusual drowsiness, refusal to drink, earache, and noisy or fast breathing

### Seek Emergency Care Immediately If Any of the Following Occur

- Difficulty breathing, chest tightness, or swelling in the back of the throat
- Purple spots, headache, stiff neck, vomiting, or fever
- Rash, fever, red tongue, and enlarged lymph nodes
- Red peeling rash in rectal area

If the caller agrees with the advice given, document the call and encourage the caller to call back or see PCP if the problem worsens. If the caller does not agree with the advice given, reevaluate and advise the caller to follow up with PCP, Clinic, or ED.

# Rectal Bleeding

 **Key Questions**  Name, Age, Onset, Medications, History

 **Other Protocols to Consider**  Abdominal Pain (1); Constipation (114); Diarrhea (143); Foreign Body, Rectum (209); Vomiting (492); Stools, Abnormal (429); Stool, Incontinence (427).

> *Nurse Alert:* Rectal bleeding includes black, maroon, or tarry stools, bright-red blood on toilet tissue, on the surface of stool, mixed with formed or diarrheal stool, or passed separately.

*Reminder:* Document caller response to advice, home care instructions, and when to call back.

| ASSESSMENT | ACTION |
|---|---|
| **A. Is abdominal pain present?** | |
| | **YES**  Go to Abdominal Pain protocol (1) |
| | **NO**  Go to B |
| **B. Are any of the following present?** | |
| • Light-headedness or fainting<br>• Vomiting blood or coffee-grounds–like emesis<br>• Intermittent abdominal pain<br>• Frequent black tarry stools<br>• Large amount of bright-red blood mixed in the stool or passing of blood clots | **YES**  "Seek emergency care now"<br><br>**NO**  Go to C |
| **C. Is the following present?** | |
| • Use of blood thinners, steroids, or nonsteroidal anti-inflammatory medications | **YES**  "Seek medical care within 2 to 4 hours"<br><br>**NO**  Go to D |

R

## D. Are any of the following present?

- Recent history of cancer
- Temperature >100°F (37.7°C)

**YES** "Seek medical care within 2 to 4 hours"

**NO** Go to E

## E. Are any of the following present?

- Stool streaked with red blood
- Blood on toilet tissue after wiping
- Constipation or hemorrhoids
- Bleeding persists >2 to 3 days after constipation improves
- Taking iron preparations or bismuth subsalicylate (Pepto-Bismol)
- Recent ingestion of beets or spinach

**YES** "Call back or call PCP for appointment if no improvement"
and
Follow **Home Care Instructions**

**NO** Follow **Home Care Instructions**

## Home Care Instructions
## Rectal Bleeding

- Soak in a warm saline bath for 20 minutes a day to cleanse the area and promote healing. (Add 2 tbsp of salt or baking soda to the water.)
- Keep rectal area clean. May use medicated pads (Tucks) to cleanse and soothe area; follow instruction on the label. Ask pharmacist for additional product suggestions.
- If rectal area is irritated, apply OTC hydrocortisone ointment (Anusol-HC, Cortaid) or zinc oxide paste or powder.
- If hemorrhoids persist, try OTC preparations (Anusol, Nupercainal, Preparation H) to help soothe and shrink hemorrhoids. Follow instructions on the label.
- Increase fluid intake and eat a diet high in fiber: fruits, vegetables, bran, grains, and beans. Avoid constipating foods such as cheese. This is particularly important if taking narcotic pain medications for discomfort.
- If taking iron preparations or bismuth subsalicylate (Pepto-Bismol) or eating spinach or beets, follow up with PCP for stool guaiac.

## Additional Instructions

_____

_____

_____

### Report the Following Problems to Your PCP/Clinic/ED

- No improvement in 3 days or bleeding worsens
- Abdominal pain
- Constipation or hemorrhoids persist >1 week after home treatment
- Blood mixed with stool or black stools

### Seek Emergency Care Immediately If Any of the Following Occur

- Vomiting blood or coffee-grounds–like emesis
- Light-headedness or fainting
- Intermittent abdominal pain
- Large amount of bright-red blood mixed with stool or passing of blood clots
- Frequent black tarry stools

If the caller agrees with the advice given, document the call and encourage the caller to call back or see PCP if the problem worsens. If the caller does not agree with the advice given, reevaluate and advise the caller to follow up with PCP, Clinic, or ED.

# Rectal Problems

>> **Key Questions**  Name, Age, Onset, Allergies, Medications, History, Pain Scale

>> **Other Protocols to Consider**  Constipation (114); Diarrhea (143); Foreign Body, Rectum (209); Pinworm (345); Rectal Bleeding (371); Stool, Incontinence (427).

*Reminder:* Document caller response to advice, home care instructions, and when to call back.

| ASSESSMENT | ACTION |
|---|---|

### A. Are any of the following present?

- Injury to the rectal area
- Rape or sexual abuse
- Passing more than once of black or bloody stools with clots
- Unable to remove foreign object from rectum
- Red peeling rash in rectal area

**YES** "Seek emergency care now"

**NO** Go to B

### B. Are any of the following present?

- Severe pain
- Severe bleeding

**YES** "Seek medical care within 2 to 4 hours"

**NO** Go to C

### C. Are any of the following present?

- Persistent pain or itching that is unresponsive to home care measures
- Exposure to a sexually transmitted disease
- Recent surgery
- Painless rash or lesion >24 hours
- Recent colonoscopy, sigmoidoscopy, or invasive procedure

**YES** "Seek medical care within 24 hours"

**NO** Go to D

## D. Are any of the following present?

- Intermittent rectal swelling, pain, itching, or bleeding
- Pain or bleeding for <48 hours
- First episode of rectal bleeding, swelling, pain, or itching
- Rectal itching
- Visible small worms in stools or around rectal area
- Painless rash or growth <24 hours

**YES**    "Call back or call PCP for appointment if no improvement"
and
Follow **Home Care Instructions**

**NO**    Follow **Home Care Instructions**

## Home Care Instructions
## Rectal Problems

- Soak in a warm bath for 20 to 30 minutes daily.
- Apply an OTC medication for relief of itching and discomfort.
- Avoid constipating foods (cheese and white flour products). Include fresh fruits, vegetables, and whole grains in the diet. Drink lots of water every day (unless PCP has ordered a restricted fluid intake).
- Try OTC medications for hemorrhoids.

### Additional Instructions

_____

_____

_____

### Report the Following Problems to Your PCP/Clinic/ED

- Black or bloody stools more than once
- No improvement or condition worsens

### Seek Emergency Care Immediately If Any of the Following Occur

- Black or bloody stools with clots more than once
- Red peeling rash in rectal area

If the caller agrees with the advice given, document the call and encourage the caller to call back or see PCP if the problem worsens. If the caller does not agree with the advice given, reevaluate and advise the caller to follow up with PCP, Clinic, or ED.

# Reye Syndrome, Suspected

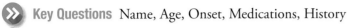 **Key Questions**  Name, Age, Onset, Medications, History

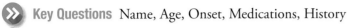 **Other Protocols to Consider**  Chickenpox (91); Confusion (107); Congestion (110); Cough (121); Fever (184).

> *Nurse Alert:*  Use this protocol if previously diagnosed with Reye syndrome or caller suspects Reye syndrome in a child or adolescent after a recent illness, taking aspirin during that illness and now has new concerning symptoms.

*Reminder:*  Document caller response to advice, home care instructions, and when to call back.

| ASSESSMENT | ACTION |
|---|---|
| **A.  Are any of the following present?** | |
| • Recent history of a viral illness such as chickenpox, the flu, or other respiratory illnesses<br>• History of taking aspirin during the illness and appearance of any of the following symptoms shortly after the viral illness:<br>  • headache, incoordination, slurred speech, confusion, lethargy, personality changes<br>  • vomiting<br>  • weakness in an arm or leg<br>  • hearing loss or double vision | **YES**  "Seek emergency care now" "Call back or call PCP for appointment if no improvement" and<br><br>**NO**  Follow **Home Care Instructions** |

R

## Home Care Instructions
## Reye Syndrome, Suspected

- In general, it is not a good idea to give children or adolescents aspirin because symptoms often do not appear until several days after a virus is contracted. Take acetaminophen for fever and discomfort.
- If the child has taken aspirin immediately before or during a viral illness, observe closely for symptoms of Reye syndrome and report to your PCP. Symptoms usually appear shortly after the acute phase of a viral illness and may progress rapidly. Symptoms include the following:
  - headache, incoordination, slurred speech, confusion, lethargy, and personality changes
  - vomiting
  - weakness in an arm or leg
  - hearing loss or double vision

## Additional Instructions

_____

_____

_____

### Report the Following Problem to Your PCP/Clinic/ED
- Suspected symptoms of Reye syndrome

### Seek Emergency Care Immediately If Any of the Following Occur
- Confusion, lethargy, and other mental changes
- Headache, incoordination, slurred speech
- Vomiting
- Weakness in an arm or leg
- Hearing loss or double vision

If the caller agrees with the advice given, document the call and encourage the caller to call back or see PCP if the problem worsens. If the caller does not agree with the advice given, reevaluate and advise the caller to follow up with PCP, Clinic, or ED.

# Roseola

» **Key Questions**  Name, Age, Onset, Known Diagnosis or Exposure, Allergies, Medications, History

» **Other Protocols to Consider**  Fever (184); Rubella (German Measles) (382); Itching (282); Rash (366).

> *Nurse Alert:*
> • Use this protocol if previously diagnosed with roseola or known exposure and child is now ill with a rash.

*Reminder:*  Document caller response to advice, home care instructions, and when to call back.

| ASSESSMENT | ACTION |
|---|---|
| **A. Diagnosed with roseola, and are any of the following present?** | |
| • Purple- or blood-colored rash or spots <br> • Child appears very ill <br> • Persistent loud crying that is unresponsive to holding and comfort <br> • Temperature >105°F (40.6°C) | **YES**  "Seek emergency care now" <br><br> **NO**  Go to B |
| **B. Are any of the following present?** | |
| • Persistent fever for >4 days <br> • Persistent rash for >3 days | **YES**  "Seek medical care within 2 to 4 hours" <br><br> **NO**  Go to C |

R

## C. Are any of the following present?

- Known or suspected exposure to roseola and no previous history of the disease
- Fine pink rash on trunk follows 3 to 4 days of fever
- Irritability
- Fever

**YES**    "Call back or call PCP for appointment if no improvement"
and
Follow **Home Care Instructions**

**NO**    Follow **Home Care Instructions**

## Home Care Instructions
## Roseola

- Give acetaminophen for fever. Do not give aspirin to a child. Avoid aspirin-like products if age <20 years. Avoid acetaminophen if liver disease is present. Avoid ibuprofen if kidney disease or stomach problems exist or in the case of pregnancy. Follow the directions on the label. Use the dosing device that comes with the medication, a measuring device, or a medicine syringe from the pharmacy. Household teaspoons often do not give the correct amount of medication.
- Ensure child is taking adequate fluids during fever.

**Additional Instructions**

_____

_____

_____

### Report the Following Problems to Your PCP/Clinic/ED

- Child refuses liquids
- Persistent fever >4 days
- Persistent rash >3 days

If the caller agrees with the advice given, document the call and encourage the caller to call back or see PCP if the problem worsens. If the caller does not agree with the advice given, reevaluate and advise the caller to follow up with PCP, Clinic, or ED.

# Rubella (German Measles)

**Key Questions**  Name, Age, Onset, Known Diagnosis or Exposure, Allergies, Medications, History, Immunization Status

**Other Protocols to Consider**  Fever (184); Itching (282); Rash (366); Rubeola (Measles) (385).

*Nurse Alert:*
- Use this protocol if previously diagnosed with Rubella or known exposure, now ill, and has a rash.

*Reminder:* Document caller response to advice, home care instructions, and when to call back.

| ASSESSMENT | ACTION |
|---|---|

### A. Diagnosed with rubella, and are any of the following present?

- Purple, flat, nonblanching rash
- Child appears very ill
- Persistent loud crying that is unresponsive to holding and comfort
- Temperature >105°F (40.6°C)

**YES** "Seek emergency care now"

**NO** Go to B

### B. Are any of the following present?

Persistent fever >3 days

Pain in joints

Pregnant with known or suspected exposure to rubella (contagious period is 7 days before and 5 days after the rash appears)

**YES** "Seek medical care within 2 to 4 hours"

**NO** Go to C

382

## C. Are any of the following present?

- Known or suspected exposure to rubella and no previous history of the disease or immunization
- Generalized red rash spreading over entire body in 24 hours
- Swollen nodes at the back of the neck
- Fever
- Persistent itching

**YES**    "Call back or call PCP for appointment if no improvement"
and
Follow **Home Care Instructions**

**NO**    Follow **Home Care Instructions**

## Home Care Instructions
## Rubella (German Measles)

- Avoid exposing pregnant women. Condition is contagious for 5 days after rash initially appears.
- Women of childbearing age should avoid pregnancy for 3 months.
- Take acetaminophen for pain. Do not give aspirin to a child. Avoid aspirin-like products if age <20 years. Avoid acetaminophen if liver disease is present. Avoid ibuprofen if kidney disease or stomach problems exist or in the case of pregnancy. Follow the directions on the label. Use the dosing device that comes with the medication, a measuring device, or a medicine syringe from the pharmacy. Household teaspoons often do not give the correct amount of medication.
- Try soda or oatmeal baths for itching.

**Additional Instructions**

_____

_____

_____

### Report the Following Problems to Your PCP/Clinic/ED

- First trimester of pregnancy and exposed to rubella
- Pain in joints
- Persistent fever >3 days
- Persistent rash >5 days

### Seek Emergency Care Immediately If Diagnosed with Rubella and Any of the Following Occur

- Purple, flat, nonblanching rash
- Child appears very ill
- Persistent loud crying that is unresponsive to holding and comfort
- Temperature >105°F (40.6°C)

If the caller agrees with the advice given, document the call and encourage the caller to call back or see PCP if the problem worsens. If the caller does not agree with the advice given, reevaluate and advise the caller to follow up with PCP, Clinic, or ED.

# Rubeola (Measles)

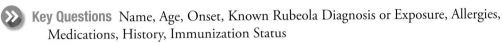 **Key Questions** Name, Age, Onset, Known Rubeola Diagnosis or Exposure, Allergies, Medications, History, Immunization Status

**Other Protocols to Consider** Cough (121); Earache, Drainage (150); Fever (184); Rash (366); Rubella (German Measles) (382); Sore Throat (420).

> **Nurse Alert:**
> ● Use this protocol if previously diagnosed with Rubeola or known exposure and now ill.

***Reminder:*** Document caller response to advice, home care instructions, and when to call back.

| ASSESSMENT | ACTION |
|---|---|
| **A. Known rubeola diagnosis or exposure, and are any of the following present?** | |
| ● Difficulty breathing <br> ● Severe headache and/or neck pain <br> ● Confusion <br> ● Difficulty awakening <br> ● Decreased level of consciousness <br> ● Seizures | **YES** "Seek emergency care now" <br><br> **NO** Go to B |
| **B. Are any of the following present?** | |
| ● Fever >4 days after onset of rash <br> ● Yellow or green nasal discharge >48 hours <br> ● Ill appearance <br> ● Unvaccinated infant, <12 months of age, who has been exposed <br> ● Unvaccinated, immunocompromised child who has been exposed | **YES** "Seek medical care within 2 to 4 hours" <br><br> **NO** Go to C |

R

## C.  Are any of the following present?

- Red, watery or itchy eyes, cough, and runny nose
- Earache
- Eyes crusted closed in the morning or yellow discharge
- Eyes sensitive to light
- Bluish-white spots in mouth
- Blotchy red rash spreads from the face down the body and persists >7 days
- Fever
- Known exposure to measles within past 12 days and no prior vaccination for measles

**YES**  "Call back or call PCP for appointment if no improvement"
and
Follow **Home Care Instructions**

**NO**  Follow **Home Care Instructions**

## Home Care Instructions
## Rubeola (Measles)

- Take acetaminophen for fever and discomfort. Do not give aspirin to a child. Avoid aspirin-like products if age <20 years. Avoid acetaminophen if liver disease is present. Avoid ibuprofen if kidney disease or stomach problems exist or in the case of pregnancy. Follow the directions on the label.
- To soothe cough, give ½ to 1 tsp corn syrup to child 4 years old or younger; give cough drops, hard candy, or cough syrup to older children. Warm clear fluids, such as apple juice and herbal teas, are soothing to the throat and can be given to children older than 4 months.
- Remove eye drainage with a wet cotton ball, which should be discarded after use. Use a separate cotton ball for each eye.
- If eyes are sensitive to light, keep the child in a darkened or dimly lit room.
- Enforce rest until fever is gone.
- Call PCP for confirmed diagnosis.
- Keep child away from others who have not had the illness or been immunized until the rash is gone (about 7 days).

## Additional Instructions

_____

_____

_____

### Report the Following Problems to Your PCP/Clinic/ED

- Earache or sore throat
- Yellow or green nasal discharge for >48 hours
- Fever for >4 days after onset of rash
- Eyes crusted closed in the morning or yellow discharge

### Seek Emergency Care Immediately If Any of the Following Occur

- Difficulty breathing
- Severe headache
- Confusion
- Difficulty awakening
- Seizures

If the caller agrees with the advice given, document the call and encourage the caller to call back or see PCP if the problem worsens. If the caller does not agree with the advice given, reevaluate and advise the caller to follow up with PCP, Clinic, or ED.

# Scabies

**Key Questions**  Name, Age, Onset, Known or Suspected Exposure to Scabies, Allergies, Medications, History

**Other Protocols to Consider**  Itching (282); Rash (366).

> **Nurse Alert:** Use this protocol if previously diagnosed with scabies, known or suspected exposure to someone with scabies, and small blisters present. Scabies is highly contagious.

**Reminder:** Document caller response to advice, home care instructions, and when to call back.

| ASSESSMENT | ACTION |
|---|---|
| **A. Are any of the following present?** | |
| • Lines of small itchy blisters:<br>  • between fingers or toes<br>  • on wrists, elbows, or armpits<br>  • on waist, buttock creases, inner thighs, or creases under breasts<br>• Other household members have same symptoms<br>• Blisters break easily when scratched<br>• Increased itching at night<br>• Signs of infection: increased discomfort, drainage, redness, red streaks from wound, or warmth |  "Seek medical care within 48 hours"<br>or<br>"Call back or call PCP for appointment if no improvement"<br>and<br>Follow **Home Care Instructions** |
| | **NO** Follow **Home Care Instructions** |

## Home Care Instructions
## Scabies

- Scabies is highly contagious, and all members of a household should be treated after exposure to diagnosed scabies. Symptoms can take 30 days to appear after exposure.
- If using crotamiton (Eurax), as prescribed by health care provider, leave on for 24 hours, then apply a second coat. Do not wash off the first coat. After 48 hours, wash off the second coat. Repeat process in 1 week. If using permethrin (Elimite) apply a thin layer of permethrin topical to all body parts from the neck down to the soles of the feet. Rub in completely. Leave the medication on for 8 to 14 hours, then wash it off completely.
- Take cool baths without soap to help relieve itching.
- Take an antihistamine (Benadryl) to help relieve itching, and follow instructions on the label.
- Wash all clothes, linens, and undergarments in hot soapy water.
- Store blankets and stuffed animals for 3 to 4 days. Scabies cannot live if separated from a host body.
- Use OTC or prescribed medications as directed by your PCP or pharmacist.

## Additional Instructions

_____

_____

_____

### Report the Following Problems to Your PCP/Clinic/ED

- Rash shows signs of infection: redness, swelling, drainage, red streaks, or pain
- Persistent rash after two treatments or 3 weeks
- Condition worsens

If the caller agrees with the advice given, document the call and encourage the caller to call back or see PCP if the problem worsens. If the caller does not agree with the advice given, reevaluate and advise the caller to follow up with PCP, Clinic, or ED.

# Scrotal Problems

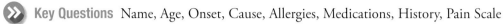

**Key Questions**  Name, Age, Onset, Cause, Allergies, Medications, History, Pain Scale

**Other Protocols to Consider**  Genital Lesions (226); Penis Problems (331); Piercing Problems (338); Sexually Transmitted Infection (STI) (403); Urination, Painful (477).

*Reminder:*  Document caller response to advice, home care instructions, and when to call back.

---

| ASSESSMENT | ACTION |
|---|---|

**A. Severe testicular pain and swelling and are any of the following present?**

- Injury to genitals <48 hours ago
- No known injury, sudden onset of pain, swelling, fever, nausea, vomiting
- Scrotum black, blue, or bright red

**YES** "Seek emergency care now"

**NO** Go to B

**B. Are any of the following present?**

- Injury to genitals >48 hours ago with pain and swelling
- Gradual onset of pain, fever, or swelling
- One enlarged testicle
- Unable to reduce scrotal swelling in infant in whom fever, vomiting, and irritability are present

**YES** "Seek medical care within 2 to 4 hours"

**NO** Go to C

**C. Are any of the following present?**

- Painless lump or swelling
- Sores or painful red rash on scrotal sac
- Signs of infection: pain, swelling, redness, warmth, red streaks, or drainage
- Scrotal itching, redness, swelling, or discomfort

**YES** "Seek medical care within 24 hours"

**NO** Go to D

## D. Is the following present?

- Painless rash <24 hours

**YES** "Call back or call PCP for appointment if no improvement"
and
Follow **Home Care Instructions**

**NO** Follow **Home Care Instructions**

## Home Care Instructions
## Scrotal Problems

- While waiting for appointment or visit, support scrotum on rolled towel, apply ice pack to area, and wear supporter.
- Take your usual pain medication (acetaminophen, ibuprofen) for discomfort. Do not give aspirin to a child. Avoid aspirin-like products if age <20 years. Avoid acetaminophen if liver disease is present. Avoid ibuprofen if kidney disease or stomach problems exist or in the case of pregnancy. Follow the directions on the label.

### Additional Instructions

_____

_____

_____

### Report the Following Problems to Your PCP/Clinic/ED

- Any lump
- No improvement after 48 hours or condition worsens
- Signs of infection: pain, swelling, redness, warmth, red streaks, or drainage
- Pain for >2 weeks
- Pain with urination
- Fever

### Seek Emergency Care Immediately If the Following Occurs

- Testicles turn black, blue, or bright red

If the caller agrees with the advice given, document the call and encourage the caller to call back or see PCP if the problem worsens. If the caller does not agree with the advice given, reevaluate and advise the caller to follow up with PCP, Clinic, or ED.

# Seizure, Febrile

>> **Key Questions**  Name, Age, Onset, History of Seizures, Temperature (if Known), Does Child Feel Hot, Allergies, Medications, History

>> **Other Protocols to Consider**  Altered Mental Status (526); Confusion (107); Fever (184); Head Injury (242).

*Reminder:*  Document caller response to advice, home care instructions, and when to call back.

| ASSESSMENT | ACTION |
|---|---|

### A. Are any of the following present?

- Multiple seizures
- Difficulty breathing or breathing stopped >60 seconds
- Seizure lasts >5 minutes

**YES** "Call ambulance"
and
"Begin rescue breathing if child is not breathing"

**NO** Go to B

### B. Are any of the following present?

- First-time seizure
- Child younger than 6 months or older than 5 years
- Severe headache, stiff or painful neck

**YES** "Seek emergency care now"

**NO** Go to C

### C. Is the following present?

- Persistent temperature >102°F (38.9°C) that is unresponsive to fever-reducing measures

**YES** "Seek medical care within 24 hours"

**NO** Go to D

## D. Are any of the following present?

- Alert and oriented after seizure
- Child wants to sleep after seizure, but can be aroused without irritability

**YES** "Call back or call PCP for appointment if no improvement"
and
Follow **Home Care Instructions**

**NO** Follow **Home Care Instructions**

## Home Care Instructions
## Seizure, Febrile

### Protect the Airway
- Lay the victim on side or stomach, with the head turned toward the side to prevent choking on secretions or vomit.
- If there is any noisy breathing, pull the jaw and chin forward. Do not put your fingers, medication, or any other object in the seizing person's mouth.
- Loosen clothing.

### Protect from Injury
- Move the seizing person to a safe area away from objects that could cause injury.
- Protect the head from hitting a hard surface.
- Do not try to hold the person and restrict movement. Allow the seizure to run its course.

### Postictal Phase
- Expect drowsiness. Allow rest in a cool room. Lightly dress the victim in undergarments.
- Do not give anything by mouth until fully awake.

### Reduce High Fever After the Seizure
- Remove clothing to help cooling process. Do not bathe with alcohol rubs.
- Apply cool compresses to the forehead, face, and neck.
- Give acetaminophen or ibuprofen for fever. Use acetaminophen suppositories if person is still groggy. Do not give aspirin to a child. Avoid aspirin-like products if age <20 years. Avoid acetaminophen if liver disease is present. Avoid ibuprofen if kidney disease or stomach problems exist or in the case of pregnancy. Follow the directions on the label. Use the dosing device that comes with the medication, a measuring device, or a medicine syringe from the pharmacy. Household teaspoons often do not give the correct amount of medication.

## Additional Instructions

_____

_____

_____

## Report the Following Problems to Your PCP/Clinic/ED

- Repeated seizure activity
- No improvement or condition worsens
- Fever unresponsive to fever-reducing measures

## Seek Emergency Care Immediately If Any of the Following Occur

- Difficulty breathing or breathing stops >60 seconds
- Seizure lasts >5 minutes
- Face, lips, or nails turn blue
- Injury occurs during seizure
- Persistent confusion
- Severe headache, stiff or painful neck

If the caller agrees with the advice given, document the call and encourage the caller to call back or see PCP if the problem worsens. If the caller does not agree with the advice given, reevaluate and advise the caller to follow up with PCP, Clinic, or ED.

# Seizure, Nonfebrile

 **Key Questions** Name, Age, Onset, History of Seizures, Allergies, Medications, History

 **Other Protocols to Consider** Alcohol Problems (9); Confusion (107); Fever (184); Head Injury (242); Seizure, Febrile (393).

*Reminder:* Document caller response to advice, home care instructions, and when to call back.

| ASSESSMENT | ACTION |
|---|---|
| **A. Are any of the following present?** | |
| <ul><li>Multiple seizures</li><li>Difficulty breathing</li><li>Seizure lasts >5 minutes</li><li>Severe headache</li><li>Persistent unusual lethargy</li><li>History of recent head injury</li><li>History of recent drug ingestion</li><li>First-time seizure</li><li>Pregnancy</li></ul> | **YES** "Call ambulance" or "Seek emergency care now" <br><br> **NO** Go to B |
| **B. Are any of the following present?** | |
| <ul><li>Injury during seizure</li><li>History of habitual heavy alcohol or drug use and recently quit drinking or taking drugs</li><li>High fever</li><li>Frequent seizures while on seizure medication</li></ul> | **YES** "Seek medical care within 2 hours" <br><br> **NO** Go to C |
| **C. Are any of the following present?** | |
| <ul><li>Stopped taking seizure medication</li><li>History of diabetes, cancer, or cardiovascular or neuromuscular disease</li></ul> | **YES** "Seek medical care within 24 hours" <br><br> **NO** Go to D |

## D. Is the following present?

- History of seizures and alert and oriented after waking up from the seizure

**YES** "Call back or call PCP for appointment if no improvement" and Follow **Home Care Instructions**

**NO** Follow **Home Care Instructions**

## Home Care Instructions
## Seizure

### Protect the Airway
- Lay the victim on side or stomach, with the head turned toward the side to prevent choking on secretions or vomit.
- If there is noisy breathing, pull the jaw and chin forward. Do not put your fingers, medication, or any other object in the seizing person's mouth.
- Loosen tie or other restrictive clothing.

### Protect from Injury
- Move the seizing person to a safe area away from objects that could cause injury.
- Protect the head from hitting a hard surface.
- Do not try to hold the person and restrict movement. Allow the seizure to run its course.

### Postictal Phase
- Expect the person to sleep approximately 30 minutes after the seizure and slowly awaken.
- Do not allow person to drive after a seizure.
- Do not give anything by mouth until fully awake.

## Additional Instructions

_____

_____

_____

### Report the Following Problems to Your PCP/Clinic/ED
- Repeated seizure activity
- No improvement or condition worsens
- Fever unresponsive to fever-reducing measures after a seizure

### Seek Emergency Care Immediately If Any of the Following Occur
- Difficulty breathing
- Severe headache, stiff or painful neck
- Persistent confusion

If the caller agrees with the advice given, document the call and encourage the caller to call back or see PCP if the problem worsens. If the caller does not agree with the advice given, reevaluate and advise the caller to follow up with PCP, Clinic, or ED.

# Sexual Assault

 **Key Questions** Name, Age, Onset, Medications, History

 **Other Protocols to Consider** Child Abuse (94); Foreign Body, Rectum (209); Foreign Body, Vagina (216); Rectal Problems (374); Sexually Transmitted Infection (STI) (403); Vaginal Bleeding (484); Vaginal Discharge/Pain/Itching (486).

*Nurse Alert:* Many sexual assault victims are confused about what to do after an assault. Encourage to go to the ED where a sexual assault examination can be performed by staff specially trained in sexual assault evidence collection, examination, support, and follow-up. Instruct not to shower before going to the ED. In some states, the RN sexual assault examiner can examine victims and collect evidence in locations other than the ED. Refer to the services available in your local area.

*Reminder:* Document caller response to advice, home care instructions, and when to call back.

| ASSESSMENT | ACTION |
|---|---|

### A. Are any of the following present?

- Sexual assault is in process at time of call
- Victim is seriously injured, unconscious, or dead

**YES** "Call ambulance and local police"

**NO** Go to B

### B. Sexual assault has occurred and are any of the following present?

- Vaginal or anal tearing or bleeding
- Suspected fractures or dislocations
- Abrasions, lacerations, bruising, discoloration, or swelling
- Difficulty breathing, chest pain, or abdominal pain
- Victim requests an examination and collection of evidence
- Victim is a minor

**YES** "Seek emergency care now" and Follow **Home Care Instructions**

**NO** Go to C

**C. Sexual assault has occurred and victim requests a medical examination without collection of evidence or has questions and concerns. Ask the following questions:**

- Are you in a safe environment now?
- Are you alone?
- Where is the abuser now?
- Do you have family or friends who can help you?
- Have you called the police?
- Have you called a rape crisis center or rape hotline?

| YES | "Seek medical care within 24 hours" and Follow **Home Care Instructions** |

| NO | Follow **Home Care Instructions** |

S

# Home Care Instructions
# Sexual Assault

- Advise the victim to stay in a safe and supportive environment.
- Encourage the victim to have a medical examination with testing for STDs and pregnancy.
- Encourage the victim to report the incident to the police.
- Encourage the victim to call a rape crisis center or rape hotline.
- Advise caller not to shower or change clothes before the medical examination.

## Referral Telephone Numbers

## Additional Instructions

## Report the Following Problems to Your PCP/Clinic/ED

- Pain or bleeding persists or worsens
- Feelings of anger, depression, suicidal thoughts, or uncontrollable crying
- Fever, discharge, or sores develop

If the caller agrees with the advice given, document the call and encourage the caller to call back or see PCP if the problem worsens. If the caller does not agree with the advice given, reevaluate and advise the caller to follow up with PCP, Clinic, or ED.

# Sexually Transmitted Infection (STI)

>> **Key Questions**  Name, Age, Onset, Suspected STD, Known or Suspected Exposure to STD, Medications, History

>> **Other Protocols to Consider**  Genital Lesions (226); Penis Problems (331); Sexual Assault (400); Urination, Painful (477); Vaginal Discharge/Pain/Itching (486).

> *Nurse Alert:* Use this protocol if known STD, exposure or suspected exposure to STD.

*Reminder:*  Document caller response to advice, home care instructions, and when to call back.

| ASSESSMENT | ACTION |
|---|---|
| **A. Are any of the following present?** | |
| • Victim of sexual assault<br>• Unprotected sex with known HIV carrier<br>• Unprotected anal, oral, or vaginal sex with suspected HIV carrier | **YES** "Seek medical care now to discuss options"<br><br>**NO** Go to B |
| **B. Are any of the following present?** | |
| • Suspected or known exposure to STD<br>• Vaginal or penile discharge<br>• Vaginal, penile, or perineal lesions<br>• Pelvic pain with or without fever | **YES** "Seek medical care within 24 hours to discuss options"<br><br>**NO** Go to C |
| **C. Are any of the following present?** | |
| • Possible vaginal yeast infection<br>• Known genital herpes | **YES** "Call back or call PCP for appointment if no improvement"<br>and<br>Follow **Home Care Instructions**<br><br>**NO** Follow **Home Care Instructions** |

## Home Care Instructions
## Sexually Transmitted Infection (STI)

- A warm bath may ease discomfort of herpes but will not cure it. Avoid sex when open sores are present. Use latex condoms at all times.
- If unprotected sex has occurred with multiple partners or with a person who is known to have or is suspected of having HIV, obtain a laboratory test for HIV infection immediately and then 3 and 6 months after the initial exposure. Avoid the potential of infecting others and yourself by using a condom or abstaining from sex. Contact PCP or Health Department Clinic for testing. Possible medical treatment is available immediately after contact.
- Both partners should be tested and treated for STDs and should avoid unprotected sexual contact.
- Discuss STD and HIV exposure history with a new partner before engaging in sexual intimacy.
- Use latex condoms (unless an allergy to latex exists).

## Additional Instructions

_____

_____

_____

## Report the Following Problems to Your PCP/Clinic/ED

- At risk for HIV infection and persistent illness, fatigue, weight loss, diarrhea, swollen glands, sores, dry cough, or night sweats
- Suspected exposure to STD
- Unusual vaginal or penile discharge, genital lesions, or genital pain
- Known genital herpes and unable to tolerate persistent discomfort
- Pelvic pain with or without fever

If the caller agrees with the advice given, document the call and encourage the caller to call back or see PCP if the problem worsens. If the caller does not agree with the advice given, reevaluate and advise the caller to follow up with PCP, Clinic, or ED.

# Shoulder Pain/Injury

 **Key Questions**  Name, Age, Onset, Cause, Allergies, Medications, History, Pain Scale

 **Other Protocols to Consider**  Abdominal Pain (1); Chest Pain (85); Extremity Injury (163); Joint Pain/Swelling/Injury (287).

***Reminder:***  Document caller response to advice, home care instructions, and when to call back.

| ASSESSMENT | ACTION |
|---|---|
| **A. Are any of the following present?** | |
| • Sudden pain in shoulder and neck, jaw, or chest and shortness of breath or sweating<br>• Deformity, bruising, and limited movement in shoulder after an injury<br>• Sudden shoulder and abdominal pain in female with menses >4 weeks late | **YES** "Call ambulance"<br>or<br>"Seek emergency care now"<br><br>**NO** Go to B |
| **B. Are any of the following present?** | |
| • Recent history of blunt trauma to shoulder, abdomen, or back<br>• Fever, joint swollen, red, or warm, and recent illness<br>• Unable to raise arm or move shoulder<br>• Abdominal pain radiating to shoulder | **YES** "Seek medical care within 2 to 4 hours"<br><br>**NO** Go to C |
| **C. Are any of the following present?** | |
| • Sudden onset of pain in other joints<br>• Recent shoulder injury and no improvement in pain after >3 days of ice, heat, and rest | **YES** "Seek medical care within 24 hours"<br><br>**NO** Go to D |

## D. Are any of the following present?

- Progressive soreness in shoulder, increased with movement
- Progressive pain and stiffness
- Pain worsens by end of day and repetitive use or reaching to the side

**YES** "Call back or call PCP for appointment if no improvement"
and
Follow **Home Care Instructions**

**NO** Follow **Home Care Instructions**

## Home Care Instructions
## Shoulder Pain/Injury

- After initial injury, apply ice pack every 20 to 30 minutes, 4 to 6 times a day, for 24 to 48 hours, then apply moist heat. Rest shoulder for 24 to 48 hours. Do not apply ice directly on skin. Do not sleep on a heating pad.
- No lifting, pulling, or pushing.
- For pain (no injury) apply moist heat to area every 20 to 30 minutes, 4 to 6 times a day.
- If no known injury, exercise joint with slow, gradual stretching, raising arm as high as tolerated. Reach down, forward, up, and to each side.
- Take usual OTC pain reliever (acetaminophen, ibuprofen) for discomfort. Do not give aspirin to a child. Avoid aspirin-like products if age <20 years. Avoid acetaminophen if liver disease is present. Avoid ibuprofen if kidney disease or stomach problems exist or in the case of pregnancy. Follow the directions on the label. Use the dosing device that comes with the medication, a measuring device, or a medicine syringe from the pharmacy. Household teaspoons often do not give the correct amount of medication.
- If working at a computer or other repetitive movement activity, consider having an ergonomic assessment of workstation if shoulder pain consistently worsens at the end of the day.

## Additional Instructions

_____

_____

_____

### Report the Following Problems to Your PCP/Clinic/ED
- Pain persists or worsens
- New symptoms

### Seek Emergency Care Immediately If the Following Occur
- Recurring or sudden pain in shoulder and neck, jaw, or chest and shortness of breath or sweating

If the caller agrees with the advice given, document the call and encourage the caller to call back or see PCP if the problem worsens. If the caller does not agree with the advice given, reevaluate and advise the caller to follow up with PCP, Clinic, or ED.

# Sickle Cell Disease Problems

 **Key Questions** Name, Age, Onset, Medications, Pain Scale, History

 **Other Protocols to Consider** Abdominal Pain (1); Breathing Problems (68); Chest Pain (85); Jaundice (285); Joint Pain/Swelling/Injury (287); Urine, Abnormal Color (480).

*Nurse Alert:* Use the protocol if known sickle cell disease and problems or questions.

*Reminder:* Document caller response to advice, home care instructions, and when to call back.

| ASSESSMENT | ACTION |
|---|---|
| **A. Are any of the following present?** | |
| • Fever >101°F (38.3°C) <br> • Chest pain with or without cough <br> • Severe abdominal pain <br> • Severe joint or bone pain <br> • Syncope <br> • Difficulty breathing <br> • Nonblanching dark red or purple rash <br> • Severe headache <br> • Persistent erection of the penis <br> • Altered mental status <br> • Transient neurologic symptoms <br> • Worst-pain crisis | **YES** "Call ambulance" or "Seek emergency care now" <br><br> **NO** Go to B |
| **B. Are any of the following present?** | |
| • Moderate pain not responsive to normal pain management <br> • Blood in urine <br> • Difficulty walking <br> • Joint swelling, redness, or warmth <br> • Pallor <br> • Vomiting <br> • Jaundice <br> • Tachycardia | **YES** "Seek medical care immediately" <br><br> **NO** Go to C |

## C. Are any of the following present?

- Fatigue
- Persistent sore unresponsive to treatment

**YES**  "Seek medical care within 24 hours"

**NO**  Go to D

## D. Are any of the following present?

- Fever
- Worsening pain

**YES**  "Call back or call PCP for appointment if no improvement" and Follow **Home Care Instructions**

**NO**  Follow **Home Care Instructions**

## Home Care Instructions
## Sickle Cell Disease Problems

- Rest.
- Increase oral hydration. Drink lots of fluids.
- Apply topical heat to affected area for first 24 to 48 hours.
- Do not smoke.
- Take medications as directed.

**Additional Instructions**

_____

_____

_____

### Report the Following Problems to Your PCP/Clinic/ED

- Fever
- Worsening pain
- Decreased range of motion
- Increased swelling
- Blood in urine
- Increased difficulty walking, joint swelling, redness, or warmth
- Increased vomiting or jaundice

### Seek Emergency Care Immediately If Any of the Following Occur

- Chest pain with or without cough, syncope, or difficulty breathing
- Severe abdominal pain
- Severe joint or bone pain
- Nonblanching dark red or purple rash
- Severe headache or altered mental status
- Persistent erection of the penis

If the caller agrees with the advice given, document the call and encourage the caller to call back or see PCP if the problem worsens. If the caller does not agree with the advice given, reevaluate and advise the caller to follow up with PCP, Clinic, or ED.

# Sinus Problems

**» Key Questions**  Name, Age, Onset, Allergies, Medications, Prior Sinus Problems, History, Pain Scale

**» Other Protocols to Consider**  Breathing Problems (68); Common Cold Symptoms (103); Congestion (110); Cough (121); Earache, Drainage (150); Facial Problems (172); Fever (184); Headache (238); Sore Throat (420).

> *Nurse Alert:* Use the protocol if history of sinus problems or under current treatment for a sinus condition.

*Reminder:* Document caller response to advice, home care instructions, and when to call back.

| ASSESSMENT | ACTION |
|---|---|
| **A. Are any of the following present?** | |
| • Redness and swelling in cheek, forehead, or eyelid<br>• Vision change | **YES** "Seek medical care within 2 to 4 hours"<br>**NO** Go to B |
| **B. Are any of the following present?** | |
| • Persistent fever and sinus congestion or facial pain >2 to 3 days<br>• Yellow or green nasal discharge >3 to 5 days<br>• Persistent dull ache or tenderness around eyes or cheekbones<br>• No improvement after 48 hours of antibiotic therapy<br>• Pain worsens when bending over | **YES** "Seek medical care within 24 hours"<br>**NO** Go to C |

## C. Are any of the following present?

- Some sinus discomfort and clear nasal discharge
- Recent cold
- History of allergies
- Postnasal drainage
- Chronic cough

**YES** "Call back or call PCP for appointment if no improvement"
and
Follow **Home Care Instructions**

**NO** Follow **Home Care Instructions**

## Home Care Instructions
## Sinus Problems

- Use a vaporizer or humidifier to keep air moist, especially at night, and change the water daily.
- Breathe steam several times a day to help promote sinus drainage. Sit in a steam-filled bathroom for 10 to 20 minutes or cover head with a towel and breathe steam from a tea kettle or basin filled with hot water. Younger children should be accompanied in the bathroom by a parent at all times when breathing steam from shower.
- Apply hot packs to area around the eyes and cheekbones. Diabetics should use heat with caution.
- Take OTC decongestant of choice, and follow instructions on the label. If hypertensive or pregnant, such medications may not be appropriate. Check label on container before taking such medications. Do not give decongestants to children less than 12 years of age.
- For nasal congestion, use saline nose drops or spray.
- For postnasal drainage and age 12 years or older, may try phenylephrine (Neo-Synephrine) or oxymetazoline nasal (Afrin) nose drops for as long as 3 days. Then discontinue use. Prolonged use may worsen congestion when use of spray is discontinued. Do not take if cardiac disease, hypertension, or prostate problems are present.
- Take your usual pain medication (acetaminophen, ibuprofen) as tolerated for discomfort. Do not give aspirin to a child. Avoid aspirin-like products if age <20 years. Avoid acetaminophen if liver disease is present. Avoid ibuprofen if kidney disease or stomach problems exist or in the case of pregnancy. Follow the directions on the label.
- Avoid dairy products.
- Drink at least six 8-ounce glasses of liquids a day, unless on fluid restriction diet.

## Additional Instructions

_____

_____

_____

### Report the Following Problems to Your PCP/Clinic/ED
- Yellow or green nasal discharge for >3 to 5 days
- No improvement after 48 hours of antibiotic therapy
- Redness and swelling in cheek, forehead, or eyelid
- No improvement after 5 days or condition worsens

If the caller agrees with the advice given, document the call and encourage the caller to call back or see PCP if the problem worsens. If the caller does not agree with the advice given, reevaluate and advise the caller to follow up with PCP, Clinic, or ED.

# Skin Lesions: Lumps, Bumps, and Sores

 **Key Questions** Name, Age, Onset, Allergies, Medications, History

 **Other Protocols to Consider** Bedbug Exposure or Concerns (37); Eye Problems (169); Facial Skin Problems (175); Genital Lesions (226); Impetigo (270); Itching (282); Mouth Problems (302); Penis Problems (331); Piercing Problems (338); Rash (366); Scabies (388); Tattoo Problems (456); Vaginal Discharge/Pain/Itching (486).

*Reminder:* Document caller response to advice, home care instructions, and when to call back.

| ASSESSMENT | ACTION |
|---|---|

### A. Are any of the following present?

- New large lesion on the face or near the eyes, rectum, or genitals
- Severe pain
- Painful blisters
- Fever
- Recent use of sulfa drugs
- Diabetic or weakened immune system and signs of infection in the lesion
- Age <1 month and new-onset pimples or small blisters

 **YES** "Seek medical care within 2 to 4 hours"

**NO** Go to B

### B. Are any of the following present?

- Lesion located near upper lip, on tip or opening of nose, on eye or eyelid
- Temperature >100°F (37.8°C)
- Recent rapid change in color, shape, or size of a mole
- Painful or bleeding mole
- Signs of infection: pain, swelling, redness, drainage, red streaks, or warmth
- Lesion on bottom of foot that makes walking painful
- Persistent tender lesion after 48 to 72 hours of home care treatment
- Bumps under armpit
- New lesions develop on other parts of the body

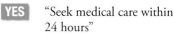 **YES** "Seek medical care within 24 hours"

**NO** Go to C

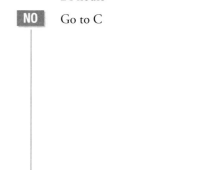

## C. Are any of the following present?

- Warts or moles that protrude so far they are frequently bumped or in the way
- Request for wart removal
- History of frequently occurring boils, warts, or lesions
- Infant and new onset of scaly or crusty lesions on scalp
- New warts develop after 2 weeks of treatment
- Persistent wart after 8 weeks of treatment
- New onset of pimples
- Circular, raised, rough pink patch with clear center ½ to 1 inch and itchy
- Circular, raised, rough pink patch on scalp with clear center ½ to 1 inch and itchy
- Concern for possible sexually transmitted disease
- Persistent painless lesion after 10 days of home care treatment
- Recurring lesion and person requests prescription to prevent future breakouts

**YES** "Call back or call PCP for appointment if no improvement" and Follow **Home Care Instructions**

**NO** Follow **Home Care Instructions**

S

## Home Care Instructions
## Skin Lesions

- Do not pick at or irritate the lesion. Do not squeeze boils.
- Apply warm soaks for 10 to 15 minutes, 4 to 6 times a day, to tender lesions or if there are signs of infection. Boils usually drain after a few days of heat treatment. People with diabetes should use heat with caution.
- Examine lesions frequently that are often irritated or rubbed by clothing.
- Take acetaminophen, or ibuprofen as tolerated for discomfort. Do not give aspirin to a child. Avoid aspirin-like products if age <20 years. Avoid acetaminophen if liver disease is present. Avoid ibuprofen if kidney disease or stomach problems exist or in the case of pregnancy. Follow the directions on the label. Use the dosing device that comes with the medication, a measuring device, or a medicine syringe from the pharmacy. Household teaspoons often do not give the correct amount of medication.
- Wash pimples with antibacterial soap and apply OTC or prescription antibiotic ointment 3 times a day.
- Provide reassurance that thick yellow scaly or crusty lesions on scalp will eventually disappear. To hasten the healing process, apply baby oil 15 minutes before shampooing scalp with an OTC dandruff shampoo followed by brushing with a soft brush or washcloth for 5 minutes.

### For Warts

- Follow instructions on the OTC wart removal preparations. Do not use if the person has diabetes or circulatory problems, or the wart is on the face.
  - Apply an OTC product (salicylic acid preparation) and follow the instructions on the package. Do not apply these products if diabetes or impaired circulation is present. Consult a pharmacist or PCP for product suggestions.
  - Alternative home remedy: Apply clear nail polish or a small piece of duct tape to wart daily for a few weeks. The wart will stop growing from lack of oxygen.

### For Cold Sores

- Apply OTC cream (i.e., Abreva) 5 times a day until healed. Ask a pharmacist or PCP for product suggestions and follow the instructions on the package. Begin using OTC or prescription cream at first sign of outbreak.
- Sores are contagious until dry. Avoid spreading them to another person's eyes, lips, or genitals or exposing a person with a weakened immune system.

### For Abscesses

- Lanced or unlanced abscesses are highly resistant to antibiotics and susceptible to MRSA infections.
  - Wash hands with microbial cleanser >3 times per day or more often when soiled.
  - Shower immediately with hot water as tolerated after activity.
  - Advise others in close contact to wash their hands with microbial cleanser.
  - Keep wounds covered with clean, dry bandages, particularly if drainage is present.

- Disinfect all towels, sheets, and surfaces in contact with wound with a solution of 1:100 of household bleach to water.
- Wash and dry clothes, linens, and towels in a setting as hot as possible. Make sure all items are dry before removing them from the drier.
- Avoid participating in contact sports or skin-to-skin contact with others until the infection has healed.
- Use a skin antiseptic to treat MRSA on the skin in combination with antibiotics prescribed by the PCP.
- Avoid hot tubs.
- Do not share bars of soap, razors, towels, or athletic gear.
- Call PCP if the condition worsens or fails to improve with home care and treatment.

**Additional Instructions**

_____

_____

_____

### Report the Following Problems to Your PCP/Clinic/ED

- Persistent growth, change, bleeding, color change, pain, or poor healing after 72 hours of home care treatment
- Signs of infection: pain, swelling, redness, drainage, red streaks, or warmth
- Requests for skin tag, mole, or wart removal

If the caller agrees with the advice given, document the call and encourage the caller to call back or see PCP if the problem worsens. If the caller does not agree with the advice given, reevaluate and advise the caller to follow up with PCP, Clinic, or ED.

# Sleep Apnea, Infant

 **Key Questions** Name, Age, Onset, Medications, History

 **Other Protocols to Consider** Newborn Problems (315); Spitting Up, Infant (424).

*Reminder:* Document caller response to advice, home care instructions, and when to call back.

| ASSESSMENT | ACTION |
|---|---|
| **A. Are any of the following present?** | |
| • Infant not breathing<br>• Skin turning blue | **YES** "Call ambulance"<br>and<br>"Start CPR" |
| | **NO** Go to B |
| **B. While infant was sleeping, did the following occur?** | |
| • Lapse in breathing for 1 minute<br>• Skin turned gray or blue but is normal color now<br>• Abnormal breathing after the episode<br>• Rescue breathing was necessary | **YES** "Seek medical care immediately" |
| | **NO** Go to C |
| **C. While infant was sleeping, did the following occur?** | |
| • Lapse in breathing <1 minute<br>• No change in skin color<br>• Infant breathing normally after episode<br>• Rescue breathing was not necessary | **YES** "Seek medical care within 24 hours" |
| | **NO** Follow **Home Care Instructions** |

## Home Care Instructions
## Sleep Apnea, Infant

- Provide reassurance. Some infants have a pause in breathing of <15 seconds after several rapid respirations.
- Reinforce importance of placing child on back for sleep.
- Discuss use of a respiration monitor with PCP.
- Obtain CPR training. Rapid identification of apnea and prompt CPR can successfully revive an infant without serious problems.

## Additional Instructions

_____

_____

_____

### Report the Following Problem to Your PCP/Clinic/ED
- Persistent episodes of apnea

### Call Ambulance Immediately If Any of the Following Occur
- Infant not breathing
- Skin turning blue
- CPR in progress

If the caller agrees with the advice given, document the call and encourage the caller to call back or see PCP if the problem worsens. If the caller does not agree with the advice given, reevaluate and advise the caller to follow up with PCP, Clinic, or ED.

# Sore Throat

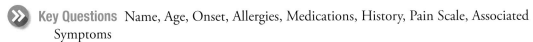

**»** **Key Questions**  Name, Age, Onset, Allergies, Medications, History, Pain Scale, Associated Symptoms

**»** **Other Protocols to Consider**  Allergic Reaction (13); Congestion (110); Cough (121); Earache, Drainage (150); Fever (184); Hoarseness (261); Mouth Problems (302); Swallowing Difficulty (442).

*Reminder:*  Document caller response to advice, home care instructions, and when to call back.

| ASSESSMENT | ACTION |
|---|---|

### A. Are any of the following present?

- Difficulty breathing (for reasons other than nasal congestion)
- Excessive drooling by a small child
- Stridor
- Inability to swallow own saliva
- Inability to open mouth fully
- Stiff neck and fever (pain bending head forward)

**YES**  "Seek emergency care now"

**NO**  Go to B

### B. Are any of the following present?

- Significant difficulty swallowing because of pain
- Temperature >104°F (40°C)
- Temperature >101°F (38.3°C) and immunosuppressed
- Difficulty moving neck and no fever
- Has two or more signs of dehydration
  - infrequent urination (<1 void in >12 hours) (<1 void in >8 hours in an infant)
  - dark yellow urine
  - sunken eyes or fontanelle
  - pinched skin does not spring back
  - excessive thirst
  - dry mouth or mucous membranes
  - Capillary refill >2 seconds
  - infant cries without tears
- Child <2 years of age

**YES**  "Seek medical care within 2 to 4 hours"

**NO**  Go to C

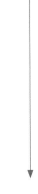

## C. Are any of the following present?

- History of rheumatic fever, mitral valve prolapse, or other heart valve problem
- Skin rash
- Close contact with someone with strep throat within the past 2 weeks
- Yellow pus or white mucus at back of throat
- Red or enlarged tonsils
- Fever and persistent sore throat >2 days
- Persistent sore throat >3 days and no fever
- Ear pain
- Fever or chills unresponsive to fever-reducing measures
- Diabetes, or immunosuppressed
- Dizziness/faintness
- Foul-smelling breath

**YES** "Seek medical care within 24 hours"
and
Follow **Home Care Instructions**

**NO** Go to D

## D. Are any of the following present?

- Nasal congestion
- Cough or sneezing
- Feeling of fullness in ear

**YES** "Call back or call PCP for appointment if no improvement"
and
Follow **Home Care Instructions**

**NO** Follow **Home Care Instructions**

S

## Home Care Instructions
## Sore Throat

- Take your usual pain medication (acetaminophen, ibuprofen) for headache or fever. Do not give aspirin to a child. Avoid aspirin-like products if age <20 years. Avoid acetaminophen if liver disease is present. Avoid ibuprofen if kidney disease or stomach problems exist or in the case of pregnancy. Follow the directions on the label. Use the dosing device that comes with the medication, a measuring device, or a medication syringe from the pharmacy. Household teaspoons often do not give the correct amount of medication.
- Gargle with salt water several times a day for throat discomfort (¼ tsp regular salt to ½ cup warm water) or sip warm chicken broth or apple juice. Use frozen cough drops or hard candy for additional relief if age >6 years.
- Increase fluids; try warm tea with lemon and honey, apple juice, gelatin, or sucking on flavored ice. Take frequent small sips if it is painful to swallow. Do not give honey to a child <1 year old.
- If you smoke, decrease or stop smoking.
- Use a vaporizer or humidifier to keep the air moist, especially at night, or put a pot of water near the heat source.
- If age >12 years, may take decongestants to help relieve congestion, unless there is a history of hypertension or pregnancy. Do not use for more than 3 days. Discuss with PCP or pharmacist.

## Additional Instructions

_____

_____

_____

## Report the Following Problems to Your PCP/Clinic/ED

- Fever >101°F (38.3°C) for several days
- Sore throat persists >3 days or worsens
- Earache
- No improvement or condition worsens
- Drooling
- Signs of dehydration

S

## Seek Emergency Care Immediately If Any of the Following Occur

- Unable to swallow own saliva
- Difficulty breathing/stridor
- Chest pain
- Excessive drooling
- Unable to open mouth fully

If the caller agrees with the advice given, document the call and encourage the caller to call back or see PCP if the problem worsens. If the caller does not agree with the advice given, reevaluate and advise the caller to follow up with PCP, Clinic, or ED.

# Spitting Up, Infant

 **Key Questions**  Name, Age, Onset, Medications, History

 **Other Protocols to Consider**  Bottle-Feeding Problems (59); Breast-Feeding Problems (63); Dehydration (132); Vomiting (492).

*Reminder:*  Document caller response to advice, home care instructions, and when to call back.

| ASSESSMENT | ACTION |
|---|---|
| **A. Are any of the following present?** | |
| <ul><li>Difficulty breathing</li><li>Blue or gray face, lips, fingernails, or earlobes</li><li>Lethargy</li></ul> | **YES** "Call ambulance" or "Seek emergency care now" |
| | **NO** Go to B |
| **B. Are any of the following present?** | |
| <ul><li>Persistent vomiting</li><li>Choking or coughing afterward</li><li>Blood or dark green bile in spit-up material</li><li>Fever >100.4°F (38°C) and age <3 months</li><li>Signs of dehydration:<ul><li>decreased urine</li><li>sunken eyes</li><li>poor skin elasticity (does not spring back when pinched)</li><li>excessive thirst or dry mouth</li><li>crying without tears</li></ul></li><li>Sunken soft spot</li><li>No stools in newborn</li><li>Projectile vomiting</li></ul> | **YES** "Seek medical care within 2 hours" |
| | **NO** Go to C |

424

## C. Are any of the following present?

- Persistent irritability
- Diarrhea
- Parent concerned about infant's lack of weight gain

YES    "Seek medical care within 24 hours"

NO    Go to D

## D. Are any of the following present?

- Fever and age >3 months
- Spitting up frequently occurs after infant consumes volumes larger than 1 to 2 mouthfuls
- Weight loss
- Increasing constipation
- Persistent spitting up
- Parent concerned

YES    "Call back or call PCP for appointment if no improvement"
and
Follow **Home Care Instructions**

NO    Follow **Home Care Instructions**

## Home Care Instructions
## Spitting Up, Infant

- Remember that nonforceful spitting up of a small amount of stomach contents shortly after feeding is a common condition of infants. The infant should outgrow this after starting to sit up.
- Burp the baby several times during the feedings.
- Give small frequent feedings and avoid overfeeding or feeding too quickly.
- Place infant in an upright position in a swing or baby carrier after feeding. Avoid hugging or bouncing the infant after feeding.
- Elevate the head of the bed and position infant on side if awake.
- Avoid tight diapers or binding infant when changing diapers.
- If breast-feeding, try feeding one side at a time and pump the other side. Avoid pacifiers.

## Additional Instructions

_____

_____

_____

### Report the Following Problems to Your PCP/Clinic/ED

- No improvement with home care measures or condition worsens
- Weight loss or failure to gain weight normally
- Increasing constipation
- Persistent spitting up
- Blood or dark green bile in spit-up material
- Signs of dehydration

### Seek Emergency Care Immediately If Any of the Following Occur

- Difficulty breathing
- Lethargy
- Blue or gray face, lips, fingernails, or earlobes

If the caller agrees with the advice given, document the call and encourage the caller to call back or see PCP if the problem worsens. If the caller does not agree with the advice given, reevaluate and advise the caller to follow up with PCP, Clinic, or ED.

# Stool, Incontinence

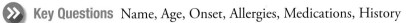 **Key Questions**  Name, Age, Onset, Allergies, Medications, History

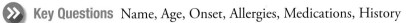 **Other Protocols to Consider**  Abdominal Pain (1); Constipation (114); Diarrhea (143); Rectal Bleeding (371); Rectal Problems (374); Stools, Abnormal (429).

**Reminder:**  Document caller response to advice, home care instructions, and when to call back.

| ASSESSMENT | ACTION |
|---|---|
| **A. Are any of the following present?** | |
| • Incontinence of urine and stool after a seizure, faint, or loss of consciousness | **YES** "Call ambulance" |
| • Sudden loss of bowel control and slurred speech, muscle weakness, blurred or double vision, or decreased level of consciousness | **NO** Go to B |
| **B. Are several of the following present?** | |
| • Recent back injury, trauma, or fall, severe pain, and several episodes of incontinence | **YES** "Seek emergency care now" |
| • Black or bloody stool with clots | **NO** Go to C |
| **C. Are any of the following present?** | |
| • Recent history of childbirth, vaginal or rectal surgery, hemorrhoids, or anal fistula or fissure | **YES** "Seek medical care within 24 hours" |
| • Abdominal pain | |
| • Several incontinent episodes | **NO** Go to D |
| **D. Are any of the following present?** | |
| • Lump felt inside anal opening | **YES** "Call back or call PCP for appointment if no improvement" and Follow **Home Care Instructions** |
| • Sudden onset of diarrhea and unable to make it to the toilet | |
| • Frequent involuntary seepage of stool and recent history of no bowel movements or several hard stools | |
| • Recurrence of stool incontinence in child previously toilet-trained | **NO** Follow **Home Care Instructions** |

427

## Home Care Instructions
## Stool, Incontinence

- Avoid constipation. Increase fiber, bulk, and fluids (fresh fruit, vegetables, whole grains, cereals, and brown rice). Try Metamucil to add bulk. Drink 6 to 8 glasses of water daily. Exercise regularly.
- In a child previously toilet-trained:
  - Allow child to determine time for toileting. Do not force child to sit on toilet.
  - Provide praise when toilet is used.
  - Discuss with child a reward for staying clean all day.
  - If child is soiled, have the child clean self and change clothes (if old enough).
  - Do not scold or punish for accidents or allow other siblings to tease the child.
- Consider renting or buying a portable toilet for use when sudden diarrhea attacks occur.
- Review diet and medications, such as use of laxatives, new medications, prune juice, or castor oil.

## Additional Instructions

_____

_____

_____

## Report the Following Problems to Your PCP/Clinic/ED

- Bloody stool
- Abdominal pain
- Several incontinent episodes
- No improvement or condition worsens

If the caller agrees with the advice given, document the call and encourage the caller to call back or see PCP if the problem worsens. If the caller does not agree with the advice given, reevaluate and advise the caller to follow up with PCP, Clinic, or ED

# Stools, Abnormal

>> **Key Questions**  Name, Age, Onset, Recent Dietary Habits, Medications, History

>> **Other Protocols to Consider**  Abdominal Pain (1); Constipation (114); Diarrhea (143); Rectal Bleeding (371); Stools, Incontinence (427).

*Reminder:*  Document caller response to advice, home care instructions, and when to call back.

| ASSESSMENT | ACTION |
|---|---|

### A. Is there abdominal pain?

**YES**  Go to Abdominal Pain (1) protocol

**NO**  Go to B

### B. Is there diarrhea?

**YES**  Go to Diarrhea (143) protocol

**NO**  Go to C

### C. Are any of the following present?

- Black or dark stools for more than two bowel movements and light-headedness or dizziness
- Vomiting blood or dark coffee-grounds–like emesis
- Passing blood clots

**YES**  "Seek emergency care now"

**NO**  Go to D

### D. Are any of the following present?

- Black tarry stools without recent ingestion of iron pills, beets, bismuth salicylate (Pepto-Bismol), or spinach
- Large amount of bright red blood mixed in the stool
- Bloody stool, fever, vomiting, ill feeling
- Age <12 weeks, fever, and bloody stools

**YES**  "Seek medical care within 2 to 4 hours"

**NO**  Go to E

### E. Are any of the following present?

- Pale stool, yellow skin and eyes
- Pale, foamy, bulky, foul-smelling stool
- Blood mixed in stool or black stools for more than two consecutive bowel movements
- Persistent weight loss and thin, pencil-like stools

**YES** "Seek medical care within 24 hours"

**NO** Go to F

### F. Are any of the following present?

- Stool streaked with red blood
- Blood on toilet tissue after wiping
- Discolored stool and recent ingestion of iron pills, beets, Pepto-Bismol, spinach, tomatoes, or peppers, or stool is color of recently ingested food
- Persistent discoloration
- Persistent bleeding >3 days
- Constipation or hemorrhoids

**YES** "Call back or call PCP for appointment if no improvement"
and
Follow **Home Care Instructions**

**NO** Follow **Home Care Instructions**

## Home Care Instructions
## Stools, Abnormal

- In newborns, the quality and the color of the stools may change from day 1 to day 5 of life. The stools will progress from a dark green sticky, pasty consistency to a soft, yellow seedy texture. The stools may also increase in frequency. Newborns may stool after each feeding. For hemorrhoids, soak in a warm saline bath for 20 minutes a day (add 2 tbsp of salt or baking soda to the water).
- Keep rectal area clean.
- If rectal area is irritated, apply OTC hydrocortisone ointment (for nondiapered children) or zinc oxide paste or powder.
- If hemorrhoids persist, try OTC preparations to help soothe and shrink hemorrhoids.
- Increase fluid intake and eat a diet high in fiber: fruits, vegetables, bran, grains, and beans. Avoid constipating foods such as cheese. Note which foods change the color of the stool.
- Remember the color of the stool should return to normal within 24 hours if the discoloration is caused by a change in diet.
- Use products with witch hazel (Tucks) to reduce discomfort.

## Additional Instructions

_____

_____

_____

### Report the Following Problems to Your PCP/Clinic/ED

- No improvement in 3 days or condition worsens
- Abdominal pain
- Bloody stool, fever, vomiting, ill feeling
- Pale stool, yellow skin and eyes
- Pale, foamy, bulky, foul-smelling stool
- Persistent weight loss and thin, pencil-like stools

### Seek Emergency Care Immediately If Any of the Following Occur

- Black or dark stools for more than two consecutive bowel movements and light-headedness or dizziness
- Vomiting blood or dark coffee-grounds–like emesis
- Passing bloody stools

If the caller agrees with the advice given, document the call and encourage the caller to call back or see PCP if the problem worsens. If the caller does not agree with the advice given, reevaluate and advise the caller to follow up with PCP, Clinic, or ED.

# Stye

 **Key Questions**  Name, Age, Onset, Medications, History

 **Other Protocols to Consider**  Eye Injury (166); Eye Problems (169).

> *Nurse Alert:* Use this protocol if previously diagnosed with a stye and has questions or concerns.

*Reminder:*  Document caller response to advice, home care instructions, and when to call back.

| ASSESSMENT | ACTION |
|---|---|
| **A. Are any of the following present?**<br>• Lump interferes with vision<br>• Several lumps suddenly appear at once<br>• Persistent pain unresponsive to home care measures<br>• New onset of red, tender, swollen area on bottom eyelid or near nose<br>• Drainage from lesion and temperature >100.5°F (38.1°C)<br>• Bloody drainage | **YES** "Seek medical care within 24 hours"<br><br>**NO** Go to B |
| **B. Are any of the following present?**<br>• Red pimple-like lump persists on upper or lower eyelid or near it >48 hours after home treatment<br>• Lumps frequently appear<br>• Lump breaks open and drains | **YES** "Call back or call PCP for appointment if no improvement"<br>and<br>Follow **Home Care Instructions**<br><br>**NO** Follow **Home Care Instructions** |

## Home Care Instructions
## Stye

- Avoid rubbing the affected eye.
- Apply warm compresses to the area for 20 minutes, 4 to 6 times a day or more if possible.
- Do not share washcloths and towels with other household members. Sties may be contagious.
- Allow the stye to break open; do not squeeze the lump.
- Avoid eye makeup or contact lenses until the stye heals.
- Apply OTC treatments and follow the instructions on the package (Stye, Bausch & Lomb Eye Wash, Collyrium Eye Wash, OCuSOFT Lid Scrub, and Stygiene, which are available as ointments, solutions, and medicated pads). Ask the pharmacist for other product suggestions.
- If antibiotic ointment is prescribed, apply to the stye at bedtime.
- Do not touch the tip of the applicator with the hand or eye surface.
- To apply eye drops, pull the lower lid down with two fingers. Put drops in the area between the eyelid and eyeball. Close eyes for 30 to 60 seconds.
- Wash hands often and before putting medications into the eye.

## Additional Instructions

_____

_____

_____

### Report the Following Problems to Your PCP/Clinic/ED

- No improvement in 48 hours or condition worsens
- Several more lumps appear
- Drainage from lesion, and temperature >100.5°F (38.1°C)
- Bloody drainage

If the caller agrees with the advice given, document the call and encourage the caller to call back or see PCP if the problem worsens. If the caller does not agree with the advice given, reevaluate and advise the caller to follow up with PCP, Clinic, or ED.

# Substance Abuse, Use, or Exposure

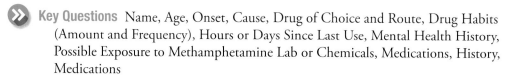 **Key Questions**  Name, Age, Onset, Cause, Drug of Choice and Route, Drug Habits (Amount and Frequency), Hours or Days Since Last Use, Mental Health History, Possible Exposure to Methamphetamine Lab or Chemicals, Medications, History, Medications

**Other Protocols to Consider**  Alcohol Problems (9); Chest Pain (85); Confusion (107); Diarrhea (143); Overdose (328); Poisoning, Suspected (347); Suicide Attempt, Threat (437).

> *Nurse Alert:*  If overdosed on prescription, nonprescription, recreational drugs, alcohol, or any chemical agent, go to Overdose Protocol (328). If suicide attempt/gesture or threat to hurt self or others, go to Suicide Attempt/Threat protocol (437).

*Reminder:*  Document caller response to advice, home care instructions, and when to call back.

| ASSESSMENT | ACTION |
|---|---|

### A. Are any of the following present?

- Altered mental status
- Apnea or difficulty breathing
- Pale, diaphoretic, and light-headed or weak
- Suicidal or homicidal ideation
- Unresponsive
- Face, lips, or tongue blue or gray
- Seizures

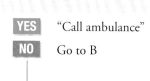 **YES**  "Call ambulance"

**NO**  Go to B

S

## B. Are any of the following present?

- Adolescent with speech slurring, confusion, poor coordination after use of drugs or alcohol
- Chest pain
- Dizziness, difficulty breathing, shakiness
- Possible overdose
- Hallucinations
- Extreme anxiety, agitation, paranoia, or terror
- Signs of withdrawal: rapid or irregular heart rate, tremors, high blood pressure, vomiting, restlessness, diaphoresis
- Exposure to methamphetamine vapors during cooking process

**YES**  "Seek emergency care now" and See **Home Care Instructions**

**NO**  Go to C

## C. Are any of the following present?

- 24 to 48 hours after cessation of substance and hallucinations: auditory (voices, buzzing, clicks), sensory (bug crawling), or visual hallucinations
- Fever
- Difficulty performing simple tasks
- Suicide thoughts but no action
- Suspected ingestion of unknown drug, inability to recall events, possible sexual contact

**YES**  "Seek medical care within 2 to 4 hours"

**NO**  Go to D

## D. Are any of the following present?

- Request for addiction services
- History of intermittent use and has concerns
- Ongoing vomiting, diarrhea, heartburn after exposure
- Postexposure eye or skin irritation
- Acute anxiety

**YES**  "Seek medical care within 24 hours"

**NO**  Go to E

## E. Are any of the following present?

- No other symptoms or problems but parent or person concerned
- 12 hours after cessation and mild tremors, anxiety, anorexia, nausea or vomiting, weakness, myalgias

**YES**  "Call back or call PCP for appointment if no improvement" and Follow **Home Care Instructions**

**NO**  Follow **Home Care Instructions**

## Home Care Instructions
## Substance Abuse, Use, or Exposure

- For chemical exposure, immediately wash exposed skin surfaces.
- Call Poison Control (1-800-222-1222) for exact care of exposure to methamphetamine-processing chemicals.
- Contact local resources for assistance: counseling, detoxification centers, inpatient and outpatient treatment programs, AA, and Al-Anon.
- Take usual pain medication for discomfort. Do not give aspirin to a child. Avoid aspirin-like products if age <20 years. Avoid acetaminophen if liver disease is present. Avoid ibuprofen if kidney disease or stomach problems exist or in the case of pregnancy. Follow the directions on the label.

**Additional Instructions**

_____

_____

_____

### Report the Following Problems to Your PCP/Clinic/ED

- Fever
- Difficulty performing simple tasks
- Dizziness
- Persistent vomiting or diarrhea

### Seek Emergency Care Immediately If Any of the Following Occur

- Signs of withdrawal: rapid heart rate, tremors, high blood pressure, vomiting, restlessness, sweating
- Seizures
- Black or tarry stools
- Dark coffee-grounds–like emesis
- Suicidal or homicidal ideation
- Chest pain
- Dizziness
- Hallucinations
- Extreme anxiety, agitation, or paranoia
- Exposure to methamphetamine vapors during cooking process

If the caller agrees with the advice given, document the call and encourage the caller to call back or see PCP if the problem worsens. If the caller does not agree with the advice given, reevaluate and advise the caller to follow up with PCP, Clinic, or ED.

# Suicide Attempt, Threat

**Key Questions** Name, Age, Onset, Cause, Address, Telephone Number, Medications, History

**Other Protocols to Consider** Alcohol Problems (9); Anxiety (18); Breathing Problems (68); Confusion (107); Depression (135); Laceration (290); Overdose (328); Substance Abuse, Use, or Exposure (434).

**Reminder:** Document caller response to advice, home care instructions, and when to call back.

| ASSESSMENT | ACTION |
|---|---|
| **A. Are any of the following present?** | |
| • Unconsciousness <br> • Severe respiratory distress, chest pain, or abdominal pain <br> • Suicide attempt, such as physical injury or overdose <br> • Suicide attempt in progress <br> • Threat to harm self or others <br> • Suicidal thoughts with a specific plan (available method such as weapons or pills) <br> • New onset of confusion or delusional thinking | **YES** "Call ambulance" or "Seek emergency care now" and Contact police if necessary <br><br> **NO** Go to B |
| **B. Are any of the following present?** | |
| • Refusal to talk anymore and considered at high risk for suicide <br> • History of prior suicide attempts <br> • Depression <br> • Intoxication <br> • Suicidal thoughts but no plan or injury <br> • Recent change in medication | **YES** "Seek medical care now" and Contact mental health professional now or call police if necessary and Follow **Home Care Instructions** <br><br> **NO** Follow **Home Care Instructions** |

## Home Care Instructions
## Suicide Attempt, Threat

- All calls dealing with suicidal thoughts should be referred to an appropriate mental health professional.
- If the caller is alone and high risk, maintain telephone contact as long as possible or transfer the call to a suicide hotline without losing the connection. Trace the call as necessary. Obtain the caller's address and telephone number.
- All calls indicating suicidal thoughts should be considered emergent until cleared by a mental health professional or ED physician.
- Note background noises.

**Additional Instructions**

_____

_____

_____

## Seek Emergency Care or Call Police Immediately If Any of the Following Occur

- Continued suicidal thoughts
- Suicidal thoughts with a specific plan (available method: weapons or pills)
- Suicide attempt (physical injury or overdose)

If the caller agrees with the advice given, document the call and encourage the caller to call back or see PCP if the problem worsens. If the caller does not agree with the advice given, reevaluate and advise the caller to follow up with PCP, Clinic, or ED.

# Sunburn

>> **Key Questions**  Name, Age, Onset, Allergies, Medications, Tetanus Immunization Status, History

>> **Other Protocols to Consider**  Dehydration (132); Eye Problems (169); Heat Exposure Problems (252); Rash (366); Skin Lesions: Lumps, Bumps, and Sores (414).

*Reminder:*  Document caller response to advice, home care instructions, and when to call back.

| ASSESSMENT | ACTION |
|---|---|

### A. Are any of the following present?

- Cool skin, dizziness, faintness
- Dry, hot skin, faintness when temperature >105°F (40.6°C)
- Confusion
- Significant decrease in urine output
- Loss of consciousness or altered mental status

**YES** "Seek emergency care now"

**NO** Go to B

### B. Are any of the following present?

- Vision changes
- Severe swelling
- Blisters on hands or genitals
- Burn circles around a digit or limb
- Burns on joints

**YES** "Seek medical care within 2 to 4 hours"

**NO** Go to C

### C. Are any of the following present?

- Multiple blisters
- Open blisters
- Signs of infection: pain, swelling, pus, or red streaks extending from blistered area
- Eye pain, decreased vision, light sensitivity

**YES** "Seek medical care within 24 hours"

**NO** Go to D

439

### D. Are any of the following present?

- Skin reddened and no blisters
- Pain unresponsive to OTC pain relievers
- Pain >48 hours
- A few blisters

**YES**  "Call back or call PCP for appointment if no improvement" and Follow **Home Care Instructions**

**NO**  Follow **Home Care Instructions**

## Home Care Instructions
## Sunburn

- Apply cold compresses to burn or take a cool bath for 10 minutes 4 times a day. May add Aveeno or ½ cup baking soda to water. Be careful area does not become numb; frostbite can occur. Do not apply ice to the skin.
- Expect some discomfort for as long as 48 hours. Use your usual pain medication (acetaminophen, ibuprofen). Do not give aspirin to a child. Avoid aspirin-like products if age <20 years. Avoid acetaminophen if liver disease is present. Avoid ibuprofen if kidney disease or stomach problems exist or in the case of pregnancy. Follow the directions on the label. Use the dosing device that comes with the medication, a measuring device, or a medicine syringe from the pharmacy. Household teaspoons often do not give the correct amount of medication.
- Do not apply greasy substance or toothpaste to burn area.
- After cooling with water, and if no open blisters are present, apply topical antibiotic, aloe vera, or a mixture of Benadryl elixir and milk of magnesia in equal amounts to burned area for a soothing effect.
- During the drying stage, apply moisturizing lotion to the skin. Peeling usually occurs in 3 to 10 days.
- For painful and swollen eyes, stay in a darkened room, apply cool compresses to the eyes, and rest.
- Increase fluid intake.
- Avoid sun exposure if taking phototoxic medications such as sulfas, tetracycline, phenothiazines, or thiazides. Always read the warning label on medications before taking them.

**Additional Instructions**

_____

_____

_____

### Report the Following Problems to Your PCP/Clinic/ED
- Signs of infection
- Severe swelling
- No improvement or if condition worsens

### Seek Emergency Care Immediately If Any of the Following Occur
- Significant decrease in urine output
- Confusion
- Cool skin, dizziness, fainting

If the caller agrees with the advice given, document the call and encourage the caller to call back or see PCP if the problem worsens. If the caller does not agree with the advice given, reevaluate and advise the caller to follow up with PCP, Clinic, or ED.

# Swallowing Difficulty

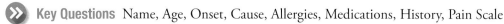

**Key Questions** Name, Age, Onset, Cause, Allergies, Medications, History, Pain Scale

**Other Protocols to Consider** Foreign Body, Swallowing of (214); Heartburn (245); Neurologic Symptoms (312); Piercing Problems (338); Sore Throat (420); Weakness (496).

> *Nurse Alert:* Sudden changes in ability to swallow; vision, speech, or mental status; weakness; and numbness may be signs of a serious neurologic disorder. Prompt treatment may prevent extensive damage to the brain or reduce permanent disability.

*Reminder:* Document caller response to advice, home care instructions, and when to call back.

| ASSESSMENT | ACTION |
|---|---|
| **A. Are any of the following present?** | |
| • Weakness of neck, chest, and limbs<br>• Double or blurred vision, drooling, or drooping eyelids<br>• Excessive drooling in small child who appears ill<br>• Sudden swelling in face, tongue, or throat or itching, hives, or wheezing<br>• Difficulty breathing<br>• Pain in jaw, throat, neck, shoulders, chest, or arms<br>• Inability to swallow own saliva | **YES** "Call ambulance" or "Seek emergency care now"<br><br>**NO** Go to B |
| **B. Is the following present?** | |
| • Sensation that bone or food is stuck in throat or esophagus | **YES** "Seek medical care within 2 to 4 hours"<br><br>**NO** Go to C |

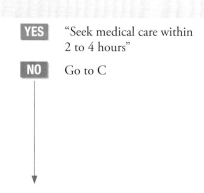

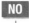

## C. Is the following present?

● Unexplained weight loss       **YES**   "Seek medical care within 24 hours"

                                                      **NO**   Go to D

## D. Are any of the following present?

● Difficulty swallowing because of sore throat      **YES**   "Call back or call PCP
● Intermittent chest pain on bending forward or lying                  for appointment if no
  down                                                     improvement"
● Throat feels tight after swallowing                             and
● Recent increase in stress                                     Follow **Home Care Instructions**

                                                      **NO**   Follow **Home Care Instructions**

## Home Care Instructions
## Swallowing Difficulty

- Take your usual pain medication (acetaminophen, ibuprofen) as tolerated for fever and discomfort. Do not give aspirin to a child. Avoid aspirin-like products if age <20 years. Avoid acetaminophen if liver disease is present. Avoid ibuprofen if kidney disease or stomach problems exist or in the case of pregnancy. Follow the directions on the label.
- Gargle with salt water several times a day for throat discomfort (¼ tsp regular salt to ½ cup warm water) or sip warm chicken broth or apple juice. Use frozen cough drops or hard candy for additional relief if age >6 years.
- Increase fluids; try warm tea with lemon and honey, apple juice, gelatin, or sucking on flavored ice. Take frequent small sips if it is painful to swallow. Do not give honey to a child <1 year old.
- Swallow bread or soft foods, as tolerated.
- Try OTC antacids, such as Gelusil, Maalox, Mylanta, Riopan, and Tums, and follow instructions on the label.
- Do not lie down, bend over, or exercise soon after eating.
- Eat small, frequent meals.
- Avoid spicy foods, alcohol, coffee, smoking, chocolate, vinegar, fatty foods, and carbonated beverages.

## Additional Instructions

_____

_____

_____

### Report the Following Problems to Your PCP/Clinic/ED

- No improvement after 3 days or condition worsens
- Burping or vomiting blood or dark coffee-grounds–like emesis
- Excessive drooling
- Persistent fever unresponsive to home care measures

### Seek Emergency Care Immediately If Any of the Following Occur

- Weakness of neck, chest, and limbs
- Double or blurred vision, drooling, or drooping eyelids
- Excessive drooling in small child who appears ill
- Sudden swelling in face, tongue, or throat or itching, hives, or wheezing
- Difficulty breathing
- Pain in jaw, throat, neck, shoulders, chest, or arms
- Inability to swallow own saliva

If the caller agrees with the advice given, document the call and encourage the caller to call back or see PCP if the problem worsens. If the caller does not agree with the advice given, reevaluate and advise the caller to follow up with PCP, Clinic, or ED.

# Sweating, Excessive

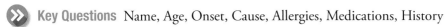

>> **Key Questions**  Name, Age, Onset, Cause, Allergies, Medications, History

>> **Other Protocols to Consider**  Alcohol Problems (9); Anxiety (18); Breathing Problems (68); Chest Pain (85); Diabetes Problems (138); Fever (184); Heat Exposure Problems (252); Poisoning, Suspected (347); Substance Abuse, Use or Exposure (434).

*Reminder:*  Document caller response to advice, home care instructions, and when to call back.

| ASSESSMENT | ACTION |
|---|---|

### A. Are any of the following present?

- Pale, cool skin and rapid pulse
- Pain in chest, throat, neck, jaw, shoulders, or arms
- Difficulty breathing

**YES**  "Call ambulance"
or
"Seek emergency care now"

**NO**  Go to B

### B. Are any of the following present?

- Prolonged exposure to heat and fatigue, weakness, dizziness, or nausea
- Signs of dehydration in young children or immunosuppressed individuals:
  - decreased urine for >8 hours
  - sunken eyes or fontanelle
  - crying without tears
  - skin does not bounce back when pinched
  - excessive thirst
  - dry mouth
  - unusual lethargy

**YES**  "Seek medical care within 2 to 4 hours"

**NO**  Go to C

### C. Are any of the following present?

- Excessive sweating at night and weight loss, persistent cough, blood in sputum
- Persistent fever and fatigue
- Recent abrupt cessation of drugs (OTC, prescription, or street), alcohol, or caffeine

**YES**  "Seek medical care within 24 hours"

**NO**  Go to D

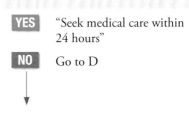

## D. Are any of the following present?

- Weight loss, increased appetite, weakness, difficulty sleeping
- Obesity
- Temperature >100°F (37.8°C)
- Sweating occurs after consuming alcohol or large doses of aspirin
- Sweating occurs when wearing synthetic clothing
- Only the hands and feet sweat
- Recent increase in stress
- Beginning signs of dehydration
- Problems with body odor

**YES** "Call back or call PCP for appointment if no improvement" and Follow **Home Care Instructions**

**NO** Follow **Home Care Instructions**

S

## Home Care Instructions
## Sweating, Excessive

- Remember that sweating often is a natural response to fever, hormonal changes, exercise, and stress.
- Sweating increases with obesity. Reduction in weight should decrease the amount of sweat.
- Take your usual pain medication (acetaminophen, ibuprofen) to reduce fever. Do not give aspirin to a child. Avoid aspirin-like products if age <20 years. Avoid acetaminophen if liver disease is present. Avoid ibuprofen if kidney disease or stomach problems exist or in the case of pregnancy. Follow the directions on the label. Use the dosing device that comes with the medication, a measuring device, or a medicine syringe from the pharmacy. Household teaspoons often do not give the correct amount of medication.
- If sweating is related to heat exposure, cool down with cold compresses, cold bath or shower, and light cotton clothing and drink cool fluids.
- For signs of dehydration, increase fluid intake: Give young children Lytren, Pedialyte, or Rehydralyte; older children should consume sports drinks, water, juice, or soft drinks.
- Wash and dry hands and feet frequently for excessive sweating. Wear cotton or other natural-fiber clothing and socks.

## Additional Instructions

_____

_____

_____

## Report the Following Problems to Your PCP/Clinic/ED

- Persistent or worsening of unexplained excessive sweating
- Excessive sweating at night and weight loss, persistent cough, blood in sputum
- Weight loss, increased appetite, weakness, difficulty sleeping
- Persistent fever and fatigue

## Seek Emergency Care Immediately If Any of the Following Occur

- Pain in chest, throat, neck, jaw, shoulders, or arms
- Pale, cool skin and rapid pulse
- Difficulty breathing

If the caller agrees with the advice given, document the call and encourage the caller to call back or see PCP if the problem worsens. If the caller does not agree with the advice given, reevaluate and advise the caller to follow up with PCP, Clinic, or ED.

# Swelling

 **Key Questions** Name, Age, Onset, No Known Injury, Medications, History

 **Other Protocols to Consider** Abdominal Pain (1); Abdominal Swelling (4); Bruising (71); Cast/Splint Problems (83); Finger and Toe Problems (189); Glands, Swollen or Tender (229); Pregnancy Problems (358); Wound Healing and Infection (509).

*Reminder:* Document caller response to advice, home care instructions, and when to call back.

| ASSESSMENT | ACTION |
|---|---|

### A. In addition to swelling in the face, ankles, or hands, are any of the following present?

- Severe respiratory difficulty, wheezing, or cough
- Swollen tongue or swelling at back of throat
- Rapid progression of swelling
- Coughing up frothy pink-tinged sputum

**YES** "Seek emergency care now"

**NO** Go to B

### B. Are any of the following present?

- Area warm, red, or tender
- Area cold or blue
- Rings cutting into skin because of increased swelling
- Vomiting or diarrhea
- Persistent painful swelling in groin or abdomen that does not disappear with pressure
- Swelling in groin or abdomen and nausea or vomiting present

**YES** "Seek medical care within 2 to 4 hours"

**NO** Go to C

449

## C. Are any of the following present?

- Recent trauma and unexpected swelling
- History of kidney disease
- Swelling and fever with no other related symptoms
- Swelling in child <3 months old
- Ankle swelling and increased difficulty breathing at night when lying flat
- History of heart disease
- Persistent swelling
- Swelling in groin or abdomen disappears with pressure or enlarges with coughing
- Persistent swelling in armpit, neck, or groin

**YES** "Seek medical care within 24 hours"

**NO** Go to D

## D. Are any of the following present?

- Intermittent recurring swelling of ankles and fingers
- Swelling interferes with activity
- Recent weight gain >5 pounds and no change in dietary or activity habits
- Swelling occurs 1 to 2 weeks before menstruation or at end of the day
- Swelling goes down after removing restrictive clothing
- High intake of salty foods or soda

**YES** "Call back or call PCP for appointment if no improvement"
and
Follow **Home Care Instructions**

**NO** Follow **Home Care Instructions**

S

# Home Care Instructions
## Swelling

- Reduce salt in the diet.
- Increase exercise, and avoid prolonged sitting or standing.
- Elevate legs at end of the day.
- Avoid restrictive clothing.
- Avoid crossing legs when sitting.
- Avoid wearing rings if fingers frequently swell.

## Additional Instructions

_____

_____

_____

### Report the Following Problem to Your PCP/Clinic/ED

- Condition persists or worsens

### Seek Emergency Care Immediately If Any of the Following Occur

- Severe respiratory difficulty, wheezing, or cough
- Swollen tongue or swelling at back of throat
- Rapid progression of swelling
- Coughing up frothy, pink-tinged sputum

If the caller agrees with the advice given, document the call and encourage the caller to call back or see PCP if the problem worsens. If the caller does not agree with the advice given, reevaluate and advise the caller to follow up with PCP, Clinic, or ED.

# Swine Flu (H1N1 Virus) Exposure

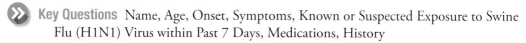 **Key Questions** Name, Age, Onset, Symptoms, Known or Suspected Exposure to Swine Flu (H1N1) Virus within Past 7 Days, Medications, History

**Other Protocols to Consider** Breathing Problems (68); Common Cold Symptoms (103); Congestion (110); Cough (121); Dehydration (132); Fever (184); Headache (238); Influenza (276); Rash (366); Sore Throat (420).

> *Nurse Alert:* Use this protocol if diagnosed with Swine Flu, known or suspected exposure to Swine Flu (H1N1) virus within past 7 days.

*Reminder:* Document caller response to advice, home care instructions, and when to call back.

| ASSESSMENT | ACTION |
|---|---|
| **A. Are any of the following present?** | |
| • Confusion, delirium, or difficulty arousing<br>• Severe difficulty breathing for reasons other than congestion<br>• Flat purple or dark red spots on the face or trunk, fever, stiff or painful neck, or headache<br>• Severe headache<br>• Skin or lips turn blue or gray<br>• Profuse sweating and light-headedness or weakness | **YES** "Call ambulance" or "Seek emergency care now"<br><br>**NO** Go to B |
| **B. Are any of the following present?** | |
| • Weakened immune system, diabetes, or bedridden and fever >101°F (38.3°C)<br>• Infant <3 months old and fever >100.4°F (38°C)<br>• Fever in a child who appears very ill, lethargic, or irritable<br>• Signs of dehydration in a young child, or persons who have a weakened immune system<br>• Age <6 weeks | **YES** "Seek medical care immediately"<br><br>**NO** Go to C |

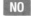

## C. Known exposure and are any of the following present?

- Fatigue, fever <103.1°F (39.5°C), dry cough, sore throat, GI symptoms, runny nose or congestion, muscle aches
- Child with fever >104.9°F (40.5°C)
- History of a weakened immune system, age 6 weeks to 23 months pregnant, asthma
- Green, brown, or yellow sputum or nasal discharge >72 hours
- Persistent signs of dehydration after home care
- Sinus pain or pressure
- Persistent earache

**YES**  "Seek medical care within 24 hours"

**NO**  Go to D

## D. Are any of the following present?

- Green, brown, or yellow sputum or nasal discharge >72 hours
- Cough >3 weeks
- Mild symptoms
- No symptoms but parent or person concerned about exposure to the swine flu virus
- Exposure to swine flu >7 days and no respiratory symptoms

**YES**  "Call back or call PCP for appointment if no improvement"
and
Follow **Home Care Instructions**

**NO**  Follow **Home Care Instructions**

## Home Care Instructions
## Swine Flu (H1N1 Virus) Exposure

- Wash hands frequently with soap and water or alcohol-based hand rubs.
- Reinforce that swine flu virus is highly contagious. Maintain good respiratory etiquette; cover the mouth and nose with a tissue when coughing or sneezing.
- Avoid contact with sick individuals.
- If sick, avoid contact with other people. Stay home for 24 hours after last fever (except for doctor appointments).
- Get a lot of rest and drink plenty of fluids.
- Take your usual pain reliever for fever or discomfort. Do not give aspirin to a child. Avoid aspirin-like products if age <20 years. Avoid acetaminophen if liver disease is present. Avoid ibuprofen if kidney disease or stomach problems exist or in the case of pregnancy. Follow the directions on the label.
- Consider antiviral medications to prevent or treat swine flu virus: oseltamivir (Tamiflu) and zanamivir (Relenza).
- Remember that the virus enters the body through the mouth and nose and can be contracted anywhere. Prevent the growth and spread of the virus whether or not you have symptoms by:
  - Resisting touching of the face as much as possible except for bathing and eating
  - Practicing frequent hand washing
  - If age >8 years, may gargle twice a day with warm salt water or Listerine to help prevent the growth of the virus in the mouth
  - Cleaning the nostrils once a day with warm salt water. Blow the nose, then swab both nostrils with warm salt water
  - Boosting immunity by consuming foods rich in vitamin C (such as citrus fruits)
  - Drinking plenty of warm fluids to help flush the virus from the throat into the stomach where the virus cannot survive

## Additional Instructions

### Report the Following Problems to Your PCP/Clinic/ED

- Persistent fever >103.1°F (39.5°C) and unresponsive to home care measures
- Fever in a child who appears very ill, lethargic, or irritable
- Signs of dehydration

### Seek Emergency Care If Any of the Following Occur

- Flat purple or dark red spots on the face or trunk, fever, headache, or stiff or painful neck
- Skin or lips turn blue or gray
- Profuse sweating and light-headedness or weakness
- Confusion, delirium, or difficulty arousing person
- Severe difficulty breathing for reasons other than congestion

If the caller agrees with the advice given, document the call and encourage the caller to call back or see PCP if the problem worsens. If the caller does not agree with the advice given, reevaluate and advise the caller to follow up with PCP, Clinic, or ED.

# Tattoo Problems

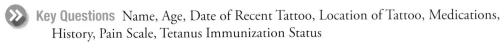 **Key Questions**  Name, Age, Date of Recent Tattoo, Location of Tattoo, Medications, History, Pain Scale, Tetanus Immunization Status

**Other Protocols to Consider**  Abrasions (7); Laceration (290); Piercing Problems (338); Wound Healing and Infection (509).

*Reminder:* Document caller response to advice, home care instructions, and when to call back.

| ASSESSMENT | ACTION |
| --- | --- |

### A. Are any of the following present?

- Rapid swelling of tongue or throat
- Difficulty swallowing or breathing
- Inability to speak

**YES** "Call ambulance"

**NO** Go to B

### B. Are any of the following present?

- Swelling and area below tattoo is cool, clammy, or painful
- Faintness or dizziness
- Rapid joint swelling near site of tattoo
- Diabetic or weakened immune system and signs of infection: pain, swelling, drainage, warmth, or red streaks extending from the tattoo
- Sudden onset of hoarseness
- Recent tattoo and pain at wound site, muscle spasms, stiff jaw and neck, or difficulty swallowing or opening mouth

**YES** "Seek emergency care now"

**NO** Go to C

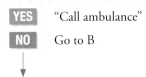

## C. Are any of the following present?

- New tattoo and chills, feeling ill, or headache
- No improvement with home care measures
- Wound <24 hours old and tetanus immunization >5 years
- Signs of infection
- Persistent bleeding after 24 hours and unresponsive to home care measures
- Swollen lymph nodes near the tattoo: neck, armpit, or groin
- Blistering around the tattoo
- Temperature >100.4°F (38°C)

**YES** "Seek medical care within 24 hours"

**NO** Go to D

## D. Are any of the following present?

- Itching around the tattoo edges
- Painless bumps around the tattoo
- Desire to have tattoo removed and requests referral to a health-care provider

**YES** "Call back or call PCP for appointment if no improvement"
and
Follow **Home Care Instructions**

**NO** Follow **Home Care Instructions**

T

## Home Care Instructions
## Tattoo Problems

- Stop bleeding by applying direct pressure to the area.
- Apply a cold pack (in 20-minute intervals) to reduce swelling, bruising, or itching. Do not put ice directly on the skin; place a cloth barrier between ice and the skin.
- Remove the bandage after 24 hours and apply antibiotic ointment (Triple Antibiotic Ointment or bacitracin). Replace with a nonstick bandage if the wound becomes dirty or irritated by clothing. Replace with a clean bandage daily and change if it gets wet.
  - If the bandage sticks to the tattoo, hold it under running water and gently remove the bandage.
- Keep the skin clean. Do not rub. Avoid strong soaps, detergents, or other chemicals. Pat dry after cleaning. Check the tattoo daily during the healing period for signs of infection.
  - Some clear, yellow, or blood-tinged drainage is normal. Report signs of infection: redness, swelling, foul drainage, red streaks, warm to touch, or increased pain.
- Leave the tattoo open to the air whenever possible during the healing period.
- Apply moisturizer several times a day and avoid sun exposure.
- Avoid hot tubs or pools for 14 days.
- Take an antihistamine (Benadryl or Chlor-Trimeton) if hives or itching is present. Follow the instructions on the label.
- Take your usual pain medication. Do not give aspirin to a child. Avoid aspirin-like products if age <20 years. Avoid acetaminophen if liver disease is present. Avoid ibuprofen if kidney disease or stomach problems exist or in the case of pregnancy. Follow the directions on the label.
- Allow up to 2 weeks for healing.
- If you are scheduled for an MRI, inform the radiologist or technician that you have a tattoo and indicate the location and colors. Some tattoos can distort imaging or react to the MRI.

## Additional Instructions

## Report the Following Problems to Your PCP/Clinic/ED

- Headache, muscle aches, general ill feeling, or fever
- No improvement or condition worsens
- Temperature >100.4°F (38°C)
- Signs of infection

## Seek Emergency Care Immediately If Any of the Following Occur

- Swelling and area below tattoo is cool, clammy, or painful
- Rapid joint swelling near the site of the tattoo
- Painful site, muscle spasms, stiff jaw and neck, or difficulty swallowing or opening mouth

If the caller agrees with the advice given, document the call and encourage the caller to call back or see PCP if the problem worsens. If the caller does not agree with the advice given, reevaluate and advise the caller to follow up with PCP, Clinic, or ED.

# Teething

 **Key Questions**  Name, Age, Onset, Medications, History

 **Other Protocols to Consider**  Crying, Excessive, in Infants (128); Earache, Drainage (150); Fever (184).

*Reminder:*  Document caller response to advice, home care instructions, and when to call back.

| ASSESSMENT | ACTION |
|---|---|
| **A. In addition to drooling, chewing, swollen and bruised gums, are any of the following present?** | |
| • Excessive irritability, intermittent lethargy, and high fever <br> • Constant crying >2 hours and unrelated to colic <br> • Persistent high fever <br> • Child appears ill | **YES** "Seek medical care within 2 to 4 hours" <br><br> **NO** Go to B |
| **B. Are any of the following present?** | |
| • Fussiness >2 days <br> • Crying interferes with child's sleep <br> • Child pulling on ears | **YES** "Seek medical care within 24 hours" <br><br> **NO** Go to C |
| **C. Are any of the following present?** | |
| • Teething, gums are red and swollen, and child is 4 to 8 months old <br> • Temperature <101°F (38.3°C) <br> • Poor appetite | **YES** "Call back or call PCP for appointment if no improvement" <br> and <br> Follow **Home Care Instructions** <br><br> **NO** Follow **Home Care Instructions** |

460

# Home Care Instructions
# Teething

- Massage the swollen or irritated gum with finger for 2 minutes.
- Give acetaminophen for discomfort. Do not give aspirin to a child. Avoid aspirin-like products if age <20 years. Avoid acetaminophen if liver disease is present. Avoid ibuprofen if kidney disease or stomach problems exist. Follow the directions on the label.
- Provide a cold teething ring, chilled banana, or chilled bagel for infant to chew.
- Avoid salty or acidic foods.
- Avoid teething gels with benzocaine, which may numb the throat and cause choking or a drug reaction.
- Remember that infants 3 to 8 months of age may have symptoms of teething (drooling, chewing) when not actually teething.
- Discuss teething remedies with PCP if no tooth or gum swelling is observed.

## Additional Instructions

_____

_____

_____

## Report the Following Problems to Your PCP/Clinic/ED

- Excessive irritability, intermittent lethargy, and high fever
- Constant crying >2 hours
- Persistent high fever
- Infant stops eating

If the caller agrees with the advice given, document the call and encourage the caller to call back or see PCP if the problem worsens. If the caller does not agree with the advice given, reevaluate and advise the caller to follow up with PCP, Clinic, or ED.

# Tongue Problems

 **Key Questions**  Name, Age, Onset, Cause, Allergies, Medications, History, Pain Scale

 **Other Protocols to Consider**  Allergic Reaction (13); Mouth Problems (302); Piercing Problems (338); Sore Throat (420); Swallowing Difficulty (442); Toothache (465).

*Reminder:*  Document caller response to advice, home care instructions, and when to call back.

| ASSESSMENT | ACTION |
|---|---|
| **A. Is the following present?** | |
| ● Sudden onset of tongue swelling and difficulty breathing | **YES** "Call ambulance" <br> **NO** Go to B |
| **B. Are any of the following present?** | |
| ● Sudden onset of tongue swelling and no difficulty breathing <br> ● Pain, swelling, drainage around piercing <br> ● Gaping laceration from torn piercing | **YES** "Seek medical care within 2 to 4 hours" <br> **NO** Go to C |
| **C. Are any of the following present?** | |
| ● Pain after taking a new medication <br> ● Pain on one side of face <br> ● Persistent hard lump on tongue or mouth <br> ● Persistent pain and diarrhea with loose, foul-smelling, bulky stools <br> ● Ulcers, cracks, redness, and persistent pain unresponsive to >3 days of home care measures <br> ● Minor tear from piercing and last tetanus shot >5 years <br> ● White patches on tongue, gums, or inner cheeks | **YES** "Seek medical care within 24 hours" <br> **NO** Go to D |

## D. Are any of the following present?

- Tongue bright red and swollen
- Red tip and edges
- Tongue appears hairy
- Ulcers
- Sore on one area of tongue
- Tongue appears black from Pepto-Bismol
- Irritation from rough tooth or braces

**YES**  "Call back or call PCP for appointment if no improvement" and Follow **Home Care Instructions**

**NO**  Follow **Home Care Instructions**

T

## Home Care Instructions
## Tongue Problems

- Drink through a straw to minimize discomfort.
- Note relationship between certain foods and tongue pain and avoid those foods in the diet. Alcohol, hot food or spices, tobacco, chocolate, citrus foods, vinegar, pickles, salted nuts, and chips may irritate the tongue. Milk, gelatin, yogurt, ice cream, and custard are soothing to the tongue.
- Rinse mouth 4 times a day with a salt or baking soda solution. Add ½ tsp salt or baking soda to 8 ounces of water.
- If irritation is caused by a rough tooth or braces, contact your dentist.
- If swelling is related to medication, discontinue use and contact PCP if it is a prescription medication.
- Increase fluid intake.

### Additional Instructions

_____

_____

_____

### Report the Following Problems to Your PCP/Clinic/ED

- No improvement or condition worsens after 3 days of home care measures
- Pain becomes intolerable
- Fever, rash, facial swelling

### Seek Emergency Care Immediately If Any of the Following Occur

- Difficulty breathing
- Swelling of the back of the mouth

If the caller agrees with the advice given, document the call and encourage the caller to call back or see PCP if the problem worsens. If the caller does not agree with the advice given, reevaluate and advise the caller to follow up with PCP, Clinic, or ED.

# Toothache

>> **Key Questions** Name, Age, Onset, Cause, Allergies, Medications, History. If injury occurred, see Tooth Injury protocol (468).

>> **Other Protocols to Consider** Chest Pain (85); Facial Problems (172); Mouth Problems (302); Teething (460); Tooth Injury (468).

*Reminder:* Document caller response to advice, home care instructions, and when to call back.

| ASSESSMENT | ACTION |
|---|---|
| **A. Is the following present?** | |
| • Gnawing pain in lower teeth and neck, chest, shoulder, or arm | **YES** "Seek emergency care now" <br> **NO** Go to B |
| **B. Are any of the following present?** | |
| • History of cardiac problems or diabetes and jaw pain (no known injury or dental problem) <br> • Temperature >100.4°F (38.0°C) | **YES** "Seek medical care within 2 hours" <br> **NO** Go to C |
| **C. Are any of the following present?** | |
| • Persistent pain and swelling over upper or lower jaw <br> • Drainage from dental abscess <br> • Broken tooth (nontraumatic) | **YES** "Seek dental care within 24 hours" <br> **NO** Go to C |

## D. Are any of the following present?

- Pain interferes with daily activities
- Red, swollen, bleeding gums
- Pain when biting food for several days
- Recent filling and pain for several days
- History of problems with same tooth (previous break or crack, hot or cold sensitivity)
- Pain without trauma, fracture, fever, or facial swelling
- Sores in mouth
- Tooth loose, chipped, or decayed
- Pain during or just after eating

 **YES**    "Call back or call dentist for appointment if no improvement"
and
Follow **Home Care Instructions**

Follow **Home Care Instructions**

## Home Care Instructions
## Toothache

- Apply ice pack for 20 minutes, 4 times a day, to reduce swelling.
- Take your usual pain medication (acetaminophen, ibuprofen) for discomfort. Do not give aspirin to a child. Avoid aspirin-like products if age <20 years. Avoid acetaminophen if liver disease is present. Avoid ibuprofen if kidney disease or stomach problems exist or in the case of pregnancy. Follow the directions on the label.
- Rinse mouth with ½ tsp baking soda or salt in a cup of warm water several times a day if sores are present.
- Brush teeth at least twice a day.
- Call a dentist for an appointment.

T

## Additional Instructions

_____

_____

_____

### Report the Following Problems to Your Dentist/PCP/Clinic

- Persistent pain unresponsive to pain medication
- Facial swelling
- Fever
- Drainage from dental abscess

### Seek Emergency Care Immediately If Any of the Following Occur

- Pain in chest, shoulder, or arms
- Gnawing pain in lower teeth and neck

If the caller agrees with the advice given, document the call and encourage the caller to call back or see PCP if the problem worsens. If the caller does not agree with the advice given, reevaluate and advise the caller to follow up with PCP, Clinic, or ED.

# Tooth Injury

 **Key Questions**  Name, Age, Onset, Cause, Allergies, Medications, History

 **Other Protocols to Consider**  Back/Neck Injury (31); Mouth Problems (302); Toothache (465).

> *Nurse Alert:* If the tooth has been knocked out, timing is critical because the success rate of reimplantation decreases significantly after 60 minutes. See home care instructions (470) for specific directions to help save the tooth.

*Reminder:*  Document caller response to advice, home care instructions, and when to call back.

| ASSESSMENT | ACTION |
|---|---|
| **A. Are any of the following present?**<br><br>• Altered mental status<br>• Severe neck pain<br>• Numbness or tingling in arms or legs | **YES**  "Call ambulance"<br><br>**NO**  Go to B |
| **B. Are any of the following present?**<br><br>• Tooth (or teeth) knocked out<br>• Tooth or teeth loose and about to fall out<br>• Tooth repositioned<br>• Unable to stop bleeding with pressure | **YES**  "Seek dental or emergency care now"<br>and<br>Follow **Home Care Instructions**<br><br>**NO**  Go to C |
| **C. After a traumatic injury to teeth, are any of the following present?**<br><br>• Severe pain and swelling over affected area<br>• Loose tooth or teeth<br>• Tooth fractured through crown or to gum line<br>• Painful cracked or chipped tooth<br>• Frenum tear or laceration<br>• Severe jaw pain | **YES**  "Seek dental or medical care within 2 to 4 hours"<br><br>**NO**  Go to D |

## D. Are any of the following present?

- Lacerated gum, cheek, or lip
- Painless cracked or chipped tooth

**YES** "Call back or call dentist for appointment if no improvement"
and
Follow **Home Care Instructions**

**NO** Follow **Home Care Instructions**

T

## Home Care Instructions
## Tooth Injury

- Find tooth, rinse gently with saliva, milk, or nonchlorinated bottle water and replace in socket as quickly as possible. Do not remove material adhered to tooth. Do not scrub tooth. Bite down on gauze pad or other material to help keep tooth in place.
- If unable to replace tooth in socket, place tooth in a cup with ¼ tsp salt and 1 cup of milk. May place tooth under tongue if victim is alert and not a young child. Child must be able to comprehend why it is important to keep tooth segment under the tongue so that there is no chance of swallowing tooth. If neither option is feasible, place the tooth in a cup and keep moist with the child's saliva and transport to dentist or emergency department.
- Bite down on a folded gauze dressing to control bleeding.
- Call dentist.
- Take your usual pain medication (acetaminophen, ibuprofen) for discomfort. Do not give aspirin to a child. Avoid aspirin-like products if age <20 years. Avoid acetaminophen if liver disease is present. Avoid ibuprofen if kidney disease or stomach problems exist or in the case of pregnancy. Follow the directions on the label. Use the dosing device that comes with the medication, a measuring device, or a medicine syringe from the pharmacy. Household teaspoons often do not give the correct amount of medication.
- Apply ice (in 20-minute intervals) to injured gum as tolerated to help control pain.

## Additional Instructions

_____

_____

_____

## Report the Following Problem to Your Dentist/PCP/Clinic
- Persistent bleeding, swelling, or pain

If the caller agrees with the advice given, document the call and encourage the caller to call back or see PCP if the problem worsens. If the caller does not agree with the advice given, reevaluate and advise the caller to follow up with PCP, Clinic, or ED.

# Umbilical Cord Care

>> **Key Questions**  Name, Age, History

>> **Other Protocols to Consider**  Newborn Problems (315); Wound Healing and Infection (509).

*Reminder:*  Document caller response to advice, home care instructions, and when to call back.

| ASSESSMENT | ACTION |
|---|---|

### A. Are any of the following present?

- Temperature <97.5°F (36.4°C) or >100.4°F (38°C)
- Signs of infection around the umbilicus: redness, pain, swelling, foul-smelling drainage, red streaks, or warmth
- Pain, vomiting, and bulging umbilicus

**YES** "Seek medical care within 2 to 4 hours"

**NO** Go to B

### B. Are any of the following present?

- Tissue in navel looks abnormal
- Bleeding longer than 3 days after cord detachment
- Moist navel after 2 days of treatment

**YES** "Seek medical care within 2 to 4 hours"

**NO** Go to C

### C. Are any of the following present?

- Newly discovered bulging umbilicus when infant cries
- Small amount of bleeding (a few drops) or discharge after cord detachment
- Cord has not fallen off within 1 month

**YES** "Call back or call PCP for appointment if no improvement" and Follow **Home Care Instructions**

**NO** Follow **Home Care Instructions**

## Home Care Instructions
## Umbilical Cord Care

- Keep the cord and surrounding area clean and dry. Do not apply alcohol to the cord. Only sponge bathe until the cord falls off.
- Keep diapers and plastic pants below umbilicus.
- Remember that the cord usually falls off in 1 to 3 weeks and a small amount of oozing blood is to be expected.
- Remember that it is common for the umbilicus to bulge when the infant cries or strains. This type of hernia will resolve with time.
- Leave the cord open to air as much as possible.
- Do not use ointments or powders on the cord.

## Additional Instructions

## Report the Following Problems to Your PCP/Clinic/ED

- Bleeding longer than 3 days after cord detachment
- Moist navel after 2 days of treatment
- Cord still attached after 3 weeks
- Condition persists or worsens
- Signs of infection inside the umbilicus

If the caller agrees with the advice given, document the call and encourage the caller to call back or see PCP if the problem worsens. If the caller does not agree with the advice given, reevaluate and advise the caller to follow up with PCP, Clinic, or ED.

# Urination, Difficult

**Key Questions**  Name, Age, Onset, Cause, Medications, History, Pain Scale

**Other Protocols to Consider**  Abdominal Pain (1); Genital Lesions (226); Urination, Painful (477); Urine, Abnormal Color (480); Urine, Incontinence (482).

*Reminder:*  Document caller response to advice, home care instructions, and when to call back.

| ASSESSMENT | ACTION |
|---|---|
| **A. Are any of the following present?** | |
| • Severe abdominal pain and inability to void >8 hours<br>• Severe abdominal pain and temperature >102°F (39°C) | **YES** "Seek emergency care"<br>**NO** Go to B |
| **B. Are any of the following present?** | |
| • Full bladder and inability to urinate >4 hours<br>• Persistent flank or low abdominal pain<br>• History of renal disease<br>• Recent urinary tract or abdominal surgery<br>• Large amount of blood in urine<br>• Recent trauma<br>• Recent back injury | **YES** "Seek medical care within 2 to 4 hours"<br>**NO** Go to C |
| **C. Are any of the following present?** | |
| • Nausea, vomiting, diarrhea<br>• Genital herpes<br>• Painful, red, and irritated perineal area<br>• Difficulty urinating after sexual activity<br>• Decreased fluid intake, excessive sweating, dark yellow or orange urine<br>• Mild discomfort<br>• New-onset incontinence<br>• Fever >102°F (39°C)<br>• Difficulty starting urination | **YES** "Call back or call PCP for appointment if no improvement"<br>and<br>Follow **Home Care Instructions**<br><br>**NO** Follow **Home Care Instructions** |

U

## Home Care Instructions
## Urination, Difficult

- Drink at least six to eight 8-ounce glasses of water a day (unless physician has ordered a fluid-restricted regimen).
- For retention problems, try urinating in a warm bath.
- For genital herpes, apply cold compresses to perineal area.
- For difficulty starting to urinate, turn on water faucet (sound of running water can help to stimulate urination), and pour warm water over perineum while sitting on toilet.

## Additional Instructions

_____

_____

_____

### Report the Following Problems to Your PCP/Clinic/ED

- Severe flank or abdominal pain
- Persistent inability to empty bladder for >12 hours
- Signs of dehydration: sunken eyes, loss of skin elasticity, excessive thirst, dry mouth or mucous membranes, infant crying without tears
- Severe nausea, vomiting, or diarrhea
- Blood in urine

### Seek Emergency Care Immediately If the Following Occur

- Severe abdominal pain and inability to void for >8 hours, or temperature >102°F (39°C)

If the caller agrees with the advice given, document the call and encourage the caller to call back or see PCP if the problem worsens. If the caller does not agree with the advice given, reevaluate and advise the caller to follow up with PCP, Clinic, or ED.

# Urination, Excessive

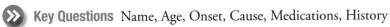

>> **Key Questions**  Name, Age, Onset, Cause, Medications, History

>> **Other Protocols to Consider**  Abdominal Pain (1); Back Pain (34); Dehydration (132);
Diabetes Problems (138); Urine, Incontinence (482).

*Reminder:*  Document caller response to advice, home care instructions, and when to call back.

| ASSESSMENT | ACTION |
|---|---|
| **A. Are any of the following present?** | |
| • Diabetic and urination greater than usual<br>• Signs of dehydration<br>  • sunken eyes or fontanelles<br>  • loose, dry skin that does not spring back when pinched<br>  • excessive thirst, dry mouth, or dry mucous membranes<br>  • crying without tears<br>• Excessive thirst | **YES** "Seek medical care within 2 to 4 hours"<br><br>**NO** Go to B |
| **B. Are any of the following present?** | |
| • History of kidney disorder<br>• Flank or back pain<br>• Abdominal pain<br>• History of parathyroid tumor or disorder<br>• Muscle cramps or weakness | **YES** "Seek medical care within 2 to 4 hours"<br><br>**NO** Go to C |
| **C. Are any of the following present?** | |
| • Increased fluid intake, especially tea, coffee, alcohol<br>• Increased stress<br>• Taking a diuretic medication (prescribed, OTC, or herbal) | **YES** "Call back or call PCP for appointment if no improvement"<br>and<br>Follow **Home Care Instructions**<br><br>**NO** Follow **Home Care Instructions** |

U

## Home Care Instructions
## Urination, Excessive

- Observe for signs of dehydration.
- Drink fluids such as electrolyte solutions without caffeine.
- If no other physical symptoms, observe for worsening of condition or new symptoms.
- If diabetic, closely monitor blood glucose levels.

**Additional Instructions**

## Report the Following Problems to Your PCP/Clinic/ED

- No improvement in 3 days or condition worsens
- Persistent fever unresponsive to fever-reducing measures
- Vomiting, diarrhea, fatigue, lethargy, or stiff neck
- Fever or swelling

If the caller agrees with the advice given, document the call and encourage the caller to call back or see PCP if the problem worsens. If the caller does not agree with the advice given, reevaluate and advise the caller to follow up with PCP, Clinic, or ED.

# Urination, Painful

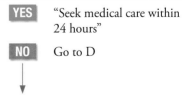

>> **Key Questions**  Name, Age, Onset, Allergies, Medications, History, Pain Scale

>> **Other Protocols to Consider**  Abdominal Pain (1); Urination, Difficult (473); Urine, Abnormal Color (480); Urine, Incontinence (482).

***Reminder:***  Document caller response to advice, home care instructions, and when to call back.

| ASSESSMENT | ACTION |
|---|---|
| **A. Are any of the following present?** | |
| • Inability to urinate <br> • Large amount of red blood in urine <br> • Back, flank, or abdominal pain and inability to urinate for >8 hours | **YES** "Seek medical care immediately" <br><br> **NO** Go to B |
| **B. Are any of the following present?** | |
| • Recent urinary tract surgery and unexpected pain or fever <br> • Recent trauma to genitalia or abdomen <br> • Use of blood-thinning medications and urine is pink or red <br> • Severe discomfort with urination <br> • Back or flank pain <br> • Fever >102°F (39°C) <br> • Severe scrotal pain or swelling <br> • Pregnancy <br> • History of lupus, glomerulonephritis, or single kidney <br> • Perineal or rectal pain <br> • Back or flank pain and fever >100.5°F (38.1°C) <br> • Inability to urinate for >4 hours | **YES** "Seek medical care within 2 to 4 hours" <br><br> **NO** Go to C |
| **C. Are any of the following present?** | |
| • Penile discharge <br> • Cloudy or foul-smelling urine <br> • Vomiting or poor fluid intake <br> • Urgency or frequency for >3 days <br> • Pain over bladder <br> • New onset of bed-wetting or daytime wetting | **YES** "Seek medical care within 24 hours" <br><br> **NO** Go to D |

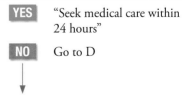

477

## D. Are any of the following present?

- Increased pain at end of urination
- Recurrent urinary tract infections
- Painful urination after sexual contact
- Frequent bubble baths or soap residue on genital area (particularly in young girls)
- Urgency or frequency of <3 days

**YES**  "Call back or call PCP for appointment if no improvement"
and
Follow **Home Care Instructions**

**NO**  Follow **Home Care Instructions**

# Home Care Instructions
# Urination, Painful

- Drink lots of fluids, especially cranberry juice.
- Avoid caffeine and alcohol.
- Urinate before and after intercourse or sexual contact.
- Wipe the perineal area from front to back.
- Wear cotton underwear.
- Avoid wearing panty hose for long periods of time.
- Young girls should avoid frequent bubble baths and wash the perineum with water only. May also soak in a tub with warm water and ¼ cup baking soda twice a day for 2 days.
- After puberty, for irritated and sore perineum, add ½ cup white vinegar to bath and soak for 20 minutes. Repeat in 2 hours and again in 12 hours.
- Take your usual pain medication (acetaminophen, ibuprofen) for discomfort. Do not give aspirin to a child. Avoid aspirin-like products if age <20 years. Avoid acetaminophen if liver disease is present. Avoid ibuprofen if kidney disease or stomach problems exist or in the case of pregnancy. Follow the directions on the label.

**U**

## Additional Instructions

_____

_____

_____

### Report the Following Problems to Your PCP/Clinic/ED

- Persistent discomfort or condition worsens after 48 hours of home care or antibiotic therapy
- Fever, back or flank pain
- Increased blood in urine
- Severe scrotal pain or swelling
- Difficulty urinating

If the caller agrees with the advice given, document the call and encourage the caller to call back or see PCP if the problem worsens. If the caller does not agree with the advice given, reevaluate and advise the caller to follow up with PCP, Clinic, or ED.

# Urine, Abnormal Color

 **Key Questions** Name, Age, Onset, Medications, History

 **Other Protocols to Consider** Abdominal Pain (1); Dehydration (132); Urination, Painful (477); Urine, Incontinence (482).

***Reminder:*** Document caller response to advice, home care instructions, and when to call back.

| ASSESSMENT | ACTION |
|---|---|
| **A. Are any of the following present?** | |
| • Pink, red, or smoky brown urine and recent trauma to back or abdomen or severe pain | **YES** "Seek medical care within 2 to 4 hours" |
| • Fever and flank or back pain | |
| • Urinary stent present and severe pain or large amount of bright red blood | **NO** Go to B |
| **B. Are any of the following present?** | |
| • Recent onset of dark brown urine, pale stools, and yellow skin and eyes | **YES** "Seek medical care within 2 to 4 hours" |
| • Blood in urine with or without pain | **NO** Go to C |
| **C. Are any of the following present?** | |
| • Dark yellow or orange urine and | **YES** "Call back or call PCP for appointment if no improvement" and Follow **Home Care Instructions** |
|   • nausea | |
|   • vomiting | |
|   • diarrhea | |
|   • fever | |
|   • exposure to a hot climate | |
|   • decreased fluid intake | |
|   • decreased urine output | **NO** Follow **Home Care Instructions** |
| • Use of medications that cause urine color changes: phenazopyridine HCl (Pyridium), phenytoin (Dilantin), phenolphthalein, metronidazole (Flagyl), or nitrofurantoin (Furadantin) | |
| • Recent ingestion of rhubarb, beets, blackberries, or other red food | |
| • New prescription | |

# Home Care Instructions
## Urine, Abnormal Color

- Increase fluid intake.
- Avoid foods that may be causing a change in urine color (rhubarb, beets, blackberries, or other red foods) and observe for change in color of urine. Urine should return to normal color within 24 hours.
- If currently taking phenazopyridine HCL (Pyridium) for a urinary tract infection, expect the urine to be red or orange.
- Blue or green urine usually is related to food or medication ingestion.

## Additional Instructions

_____

_____

_____

### Report the Following Problems to Your PCP/Clinic/ED

- Fever, pain with urination, or back pain
- Condition persists >24 hours or worsens after home care measures
- Unexpected color changes after taking a new medication
- Persistent nausea, vomiting, diarrhea, and decreased fluid intake

### Seek Emergency Care Immediately If the Following Occur

- Gross bloody urine and increased abdominal pain after a traumatic blow to the back, side, or abdomen or a fall or an accident

If the caller agrees with the advice given, document the call and encourage the caller to call back or see PCP if the problem worsens. If the caller does not agree with the advice given, reevaluate and advise the caller to follow up with PCP, Clinic, or ED.

# Urine, Incontinence

 **Key Questions**  Name, Age, Onset, Medications, History

 **Other Protocols to Consider**  Bed-Wetting (40); Pregnancy Problems (358); Seizure, Nonfebrile (397); Seizure, Febrile (393); Urination, Difficult (473); Urination, Excessive (475); Urination, Painful (477).

*Reminder:*  Document caller response to advice, home care instructions, and when to call back.

| ASSESSMENT | | ACTION |
|---|---|---|
| **A. Are any of the following present?** | | |
| • History of recent back injury or weakness in legs<br>• Sudden inability to control urination<br>• Postseizure faintness or loss of consciousness | **YES** | "Seek emergency care now" |
| | **NO** | Go to B |
| **B. Are any of the following present?** | | |
| • Signs of urinary tract infection: painful urination, frequency, or urgency<br>• Blood in urine<br>• Abdominal pain | **YES** | "Seek medical care within 24 hours" |
| | **NO** | Go to C |
| **C. Are any of the following present?** | | |
| • Leakage of urine when coughing, sneezing, lifting, straining, laughing, or running<br>• Pregnancy<br>• Obesity<br>• Sensation of heaviness in genitals<br>• Sudden urge to urinate and inability to control urine before making it to the toilet<br>• Difficulty starting urination<br>• Unable to tolerate the problem any longer | **YES** | "Call back or call PCP for appointment if no improvement"<br>and<br>Follow **Home Care Instructions** |
| | **NO** | Follow **Home Care Instructions** |

## Home Care Instructions
## Urine, Incontinence

- Practice exercises to strengthen and tighten muscles supporting the bladder and reproductive organs.
  - Tighten the muscles to stop the flow of urine midstream. Hold for a count of six, then release urine for a count of six. Stop and hold the flow of urine and count to six. Release remaining urine.
  - Practice tightening and releasing the muscles that control urine and the muscles around the anus several times a day while sitting, standing, and walking.
- Drink plenty of fluids, including cranberry juice, to help avoid urinary tract infections.
- Wear a pad or absorbent underpants.
- Observe incidence and frequency of incontinence. Avoid medications, foods, or drinks (such as caffeine or alcohol) that seem to cause or worsen incontinence.

## Additional Instructions

_____

_____

_____

### Report the Following Problems to Your PCP/Clinic/ED

- Condition persists or worsens after practicing exercises for 3 months
- Unable to tolerate the problem any longer
- Signs of urinary tract infection: painful urination, frequency, or urgency
- Blood in urine
- Sudden inability to control urination
- Abdominal pain

If the caller agrees with the advice given, document the call and encourage the caller to call back or see PCP if the problem worsens. If the caller does not agree with the advice given, reevaluate and advise the caller to follow up with PCP, Clinic, or ED.

# Vaginal Bleeding

**Key Questions** Name, Age, Onset, Number of Saturated Pads or Tampons and Size, Medications, History

**Other Protocols to Consider** Abdominal Pain (1); Pregnancy Problems (358); Sexual Assault (400); Vaginal Discharge/Pain/Itching (486).

***Reminder:*** Document caller response to advice, home care instructions, and when to call back.

| ASSESSMENT | ACTION |
|---|---|

### A. Are any of the following present?

- Recent rape or trauma
- Pregnancy >20 weeks and sudden bleeding
- Soaking more than one full-size pad in <1 hour and weakness
- Decreased level of consciousness
- Skin pale and moist
- Sudden unexpected bright red bleeding
- Soaking >2 pads or tampons per hour for >2 hours or >1 pad or tampon per hour for >6 hours

**YES** "Seek emergency care now"

**NO** Go to B

### B. Are any of the following present?

- Pelvic pain with bleeding (different from usual menstrual discomfort)
- Unusually heavy bleeding
- Dizziness or light-headedness when sitting up
- Recent abortion and increased bleeding, pain, or fever

**YES** "Seek medical care within 2 to 4 hours"

**NO** Go to C

### C. Are any of the following present?

- Small amount of bleeding:
  - after intercourse
  - during first 3 months of taking birth control pills or other hormonal contraceptives
  - missed birth control pill mid-cycle
- Bleeding >10 days

**YES** "Call back or call PCP for appointment if no improvement"
and
Follow **Home Care Instructions**

**NO** Follow **Home Care Instructions**

## Home Care Instructions
## Vaginal Bleeding

- Remember that breakthrough bleeding is not unusual at the time of ovulation, during the first 3 months of a regimen of birth control pills or other hormonal contraceptives, or with emotional crisis.
- Change tampons frequently.
- If fever, chills, or muscle aches occur while using tampons, discontinue use and notify PCP if condition persists or worsens.
- If miscarriage is suspected, do not flush toilet; save tissue and clots for physician to examine.

## Additional Instructions

_____

_____

_____

### Report the Following Problems to Your PCP/Clinic/ED

- Bleeding persists or worsens
- Severe abdominal pain
- Fever, chills, or muscle aches
- Passing tissue or large clots

### Seek Emergency Care Immediately If Any of the Following Occur

- Severe pain interferes with activity
- Soaking more than one full-size pad in <1 hour and weakness
- Decreased level of consciousness
- Skin pale and moist
- Soaking >2 pads or tampons per hour for >2 hours or 1 pad or tampon per hour for >6 hours

If the caller agrees with the advice given, document the call and encourage the caller to call back or see PCP if the problem worsens. If the caller does not agree with the advice given, reevaluate and advise the caller to follow up with PCP, Clinic, or ED.

# Vaginal Discharge/Pain/Itching

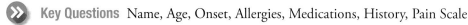

**≫ Key Questions** Name, Age, Onset, Allergies, Medications, History, Pain Scale

**≫ Other Protocols to Consider** Abdominal Pain (1); Fever (184); Genital Lesions (226); Menstrual Problems (299); Sexually Transmitted Infection (STI) (403); Vaginal Bleeding (484).

*Reminder:* Document caller response to advice, home care instructions, and when to call back.

| ASSESSMENT | ACTION |
|---|---|
| **A. Are any of the following present?** | |
| ● Severe pelvic pain interferes with activity<br>● Temperature >102.0°F (38.9°C), increased pain, chills, shakes, or vomiting<br>● Foul-smelling vaginal discharge, pain, or itching and history of recent trauma, rape, surgery, pregnancy, or abortion<br>● Last menstrual period >6 weeks ago, abdominal pain, suspicion of pregnancy | **YES** "Seek medical care within 2 to 4 hours"<br><br>**NO** Go to B |
| **B. Are any of the following present?** | |
| ● Itching interferes with activity<br>● Temperature >100.0°F (37.8°C)<br>● Foul odor and large amount of discharge<br>● Green, brown, or white cottage cheese–like discharge<br>● Exposure to venereal disease or other STI and request for an examination<br>● Painful sores or irritation on labia or vagina<br>● History of one ovary and of child-bearing age<br>● Tampon in place and unable to remove<br>● Possibility of a foreign object causing symptoms | **YES** "Seek medical care within 24 hours"<br><br>**NO** Go to C |

## C. Are any of the following present?

- Frequent use of scented feminine hygiene products
- Pain during or after intercourse
- Small amount of clear, white, or yellow discharge
- Recent prolonged sexual activity
- Concerned about possible STI and no known exposure
- Painless sore on labia or vagina
- Onset of symptoms while on antibiotics
- Exposure to chemicals or bubble bath

**YES** "Call back or call PCP for appointment if no improvement" and Follow **Home Care Instructions**

**NO** Follow **Home Care Instructions**

V

## Home Care Instructions
## Vaginal Discharge/Pain/Itching

- Note how discharge differs from usual discharge and understand that it is important that there might be a need for further investigation.

**For Swelling, Itching, or Irritation**
- Soak in a tub of warm water (avoid scented bubble baths).
- Young girls should avoid frequent bubble baths and wash the perineum with water only. May also soak in a tub with warm water and ¼ cup baking soda twice a day for 2 days.
- After puberty, for irritated and sore perineum, add ½ cup white vinegar to bath and soak for 20 minutes. Repeat in 2 hours and again in 12 hours.
- Wear loose-fitting undergarments and clothing.
- Wear underwear with cotton-lined crotch.
- Avoid scented feminine hygiene products, tampons, sanitary pads, and toilet tissue.
- Apply clotrimazole Gyne-Lotrimin cream to the area. Ask your pharmacist for other OTC product suggestions.
- Apply cool compresses to the area.

**For Discharge**
- Eat yogurt daily to help prevent infection while taking antibiotics.
- Clean the area frequently.

**For Known Infection**
- If sexually active, notify partner of infection and the need for treatment.
- Use a condom during sexual activity to help prevent cross-infection.
- Apply heating pad to abdomen for discomfort.
- Avoid sexual intercourse while symptoms are present or until examined by PCP.

## Additional Instructions

_____

_____

_____

### Report the Following Problems to Your PCP/Clinic/ED
- Temperature >102.0°F (38.9°C), shakes, chills, vomiting, or increased pain
- Symptoms persist >3 days
- Foul odor and large amount of discharge

If the caller agrees with the advice given, document the call and encourage the caller to call back or see PCP if the problem worsens. If the caller does not agree with the advice given, reevaluate and advise the caller to follow up with PCP, Clinic, or ED.

# Vision Problems

 **Key Questions**  Name, Age, Onset, Cause, Medications, History

 **Other Protocols to Consider**  Eye Injury (166); Eye Problems (169); Foreign Body, Eye (201); Neurologic Symptoms (312).

> *Nurse Alert:*
> - If eye injury or foreign body to the eye, use Eye Injury (166) or Foreign Body, Eye (201) protocols.
> - Sudden changes in vision, speech, or mental status; weakness; and numbness may be a sign of a serious neurologic disorder. Prompt treatment may prevent extensive damage to the brain or reduce permanent disability.

*Reminder:*  Document caller response to advice, home care instructions, and when to call back.

| ASSESSMENT | ACTION |
|---|---|
| **A. Are any of the following present?** | |
| • Sudden onset of severe eye pain<br>• Sudden loss of partial or total vision in one or both eyes<br>• Blood or pus in colored part of eye<br>• Pupils of unequal size<br>• History of recent head injury and vision changes<br>• Sudden or gradual increase in number of floaters, light flashes, or curtain over field of vision | **YES** "Seek emergency care now"<br>**NO** Go to B |
| **B. Are any of the following present?** | |
| • Sudden onset of blurred or double vision and eye pain<br>• Pain increases with pressure to the eye or eye movement<br>• Signs of an eye infection: pain, redness, swelling, drainage, or fever | **YES** "Seek medical care within 2 to 4 hours"<br>**NO** Go to C |

## C. Are any of the following present?

- Increased sensitivity to light
- History of flashing lights followed by a headache
- New and sudden onset of flashing lights (has not occurred in the past) preceded by a headache
- Persistent blurred or double vision
- Change in vision after a change in medication

**YES** "Seek medical care within 24 hours"

**NO** Go to D

## D. Are any of the following present?

- Intermittent episodes of blurred vision
- Difficulty seeing distant objects
- Difficulty reading
- Eyes dry and itching

**YES** "Call back or call PCP for appointment if no improvement"
and
Follow **Home Care Instructions**

**NO** Follow **Home Care Instructions**

## Home Care Instructions
## Vision Problems

- If drainage is present and eye infection is suspected, encourage family members to use separate towels and washcloths.
- Avoid rubbing or touching eyes. Wash hands frequently.
- Clean crusting or discharge with a cotton ball moistened in warm water. Discard cotton ball after use. Do not use the same cotton ball for both eyes.
- Instill saline drops in dry, itchy eyes.
- Make an appointment to have eyes checked for difficulty seeing close or distant objects.

## Additional Instructions

_____

_____

_____

V

### Report the Following Problems to Your PCP/Clinic/ED
- Sudden changes in vision
- Signs of infection
- Condition persists or worsens

### Seek Emergency Care Immediately If Any of the Following Occur
- Sudden onset of severe eye pain
- Sudden loss of partial or total vision in one or both eyes
- Pupils of unequal size
- Sudden or gradual increase in number of floaters, light flashes, or curtain over field of vision

If the caller agrees with the advice given, document the call and encourage the caller to call back or see PCP if the problem worsens. If the caller does not agree with the advice given, reevaluate and advise the caller to follow up with PCP, Clinic, or ED.

# Vomiting

 **Key Questions**  Name, Age, Onset, Suspected Cause, History, Medications, Associated Symptoms

 **Other Protocols to Consider**  Abdominal Pain (1); Confusion (107); Constipation (114); Dehydration (132); Diarrhea (143); Fever (184); Food Poisoning, Suspected (194); Headache (238); Head Injury (242); Postoperative Problems (350).

> *Nurse Alert:* There are many conditions that cause vomiting. When vomiting is associated with several other symptoms, use the protocol that is the primary concern and has the highest probability of a referral to a higher level of care.

*Reminder:* Document caller response to advice, home care instructions, and when to call back.

| ASSESSMENT | ACTION |
|---|---|
| **A. Are any of the following present?** | |
| • Altered mental status: listless, unusually irritable, confused <br> • Severe headache, stiff neck, or pain bending head forward <br> • Vomiting bright red blood or dark coffee-grounds–like emesis <br> • Recent head or abdominal injury <br> • Exposure to a poisonous substance (such as medications, plants, cleaning agents, pesticides, or wild mushrooms) <br> • Neonate <1 month of age and/or bulging fontanelle <br> • Abdomen is hard or firm when not crying | **YES** "Seek emergency care now" If poison ingestion is suspected, go to Poisoning, Suspected (347) protocol <br><br> **NO** Go to B |

## B. Are any of the following present?

- Signs of dehydration:
  - decreased urine
  - sunken eyes or fontanelle
  - dry mouth
  - crying without tears
  - unusual listlessness
- Breathing hard or fast
- Persistent or severe intermittent abdominal pain interferes with activity
- Child appears very ill
- History of diabetes and unable to control vomiting with home care measures
- Infant <3 months old and has vomited >2 times or has projectile vomiting

**YES**  "Seek medical care within 2 to 4 hours"

**NO**  Go to C

## C. Are any of the following present?

- Vomiting >12 hours
- Temperature >101°F (38.3°C) for >24 hours
- Vomited >3 times in the last 6 hours
- Persistent diarrhea
- Infant with forceful vomiting after feeding

**YES**  "Seek medical care within 24 hours"

**NO**  Go to D

## D. Are any of the following present?

- Moderate diarrhea or constipation
- History of travel out of the country or a camping trip
- Other household members are ill
- Excessive ingestion of food or fluids
- Recent ingestion of an antibiotic, pain medication, or new medication
- Earache, cold, sore throat, or fever

**YES**  "Call back or call PCP for appointment if no improvement"
and
Follow **Home Care Instructions**

**NO**  Follow **Home Care Instructions**

V

## Home Care Instructions
## Vomiting
### Infants

- Introduce 1 tsp Lytren, Pedialyte, Infalyte, or Kaolectrolyte every 5 to 15 minutes and increase as tolerated.
- If infant drinks juice, introduce 1 tsp every 5 to 15 minutes, then clear liquids as tolerated. Do not give juice if diarrhea is also present.
- If breast-feeding and infant vomits 3 or more times, offer breast for 4 to 5 minutes every 30 to 60 minutes, and offer rehydration fluids between breast-feeds, 1 tsp every 5 to 15 minutes. It should not be necessary to discontinue breast-feeding.
- If using formula, use small, frequent feedings.

### Children

- Avoid eating or drinking for 1 to 2 hours after vomiting.
- Drink 1 tsp every 5 minutes for 4 hours (fruit juice diluted with water, weak tea with sugar, clear broth, gelatin, or flavored ice). After 4 hours without vomiting, the amount of fluids offered may increase.
- Slowly introduce bland foods, such as rice, potatoes, soda cracker, pretzels, dry toast, applesauce, and bananas, as tolerated 8 hours after last emesis.

### Additional Home Care Advice

- Acetaminophen can be given for fever. Do not give aspirin to a child. Avoid aspirin-like products if age <20 years. Avoid acetaminophen if liver disease is present. Avoid ibuprofen if kidney disease or stomach problems exist or in the case of pregnancy. Follow the directions on the label. Use the dosing device that comes with the medication, a measuring device, or a medicine syringe from the pharmacy. Household teaspoons often do not give the correct amount of medication.
- If, after vomiting has subsided, diarrhea is present or continues, follow home care instructions for the treatment of diarrhea. Vomiting should always be treated first.
- Wash hands with soap and water frequently when caring for a child with vomiting and/ or diarrhea.

## Additional Instructions

_____

_____

_____

**Report the Following Problems to Your PCP/Clinic/ED**

- High fever, weakness, or abdominal pain for >2 hours
- No improvement in 48 hours or condition worsens
- Signs of dehydration

 **Seek Emergency Care Immediately If Any of the Following Occur**

- Altered mental status
- Vomiting blood or dark coffee-grounds–like emesis
- Develops a severe headache, stiff neck, or pain bending head forward
- Abdomen becomes hard or firm when not crying

If the caller agrees with the advice given, document the call and encourage the caller to call back or see PCP if the problem worsens. If the caller does not agree with the advice given, reevaluate and advise the caller to follow up with PCP, Clinic, or ED.

# Weakness

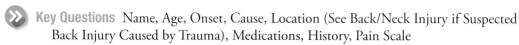 **Key Questions** Name, Age, Onset, Cause, Location (See Back/Neck Injury if Suspected Back Injury Caused by Trauma), Medications, History, Pain Scale

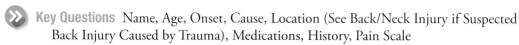 **Other Protocols to Consider** Appetite Loss (21); Back/Neck Injury (31); Back Pain (34); Confusion (107); Extremity Injury (163); Fainting (178); Fatigue (181); Heart Rate Problems (249); Heat Exposure Problems (252); Leg Pain/Swelling (293); Muscle Cramps (307); Neurologic Symptoms (312).

*Nurse Alert:* There are many conditions that can cause weakness. When weakness is associated with several other symptoms, triage with caution and note signs that may be an indication of a more serious condition.

- Sudden changes in vision, speech, or mental status; weakness; and numbness may be signs of a serious neurologic disorder. Prompt treatment may prevent extensive damage to the brain or reduce permanent disability.
- Ask how current condition is different from normal.

*Reminder:* Document caller response to advice, home care instructions, and when to call back.

| ASSESSMENT | ACTION |
|---|---|
| **A. Is chest pain present?** | |
| | **YES** Go to Chest Pain (85) protocol |
| | **NO** Go to B |
| **B. Is there difficulty breathing?** | |
| | **YES** Go to Breathing Problems (68) protocol |
| | **NO** Go to C |

## C. Is there confusion?

| | |
|---|---|
| **YES** | Go to Confusion (107) protocol |
| **NO** | Go to D |

## D. Are any of the following present?

- Inability to stand, walk, or bear weight
- Sudden onset of weakness to one side of the body
- Weakness in face, arm, or leg
- Visual disturbances
- Speech and language problems
- Irregular pulse
- Severe headache

| | |
|---|---|
| **YES** | "Call ambulance" or "Seek emergency care now" |
| **NO** | Go to E |

## E. Are any of the following present?

- Hand or foot cold or blue
- Pain, swelling, warmth, or redness in affected limb
- Severe pain interferes with normal activity

| | |
|---|---|
| **YES** | "Seek medical care within 2 to 4 hours" |
| **NO** | Go to F |

## F. Are any of the following present?

- History of dieting or use of diuretics
- History of blood clots or heart problems
- Gradual onset of numbness, tingling, or burning sensation in extremities
- Pain radiates to arm or leg
- Fever; cough; green, yellow, or brown sputum; body aches for >24 hours and unresponsive to home care measures
- Increasing difficulty with mobility

| | |
|---|---|
| **YES** | "Seek medical care within 24 hours" |
| **NO** | Go to G |

## G. Are any of the following present?

- Occasional weakness
- History of neuromuscular problems that are unresponsive to medication
- Increased exercise, activity level, or stress
- History of muscular pain
- History of eating disorder

| | |
|---|---|
| **YES** | "Call back or call PCP for appointment if no improvement" and Follow **Home Care Instructions** |
| **NO** | Follow **Home Care Instructions** |

W

## Home Care Instructions
## Weakness

- Rest and eat regular meals.
- Apply moist heat to painful swollen area (if known injury, apply ice during the first 24 hours).
- Take your usual pain medication (acetaminophen, ibuprofen). Do not give aspirin to a child. Avoid aspirin-like products if age <20 years. Avoid acetaminophen if liver disease is present. Avoid ibuprofen if kidney disease or stomach problems exist or in the case of pregnancy. Follow the directions on the label.

## Additional Instructions

### Report the Following Problem to Your PCP/Clinic/ED

- No improvement or condition worsens

### Seek Emergency Care Immediately If Any of the Following Occur

- Limb turns cold, numb, or blue
- Sudden change in ability to walk, stand, bear weight, or move
- Weakness in face, arm, or leg
- Visual disturbances
- Speech and language problems

If the caller agrees with the advice given, document the call and encourage the caller to call back or see PCP if the problem worsens. If the caller does not agree with the advice given, reevaluate and advise the caller to follow up with PCP, Clinic, or ED.

# West Nile Virus

>> **Key Questions** Name, Age, Onset, Cause, Medications, Prior History

>> **Other Protocols to Consider** Confusion (107); Fatigue (181); Fever (184); Headache (238); Neck Pain (309); Neurologic Symptoms (312); Numbness and Tingling (325); Rash (366); Weakness (496).

> *Nurse Alert:* Use this protocol only if diagnosed with West Nile virus or if caller has concerns about West Nile virus and signs and symptoms appear 2 to 15 days after known exposure to dead birds or mosquito bites.

*Reminder:* Document caller response to advice, home care instructions, and when to call back.

| ASSESSMENT | ACTION |
|---|---|
| **A. Are any of the following present?** | |
| • Altered mental status <br> • Seizures <br> • Vision loss <br> • Paralysis | **YES** "Call ambulance" <br> **NO** Go to B |
| **B. Are any of the following present?** | |
| • Neck stiffness <br> • High fever >104.9°F (40.5°C) <br> • Nonblanching purple or dark red spots <br> • Shortness of breath | **YES** "Seek emergency care now" <br> **NO** Go to C |
| **C. Are any of the following present?** | |
| • Severe headache <br> • Severe muscle weakness <br> • Numbness <br> • History of immunosuppression | **YES** "Seek medical care immediately" <br> **NO** Go to D |

W

## D. Are any of the following present?

- Body aches
- Nausea/vomiting
- Raised rash on trunk
- Swollen lymph glands
- Fatigue
- Woman currently pregnant or breast-feeding, or baby breast-feeding

**YES** "Seek medical care within 24 hours"

**NO** Go to E

## E. Is the following present?

- No other symptoms but parent or person concerned

**YES** "Call back or call PCP for appointment if no improvement"
and
Follow **Home Care Instructions**

**NO** Follow **Home Care Instructions**

## Home Care Instructions
## West Nile Virus

- Do not touch dead birds with bare hands.
- Call the local health department _____ for directions on how to report and turn over the deceased bird for testing and disposal.
- Reduce risks of West Nile virus by:
  - Applying insect repellent. Do not use insect repellents on babies younger than 2 months. Mosquito netting can be used to cover babies younger than 2 months in carriers, strollers, or cribs to protect them from mosquito bites. Do not use products containing oil of lemon eucalyptus or para-menthane-diol on children younger than 3 years. Do not apply insect repellent onto a child's hands, eyes, mouth, and any cut or irritated skin. If you are also using sunscreen, apply sunscreen first and insect repellent second
  - wearing long-sleeve shirts, long pants, and socks
  - minimizing exposed skin
  - wearing light-colored clothing
  - avoiding being outdoors at peak mosquito-biting times (from dusk to dawn)
  - using screens to cover open doors and windows and repairing or replacing any holes in the screens or ill-fitting screens
  - avoiding standing water by draining objects or areas on your property
  - cleaning clogged rain gutters
- Rest.
- Drink plenty of fluids.
- Take your usual pain medication for discomfort. Do not give aspirin to a child. Avoid aspirin-like products if age <20 years. Avoid acetaminophen if liver disease is present. Avoid ibuprofen if kidney disease or stomach problems exist or in the case of pregnancy. Follow the directions on the label. Use the dosing device that comes with the medication, a measuring device, or a medicine syringe from the pharmacy. Household teaspoons often do not give the correct amount of medication.

**W**

### Additional Instructions

_____

_____

_____

## Report the Following Problems to Your PCP/Clinic/ED

- Severe headache
- Severe muscle weakness
- Numbness
- No improvement or condition worsens

## Seek Emergency Care Immediately If Any of the Following Occur

- Altered mental status
- Neck stiffness
- Seizures
- Vision loss
- Paralysis
- High fever >104.9°F (40.5°C)
- Nonblanching dark red or purple rash

If the caller agrees with the advice given, document the call and encourage the caller to call back or see PCP if the problem worsens. If the caller does not agree with the advice given, reevaluate and advise the caller to follow up with PCP, Clinic, or ED.

# Wheezing

>> **Key Questions** Name, Age, Onset, Medications, History of Intubation, Hospitalizations, History

>> **Other Protocols to Consider** Allergic Reaction (13); Asthma (28); Breathing Problems (68); Congestion (110); Cough (121); Croup (125); Food Allergy, Known or Suspected (192); Hay Fever Problems (235).

> *Nurse Alert:* If known respiratory problems and prescribed inhalers, use $O_2$ saturation meters or peak flow meters (to measure how well air is moving out of the lungs). Assess baseline functioning, $O_2$ saturation level, and % oxygen delivered and method.
> Peak flow values are divided into three zones:
>   Green: 80% of baseline or higher (mild attack)
>   Yellow: 50% to 80% of baseline (moderate attack)
>   Red: <50% of baseline (severe attack)

*Reminder:* Document caller response to advice, home care instructions, and when to call back.

W

| ASSESSMENT | ACTION |
|---|---|

## A. Are any of the following present?

- Severe respiratory distress
- Inability to speak
- Chest retractions
- Aspiration of foreign body
- Blue lips or face
- Severe chest pain
- Sudden-onset wheezing after medication or exposure to known allergen
- Peak flow rate <50% of baseline (if asthmatic)

**YES** "Call ambulance"

**NO** Go to B

**B. Are any of the following present?**

- Unresponsive to medication treatments
- Unresponsive to home care measures
- Must sit up to breathe
- Wheezing similar to prior episodes that required hospitalization or injections
- Speaking in partial sentences
- Peak flow rate 50%–80% of baseline (if asthmatic)
- Neonate <4 weeks of age and fever >100.4°F (38.0°C)

 **YES** "Seek medical care within 2 hours"

**NO** Go to C

**C. Are any of the following present?**

- Peak flow rate >80% of baseline (if asthmatic)
- Green-, yellow-, or rust-colored sputum
- Infant, child with a chronic illness or immunosuppressed

**YES** "Seek medical care within 24 hours"

**NO** Go to D

**D. Are any of the following present?**

- First wheezing episode that resolves in short period of time
- Fever
- Speaking in full sentences

**YES** "Call back or call PCP for appointment if no improvement" and Follow **Home Care Instructions**

**NO** Follow **Home Care Instructions**

## Home Care Instructions
## Wheezing

- Take medication as directed by PCP.
- Use vaporizer with cool mist.
- Identify cause and avoid irritant.

**Additional Instructions**

_____

_____

_____

### Report the Following Problems to Your PCP/Clinic/ED

- Condition worsens
- No improvement with medication

### Seek Emergency Care Immediately If Any of the Following Occur

- Lips or face turn blue
- Fighting for air
- Decreased level of consciousness
- Inability to speak or speaking in short words
- Severe chest pain
- Peak flow rate <50% of baseline (if asthmatic)

If the caller agrees with the advice given, document the call and encourage the caller to call back or see PCP if the problem worsens. If the caller does not agree with the advice given, reevaluate and advise the caller to follow up with PCP, Clinic, or ED.

W

# Wound Care: Sutures or Staples

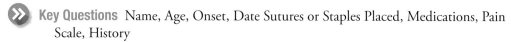

>> **Key Questions**  Name, Age, Onset, Date Sutures or Staples Placed, Medications, Pain Scale, History

>> **Other Protocols to Consider**  Piercing Problems (338); Postoperative Problems (350); Tattoo Problems (456); Wound Healing and Infection (509).

*Reminder:*  Document caller response to advice, home care instructions, and when to call back.

| ASSESSMENT | ACTION |
|---|---|
| **A. Are any of the following present?** | |
| • Altered mental status<br>• Difficulty breathing<br>• Surgical wound split or gaping and large amount of fluid, drainage, or material exposed | **YES** "Call ambulance"<br>or<br>"Seek emergency care now"<br><br>**NO** Go to B |
| **B. Are any of the following present?** | |
| • Rapidly spreading warmth, swelling, or redness around wound<br>• Recent placement of sutures/staples; headache, muscle aches, general ill feeling, or fever<br>• Fever >101.3°F (38.5°C)<br>• Wound splitting open or gaping<br>• Persistent bleeding after >10 minutes of direct pressure<br>• Numbness or swelling distal to incision<br>• Inability to move the joint distal to the incision<br>• Drain slipped from wound<br>• Loose suture or staple <48 hours since placement | **YES** "Seek medical care immediately"<br><br>**NO** Go to C |

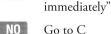

## C. Are any of the following present?

- Persistent incisional pain or discomfort
- Gradual-onset warmth, foul odor, swelling or redness around wound
- Yellow or green drainage and no fever
- History of diabetes, HIV, chronic disease, use of steroids or blood thinners, chemotherapy, and improperly healing wound

**YES**  "Seek medical care within 24 hours"

**NO**  Go to D

## D. Are any of the following present?

- Sutures/staples removed and tender to touch
- Questions about sutures/staples/glue
- Missed removal date
- Loose suture or staple and >48 hours since placement
- Itching around the edges of the wound
- Blisters around the wound

**YES**  "Call back or call PCP for appointment if no improvement"
and
Follow **Home Care Instructions**

**NO**  Follow **Home Care Instructions**

## Home Care Instructions
## Wound Care: Sutures or Staples

- Keep sutured/stapled/glued area clean and dry for at least 24 hours.
- Clean the wound gently with warm water daily and when soiled.
- Watch for signs of infection: warmth, pain, drainage, redness, or red streaks. Check the wound daily.
- Wash hands with soap and water or alcohol-based hand rub before touching the wound or changing the dressing.
- Apply antibiotic ointment to the wound 3 times a day.
- Change dressing when wet or soiled.
- If a suture or staple falls out or glue separates >48 hours after placement, keep the wound closed with tape or a butterfly bandage until ready to have the remaining sutures/staples removed.
- Keep appointment for suture/staple removal.
- Take your usual pain medication for discomfort. Do not give aspirin to a child. Avoid aspirin-like products if age <20 years. Avoid acetaminophen if liver disease is present. Avoid ibuprofen if kidney disease or stomach problems exist or in the case of pregnancy. Follow the directions on the label.
- Avoid bumping or stretching the wound for the first 2 days after suture/staple removal.
- Use sunscreen and avoid direct sun exposure to the healing wound.

## Additional Instructions

_____

_____

_____

### Report the Following Problems to Your PCP/Clinic/ED

- Signs of infection
- Fever
- Persistent bleeding
- Increasing pain
- Wound splits open
- Condition worsens or no improvement

### Seek Emergency Care Immediately If Any of the Following Occur

- Persistent bleeding with direct pressure >10 minutes
- Difficulty breathing
- Large wound splits open and body tissue is exposed
- Surgical wound opens and surgeon cannot be reached

If the caller agrees with the advice given, document the call and encourage the caller to call back or see PCP if the problem worsens. If the caller does not agree with the advice given, reevaluate and advise the caller to follow up with PCP, Clinic, or ED.

# Wound Healing and Infection

>> **Key Questions**  Name, Age, Onset, Recent Surgical Procedure, Sutures or Wound Treatment, Medications, History, Pain Scale, Wound VAC (Vacuum-Assisted Closure) Device Present

>> **Other Protocols to Consider**  Abrasions (7); Bites, Animal/Human (46); Piercing Problems (338); Laceration (290); Postoperative Problems (350); Skin Lesions: Lumps, Bumps, and Sores (414); Wound Care: Sutures or Staples (506); Tattoo Problems (456).

*Reminder:*  Document caller response to advice, home care instructions, and when to call back.

| ASSESSMENT | ACTION |
|---|---|
| **A. Are any of the following present?** | |
| • Gaping, split, jagged, or deep wound <br> • Surgical wound split or gaping, and large amount of fluid, drainage, or material protruding from wound | **YES** "Seek emergency care now" <br> **NO** Go to B |
| **B. Are any of the following present?** | |
| • Surgical wound split or gaping <br> • Healing wound and headache, muscle aches, general ill feeling, or fever <br> • Signs of infection: pain, swelling, drainage, warmth, or red streaks extending from wound <br> • Swollen lymph nodes in neck, armpit, or groin <br> • Wound caused by a bite <br> • Temperature >100.4°F (38°C) <br> • Dirty wound <br> • History of diabetes, HIV, chronic disease, use of steroids or blood thinners, chemotherapy, and a wound not healing well | **YES** "Seek medical care within 2 to 4 hours" <br> **NO** Go to C |

W

## C. Are any of the following present?

- Chills, ill feeling, or headache
- No improvement with home care measures
- Wound <24 hours old and no tetanus immunization or booster >5 years
- Blistering around wound

 **YES** "Seek medical care within 24 hours"

**NO** Go to D

## D. Are any of the following present?

- Itching around wound edges
- Wound VAC in place and concerns about
  - leaking around the tube or edges of the dressing
  - container is full
  - device has been turned off >2 hours

**YES** "Call back or call PCP for appointment if no improvement"
and
Follow **Home Care Instructions**

**NO** Follow **Home Care Instructions**

## Home Care Instructions
## Wound Healing and Infection

- Keep the wound clean and dry.
- Apply dressing if drainage is present.
- Apply moist hot packs for 20 minutes, 4 times a day.
- Check the wound daily for signs of healing.
- If no tetanus immunization or booster in <5 years, contact PCP or clinic for tetanus immunization within 72 hours of injury.
- If the wound is bleeding, lie down and apply pressure over the wound for 10 minutes; if no improvement, contact PCP.
- Monitor temperature.
- For wound VAC problems:
  - If the wound VAC is turned off >2 hours, replace the dressing with wet-to-dry dressing and notify home health (HH) nurse.
  - If the VAC is leaking around the tube or edges of the dressing, remove the VAC dressing and replace with wet-to-dry dressing and notify HH nurse.
  - If the canister is full, replace it and discard it in the garbage as directed by HH nurse.

### For Abscess
- Lanced or unlanced abscess is highly resistant to antibiotics and susceptible to MRSA infections. To prevent infection:
  - wash hands >3 times or more per day when soiled with microbial cleanser
  - shower immediately after activity with hot water as tolerated
  - advise others in close contact to wash their hands with microbial cleanser
  - keep wounds covered with clean, dry bandages, particularly if drainage is present
  - disinfect all towels, sheets, and surfaces in contact with the wound with a solution of 1:100 of household bleach to water or white vinegar
  - wash and dry clothes, linens, and towels in a setting as hot as possible; ensure all items are dry before removing them from the dryer
  - avoid participating in contact sports or skin-to-skin contact with others until the infection has healed
  - use a skin antiseptic to treat MRSA on the skin in combination with antibiotics prescribed by PCP
  - avoid hot tubs
  - do not share bars of soap, razors, towels, or athletic gear
  - call PCP if condition worsens or fails to improve with home care and treatment

W

## Additional Instructions

_____

_____

_____

### Report the Following Problems to Your PCP/Clinic/ED

- Headache, muscle aches, general ill feeling, or fever
- No improvement or condition worsens
- Temperature >100.4°F (38°C)
- Blisters develop

### Seek Emergency Care Immediately If the Following Occur

- Surgical incision opens and surgeon cannot be reached

If the caller agrees with the advice given, document the call and encourage the caller to call back or see PCP if the problem worsens. If the caller does not agree with the advice given, reevaluate and advise the caller to follow up with PCP, Clinic, or ED.

# Zika Virus

>> **Key Questions**  Name, Age, Onset, Cause, Medications, History, Pregnancy Status, Recent Travel to Area where Zika Virus Is Spreading, Recent Mosquito Bites

>> **Other Protocols to Consider**  Fever (184); Headache (238); Numbness and Tingling (325); Rash (366); Weakness (496).

> *Nurse Alert:* Use this protocol only if diagnosed with Zika virus or if caller has concerns about Zika virus and signs and symptoms appear 3 to 14 days after a mosquito bite and known travel to a Zika-infected area or exposure to an infected person through unprotected sex.

*Reminder:*  Document caller response to advice, home care instructions, and when to call back.

| ASSESSMENT | ACTION |
|---|---|
| **A. Are any of the following present?** | |
| • Shortness of breath<br>• Severe muscle weakness<br>• Severe pain<br>• Numbness<br>• History of immunosuppression | **YES** "Seek medical care immediately"<br>**NO** Go to B |
| **B. Are any of the following present?** | |
| • Muscle pain<br>• Headache<br>• Rash<br>• Joint pain<br>• Fever<br>• Red eyes<br>• Woman currently pregnant | **YES** "Seek medical care within 24 hours"<br>**NO** Go to C |

Z

## C. Is the following present?

- No other symptoms but parent or person concerned    **YES**    "Call back or call PCP for appointment if no improvement" and
Follow **Home Care Instructions**

**NO**    Follow **Home Care Instructions**

## Home Care Instructions
## Zika Virus

- Reduce risks of Zika virus by:
  - Applying insect repellent. Do not use insect repellents on babies younger than 2 months. Repellents containing 10% to 30% DEET are safe for children >2 months of age when used according to the product label. Mosquito netting can be used to cover babies younger than 2 months in carriers, strollers, or cribs to protect them from mosquito bites. Do not use products containing oil of lemon eucalyptus or para-menthane-diol on children younger than 3 years. Do not apply insect repellent onto a child's hands, eyes, mouth, and any cut or irritated skin. If you are also using sunscreen, apply sunscreen first and insect repellent second. Do not use products containing both DEET and sunscreen as reapplication of the sunscreen may result in an excessive exposure to DEET.
  - wearing long-sleeve shirts, long pants, and socks
  - minimizing exposed skin
  - wearing light-colored clothing
  - using screens to cover open doors and windows and repairing or replacing any holes in the screens or ill-fitting screens
  - avoiding standing water by draining objects or areas on your property
  - cleaning clogged rain gutters
- Avoid sexual activity with a person known to be or suspected to be infected with the Zika virus. Use condoms (male or female condoms).
- Rest.
- Drink plenty of fluids.
- Take your usual pain medication for discomfort. Do not give aspirin to a child. Avoid aspirin-like products if age <20 years. Avoid acetaminophen if liver disease is present. Avoid ibuprofen if kidney disease or stomach problems exist or in the case of pregnancy. Follow the directions on the label. Use the dosing device that comes with the medication, a measuring device, or a medication syringe from the pharmacy. Household teaspoons often do not give the correct amount of medication.
- For current information on Zika travel information and areas impacted, see CDC's website: cdc.gov/zika or wwwnc.cdc.gov/travel/page/zika-travel-information

**Additional Instructions**

_____

_____

_____

Z

### Report the Following Problems to Your PCP/Clinic/ED
- Severe pain
- Severe muscle weakness
- Numbness
- No improvement or condition worsens

### Seek Emergency Care Immediately If Any of the Following Occur
- Difficulty breathing
- Paralysis
- High fever

If the caller agrees with the advice given, document the call and encourage the caller to call back or see PCP if the problem worsens. If the caller does not agree with the advice given, reevaluate and advise the caller to follow up with PCP, Clinic, or ED.

# Appendix A: Abbreviations

| | |
|---|---|
| > | greater than |
| < | less than |
| AA | alcoholics anonymous |
| AIDS | acquired immune deficiency syndrome |
| AMS | altered mental status |
| °C | degrees Celsius |
| CDC | Centers for Disease Control |
| CPR | cardiopulmonary resuscitation |
| DPT | diphtheria, pertussis, and tetanus (immunization) |
| DTs | delirium tremens |
| ED | emergency department |
| EMS | emergency medical services |
| ER | emergency room |
| °F | degrees Fahrenheit |
| HIV | human immunodeficiency virus |
| HTN | hypertension |
| mg | milligram |
| mL | milliliter |
| MMR | measles, mumps, rubella |
| OTC | over-the-counter (medication) |
| PCP | primary care provider |
| PID | pelvic inflammatory disease |
| RLQ | right lower quadrant |
| SOB | shortness of breath |
| STI | sexually transmitted infection |
| tbsp | tablespoon |
| tsp | teaspoon |
| UTI | urinary tract infection |

# Appendix B: Sample Telephone Triage Protocol Form

**Key Questions**  Name, Age, Onset, Cause, Medications, History, Pain Scale

**Other Protocols to Consider**

*Reminder:* Document caller response to advice, home care instructions, and when to call back.

| ASSESSMENT | ACTION |
|---|---|
| **A. Are any of the following present?** | **YES** "Call ambulance" or "Seek emergency care now" <br> **NO** Go to B |
| **B. Are any of the following present?** | **YES** "Seek medical care within 2 to 4 hours" <br> **NO** Go to C |
| **C. Are any of the following present?** | **YES** "Seek medical care within 24 hours" <br> **NO** Go to D |
| **D. Are any of the following present?** | **YES** "Call back or call PCP for appointment if no improvement" and Follow **Home Care Instructions** <br> **NO** Follow **Home Care Instructions** |

## Home Care Instructions

- 
- 
- 
- 

## Additional Instructions

_____

_____

_____

### Report the Following Problems to Your PCP/Clinic/ED

- 
- 
- 
- 

### Seek Emergency Care Immediately If Any of the Following Occur

- 
- 
- 
- 

If the caller agrees with the advice given, document the call and encourage the caller to call back or see PCP if the problem worsens.
If the caller does not agree with the advice given, reevaluate and advise caller to follow up with PCP, Clinic, or ED.
• **Use this form to develop new protocols as needed to address health care needs and concerns in your care setting.**

# Appendix C: Practicing Telephone Triage Safely

## Triage Roles and Responsibilities

Roles and responsibilities of staff in managing telephone calls must be defined and clarified to ensure that only trained and qualified staff is providing the triage function. Identify who can provide triage and health information and make appointments. Clearly define the role of the receptionist, medical assistant, LPN (LVN), and RN. For example, some organizations have the receptionist take the initial call, then forward the call to the triage nurse. The triage nurse asks specific questions about a condition and advises home care, clinic appointment, or higher level of care. The organization needs to provide a list of conditions and situations that should be passed on to the nurse for triage, for example:

- Breathing problems
- Chest or abdominal pain
- Headaches
- Trauma
- Neurologic problems
- Psychiatric problems
- Drug and alcohol problems
- Symptoms that are sudden and severe
- Person sounds sick

Assign to the triage role experienced RNs who have a broad knowledge base, are trained in telephone triage, are excellent performers, and like telephone triage. Although there is some merit to training all RNs for greater flexibility within the setting, those who truly enjoy the role generally perform much better and promote better patient satisfaction and customer service. Provide a quiet environment that has the necessary resources for triage, documentation, and the discussion of sensitive issues in private.

## Protocol Structure

- All the protocols in the book follow the same format and include the following:
  - Key Questions
  - Other Protocols to Consider
  - Nurse Alert (when appropriate)
  - Reminder for Documentation
  - Assessment Questions
  - Action for the Nurse to Take
  - Home Care Instructions
  - Section to Write Additional Instructions
  - Problems to Report to Provider
  - When to Seek Emergency Care

- The **Key Questions** section prompts the nurse to ask for important information before proceeding through the protocol. This always includes asking for the caller's name, age, onset of symptoms, history, medication usage, and questions appropriate to the complaint, such as pain scale, immunization status, or frequency of symptoms. Disease-based protocols include questions about a known diagnosis, treatment, or known exposure to a disease.

- The **Other Protocols to Consider** section lists related protocols, serving as a quick resource for multiple symptoms or related conditions. After asking key questions, the nurse may determine that a different protocol is more appropriate, and can quickly select that protocol.

- A **Nurse Alert** section provides the nurse with additional important information to consider when choosing a specific protocol or when triaging the caller's concern. Referrals to additional resources are provided when appropriate to assist the nurse in gaining a better understanding of a specific condition.

- The **Reminder** text ("Document caller response to advice, home care instructions, and when to call back") prompts the nurse to document and ensure that the caller understands the advice provided.

- The **Assessment** section lists the symptoms, conditions, or combination of factors that should be assessed in determining urgency.

- **Action** is organized around yes-or-no answers to the assessment questions. If the caller answers "no" to the question, the nurse is directed to the next category of assessment questions. If the caller answers "yes," concrete advice is given regarding when and where to receive care. This advice is prioritized so that emergency actions always appear first. The terms used in the Action section instruct the nurse or the caller how to proceed. Actions the nurse should take appear in italicized type in the list below. Instructions to the caller appear in quotation marks. Action options are as follows:
  - *Go to [a related] protocol*: The nurse is directed to a related protocol that may address an emergent problem more appropriately.
  - "Call an ambulance" (911 in many areas): Emergency first aid instructions while waiting for the ambulance are also included in this section.
  - "Seek emergency care now": Refer caller to the nearest ED. Emergency first aid instructions before going to the ED may also be included here as appropriate.
  - "Seek medical care within 2 to 4 hours": Refer caller to usual care provider, clinic, or ED for urgent conditions.
  - "Seek medical care within 24 hours": Refer caller to usual care provider, clinic, or ED for less urgent conditions.
  - "Seek medical care within 24 to 48 hours": Refer caller to usual care provider, clinic, or ED for nonurgent conditions.
  - "Call back or call PCP for appointment if no improvement": Refer caller to primary care provider or clinic for nonurgent problems if no improvement occurs after following home care instructions.
  - *Follow home care instructions*: The nurse is directed to explain the information described in the Home Care Instructions section, which follows the Assessment/Action columns.

- The **Home Care Instructions** section explains what care should be given in the home before emergency help arrives, while waiting for an appointment, or if the problem can be managed at home. These guidelines can provide symptom relief, prevent a condition from worsening, and reassure the caller. Home and alternative remedies are included and offer less-expensive options for symptom relief. Drug warnings are provided whenever over-the-counter medications are suggested to help ensure medications are used in a safe manner. A warning is provided to remind the caller to ensure that the proper dosage of medication is administered. "Use the dosing device that comes with the medication, a measuring device, or a medication syringe from the pharmacy. Household teaspoons often do not give the correct amount of medication."

- An **Additional Instructions** section provides space in which the health-care professional can write customized health-care facility instructions.
- The **Report the Following Problems to Your PCP/Clinic/ED** section lists subsequent observations, symptoms, or conditions that should be reported wherever the caller generally receives ongoing health care.
- The **Seek Emergency Care Immediately** section lists subsequent observations, symptoms, or conditions that would require the caller to seek immediate emergency care. The caller is directed to watch for these symptoms and, if they occur, either call an ambulance or go directly to the ED.
- The **Advice Agreement** section prompts the nurse to ask whether or not the caller agrees with the advice given, and encourages the caller to call back or follow up with the PCP, clinic, or ED if the problem persists or worsens. This warning should be given with every call. If the caller does not agree with the advice, the nurse should reassess the advice given.

## Using Protocols Safely

Although protocol use does not replace nursing judgment, they do provide a quick, efficient, and safe way to communicate essential information. To ensure consistency and safe practice, policy should mandate that approved protocols be used for all telephone advice and then each call and advice provided documented. All protocols should be reviewed and approved by the medical provider or medical authority.

### Importance of Using Protocols When Giving Telephone Advice

- Protocols are clinical rules for managing calls and provide structure and cues to ask specific questions, starting with the most emergent concerns.
- Protocols prompt the nurse to avoid missing important facts.
- Protocols provide validity and reliability. If followed, they lead to a reasonable and safe disposition, and if given the same set of data, another nurse would reach the same disposition.
- Protocols do not replace nursing judgment. Education, training, and experience affect the nurse's knowledge base.
- When **selecting the appropriate protocol**, choose the protocol that:
  - best matches the symptom or condition;
  - will result in receiving care sooner when multiple symptoms are present;
  - is their most serious symptom or the most bothersome symptom.
- When overriding a protocol:
  - err on the side of caution;
  - upgrade rather than downgrade; do not downgrade without discussing with the provider or supervisor;
  - document the reason for choosing a different resource or overriding a protocol;
  - ensure caller is comfortable with the advice; if not, then reassess.
- **Disease-based protocols** are designed to address already diagnosed problems and should not be used to diagnose a problem. They should be used when a caller has a known diagnosis and has questions about managing his symptoms or treatment regimen. Examples of diagnosis-based protocols are diabetes problems, chickenpox, and history of an allergic reaction or a communicable disease.

- **Closure to the call** is extremely important and can significantly help to reduce liability. Each protocol includes a reminder to ensure the caller understands the advice, home care instructions, and when to call back. It is important to understand that this critical step helps to ensure that the caller:
  - verbalizes understanding of the directions and information;
  - expresses intent to comply or not comply with the advice;
  - establishes agreement with the plan of care;
  - has the opportunity to ask additional questions or address concerns;
  - addresses any concerns about appropriate transportation to the referred care center;
  - is directed to call back if condition worsens, new symptoms develop, or there is no improvement.

  Following this important step helps the nurse to determine nonunderstanding or noncompliance and provides the opportunity to reassess before ending the call.

## Medical–Legal Safeguards

A variety of methods can be used to reduce the risks of giving medical advice over the telephone. Experts in the telephone triage field agree that the use of approved protocols substantially reduces risk. Protocols establish a standard of care, and they provide a mechanism to address potentially serious conditions in a consistent manner when the nurse cannot see or touch the person.

Once telephone contact is made and the nurse has offered to help, a patient–nurse relationship has been established. Failure to follow through and provide advice could be considered abandonment, according to some experts.

Although no assurances can be made that all medical–legal problems associated with telephone triage and advice can be avoided, using the following guidelines will help in preventing them.

## Tips for Practicing Safe Telephone Triage

- Consider all calls life-threatening until proven otherwise so that all emergent questions are asked and help to prevent missing emergent problems.
- Err on the side of caution to avoid the risk in delaying treatment for potentially serious problems.
- Recognize knowledge deficits and use protocols to supplement knowledge to make appropriate triage decisions.
- Document the call and the advice given. If a lawsuit is filed a few years later claiming that the nurse did not advise a caller appropriately, the nurse's position is much more defensible if documentation shows that protocols were followed and appropriate advice was given, the caller's response to the advice, and the caller was advised to call back if no improvement or condition worsens. (See Appendix D3 and Appendix D4 for sample documentation forms.) Documentation may include a log, a note in the patient's chart, or a recording of the call.
- Establish a positive, helping relationship at the onset of the call. Good initial contact can greatly influence the caller's trust in, and satisfaction with, the telephone interaction. The average call lasts only about 6 minutes, and the effectiveness of this brief encounter depends on skillful communication.
- Use terminology the caller can understand. Avoid medical jargon as much as possible.
- Encourage the caller to briefly describe the problem and its duration, onset, and location. Be sure to obtain the age, medical history, medications, and allergies of the person with the problem. Always ask about allergies before giving medication advice.

- When advising the caller to take over-the-counter medication, give the appropriate drug warnings: Do not give aspirin to a child. Avoid aspirin-like products if age <20 years. Avoid acetaminophen if liver disease is present. Avoid ibuprofen if kidney disease or stomach problems exist or in the case of pregnancy. Follow the directions on the label. Use the dosing device that comes with the medication, a measuring device, or a medication syringe from the pharmacy. Household teaspoons often do not give the correct amount of medication.

- Know how to elicit a description of a petechiae-type rash—flat, purple, or dark red dots that do not blanch with pressure. Teach the caller how to test for blanching. Be on the alert for signs of meningitis: headache, stiff neck, fever, petechial rash, vomiting, irritability, altered mental status.

- Listen carefully to the caller and avoid jumping to conclusions. Callers may mask their real concern because of embarrassment, particularly regarding sensitive issues, such as sexually transmitted diseases, drug or alcohol problems, or mental health issues.
  **Case example:** A 16-year-old male called an emergency department asking to reserve a room for the weekend. A busy nurse hurriedly answered the call, told the patient that the emergency department does not reserve rooms, and put him on hold for the secretary to handle. In further questioning, the caller revealed that he had attempted suicide in the past, was feeling suicidal again, and was asking for help and protection from himself. He wanted to be in a safe place where he could not harm himself.

- Try to talk directly to the person with the problem, if possible. Direct communication usually is more reliable and inclusive than secondhand information.

- Assess the problem thoroughly before determining an action plan. The caller may underplay the symptoms and want reassurance that the problem is insignificant. Consider the case of a 10-year-old female who had frequent stomachaches and mom thought her daughter was trying to get out of going to school that day. She just wanted reassurance that it was okay to send her to school. Upon further questioning, it was found that the child had a high fever, severe right lower quadrant abdominal pain, and a poor appetite for 2 days. She was directed to the emergency department and found to have a ruptured appendix and rushed to surgery. A thorough assessment is essential to identify potential serious or life-threatening symptoms.

- Do not try to diagnose the caller, or let the caller self-diagnose. Assess the symptoms to determine a disposition. Chest pain, diaphoresis, and weakness may very well signal a cardiac problem, but they also may indicate pneumonia or some other condition.

- Condition-/diagnosis-specific protocols are to be used only on callers with a previously diagnosed condition or suspected or known exposure to a specific contagious condition. *Do not* try to diagnose the problem and give advice, which is outside the scope of practice for a licensed RN in most states. The focus of triage is the assessment and management of symptoms and referral to the appropriate level of care at the right time.

- You may override a protocol, but do not downgrade without discussing the case with the primary care provider. Although experience will enhance your telephone triage skills, you must always use the protocols to ensure an appropriate and safe disposition or to document the rationale for deviating from a protocol.

- Pay attention to the degree of anxiety and concern expressed by the caller. Remember, the telephone triage nurse has the disadvantage of not being able to see or touch the person. If the caller is emphatic that the person he or she is talking about is ill, encourage the caller to seek medical attention sooner than the protocols may recommend. If the caller thinks it is an emergency, it probably is. Let the EMS or ED staff determine otherwise. It is better to err on the side of caution than to miss a serious condition, such as meningitis, a head bleed after a head injury, or a ruptured appendix that can result in permanent impairment or death.

- Triage is the practice of exclusion. It is permissible to be conservative and overreact.
- When telling a parent to report specific signs and symptoms, give him or her a time period, for example, to report a change in behavior within 4 hours of onset.
- When directing the caller to call an ambulance, several avenues may be most appropriate based on the circumstances (ambulance, EMS, 911 = emergency services for that area of the country):
  ○ Caller hangs up and calls the ambulance or 911.
  ○ Caller stays on the line but calls the ambulance on a cell phone or other device.
  ○ Triage nurse calls 911 for the caller and gives address, cross streets, and telephone number.
  ○ EMS dispatch centers are trained in providing specific emergency procedure directions while waiting for an ambulance and often have GPS capability to locate the caller's location.
  ○ When there is a contagious communicable disease in question, advise not to use public transportation. Depending on the lethality of the potential contagious disease, advise to call 911 and tell dispatchers of potential contagiousness so they can prepare appropriately with personal protective equipment and transport to the appropriate facility that can manage the contagion.
- When referring a caller to the ED, give a time frame, such as "now" or "within the next 1 or 2 hours." How are they going to get there? When there is a contagious communicable disease in question, advise not to use public transportation.
- When advising a caller to seek emergency care now, consider the caller's condition and circumstances. Is there a risk of deterioration that could compromise the airway or limb, or loss of life (meningitis, head injury, traumatic injury, or allergic reaction)?
  Calls that often require emergent/urgent referral to medical care:
  ○ Confused or too weak to stand
  ○ Signs of meningitis: fever, confusion, headache, vomiting, stiff neck, or rigid body in an infant, red or blood-colored flat rash
  ○ Signs of neurologic impairment: sudden-onset numbness or tingling, difficulty walking, talking, swallowing, or thinking
- When there are repeated calls within a 12-hour period (two or more), the caller's needs may remain unmet. Ask for more information than the standard protocol. What advice was given, what has changed, get specifics and reassess. Either the caller is not satisfied with the advice or the person is sicker than described.
- Consider the time of day. If the advice is to seek medical care in 2 to 4 hours and it is 11 PM, refer the caller to the ED. If it is Friday evening and the advice is to seek medical care in 24 hours, refer the caller to a clinic or ED that is open and available within 24 hours.
  **Case example:** At 1 AM on a Saturday, a caller's son had a severe sore throat, fever, and difficulty managing secretions and was told to keep his doctor's appointment on Monday morning. He did keep his appointment and was immediately sent to the emergency department, where he was found to be critically ill from a peritonsillar abscess and sepsis.
- Treat young mothers and teenagers cautiously.
  **Case example:** A 17-year-old mother called in hysterics because her baby had a fever (felt warm) and was constipated (making grunting noises as though he needed to go to the bathroom but couldn't). She was uncooperative and wouldn't answer questions. The nurse talked to her sister and recommended a bath with baking soda to stimulate a bowel movement. The child expired from meningitis within 8 hours.
- Treat calls at the end of the day cautiously. Do not rush through them.

- Do not give advice without an opportunity for follow-up. Determine whether the caller agrees with the advice. If the caller does not agree or is not satisfied with the advice given, reassess. You may have missed something important to the caller.
- Ask the caller what he or she is going to do.
- Provide callers with an option to seek medical attention sooner if they do not agree with the advice or if their condition persists or worsens. Make sure callers know what "worse" means.

## Mental Status Challenges in Telephone Triage

A complaint of altered mental status (AMS) is frequently only one of the concerns that compel someone to seek telephone advice. Often it is paired with fever, headache, anxiety, pain, vomiting, weakness, or some other somatic concern. However, the presence of AMS, combined with another physical concern, may be enough to push the disposition into the emergent category and should not be diminished or disregarded in the telephone triage process. For example, in the protocol Headache, if there is also confusion, the disposition is to "Seek emergency care now."

Signs of AMS may include confusion; irritability; less responsive to voice or touch; drowsiness; combative, uncooperative, nonsensical verbalizing; sudden change in behavior, thinking process, or ability to communicate; auditory (voices, buzzing, clicks), sensory (bug crawling), or visual hallucinations.

- In a child, AMS may be one of the first indicators of rapidly progressing meningitis or a head injury after trauma.
- New onset of paranoia or delusional thoughts may indicate a neurologic problem, electrolyte imbalance, or suicidal ideation.
- Remember that individuals with mental health issues also have serious health conditions, requiring prompt attention.

There have been a number of lawsuits that have alleged that the telephone triage nurse failed to recognize the significance of AMS and should have referred the caller to the ED. In one case, a child had a headache, congestion, and confusion and died from meningitis. It is through listening, clarifying, and understanding that the nurse will be better equipped to apply the degree of AMS because it relates to other symptoms addressed in a protocol and reach an appropriate disposition.

## Types of Altered Mental Status

**Paranoia:** Often described as unfounded distrust in others and may be expressed as others are out to get them or are threatening harm to self or others. It is important to determine whether this is a new behavior or the person is under the influence of drugs or alcohol, taking a new medication, or has a history of mental illness.

**Confusion:** Mental state characterized by disorientation regarding time, place, person, or situation and can affect the person's ability to make decisions or perform activities of daily living. This becomes an emergency when associated with other symptoms, including fever >101°F, neck or body stiffness or rigidity, rash, head injury, flushing or dry skin, vomiting, fruity breath.

**Delusion:** Described as a false belief not shared by one's culture or incorrect beliefs not based on reality. A change from usual thinking process may indicate a more serious problem such as a stroke or other neurologic problem, substance abuse, withdrawal, poisoning, and requires further assessment and investigation.

**Delirium:** Sudden onset of confusion, disturbances in attention, disorganized thinking, or a decline in the level of consciousness occurring over a matter of hours to days. Requires emergency evaluation.

## Documentation

The purpose of documentation is to provide a clear picture of the interaction and patient condition. It provides a permanent record that serves as a resource if the caller calls back or there is a lawsuit and the call needs to be reviewed. As the saying goes, if it was not documented, it was not done, was not important, or was not considered, and this would make it difficult to recall the encounter and support the decision-making process. Use the caller's own words as much as possible, applying "quotation marks." Show evidence that questions were asked, and document denials to rule out serious conditions. Documentation policy should describe whether the documentation process is by exception, omitting negatives, or by inclusion, including negatives.

Documentation elements should include the following whether it is an electronic record or handwritten document (See Appendix D3 and Appendix D4 for sample documentation forms.):

- Caller name and relation to the patient
- Date and time of call
- Demographics per policy
- Chief complaint
- Provider
- Description of signs and symptoms, onset, and duration
- Associated symptoms
- Relevant medical history
- Medications
- Disposition and advice given
- The protocol followed and recommended time frame to seek care
- Your name and title
- Time frame to call back if no improvement

## Training Guidelines

Provide initial and ongoing training for all staff and identify how their roles are impacted by the triage process. Focus on interviewing the caller, protocol selection, application, and patient teaching. All staff should be alerted to community outbreaks such as a new widespread infestation of bedbugs or lice, or communicable diseases such as pertussis, or a new form of influenza. Post fliers from local health departments. Regularly review CDC guidelines for most current outbreaks, triage suggestions, isolation requirements, and treatment modalities.

Provide one-on-one, group training, or a combination of both. See Appendix D7 for developing an in-house training program. Take advantage of outside training sessions and workshops or bring in a trainer for a more cost-effective and tailored program. In addition to formal training, staff training should include the following elements:

- Review the preface for key features of the book and to see how the protocols are structured.
- Review triage roles and responsibilities.
- Review Practicing Telephone Triage Safely Appendix C for protocol structure elements, using protocols safely, medical–legal safeguards, mental status challenges, documentation, training guidelines, and strategies to ensure quality.

- Review policies and procedures that address how calls should be handled. Policies should clearly outline roles and responsibilities of the triage nurse and other members of the team.
- Review the protocols that address the most frequent types of calls received in your setting.
  Most common pediatric concerns:
  - Fever
  - Sore throat
  - Gastrointestinal problems
  - Respiratory problems
  - Minor trauma
  - Skin and infectious disease problems
  - Earache
  - Immunization problems
- Review and become familiar with diseases that may result in a poor outcome if diagnosis is delayed:
  - Appendicitis
  - Meningitis
  - Pneumonia
  - Head Injury
- Review and become familiar with Table of Contents By Body System (xviii–xxiii) to better understand how protocols address different body parts and systems.
- Review the emergency dispositions of the most common protocols.
- Review documentation standards and forms. (See pages (533–534) for sample forms, Appendix D3 and Appendix D4.)
- Provide structured practice and provide feedback. Guidelines for Scenario Practice; (page 538): Skills Assessment and Exercise Form (page 543). Practice scenarios with one another to gain confidence and familiarity with using the protocols. It is important to the learning process to experience both the one asking the questions and being on the receiving end and providing answers. Assess understanding and provide feedback.
- Review Appendix G (page 547): Teaching Self-Assessment. Practice with one another, asking the questions, performing the assessment techniques, and providing feedback.
- Observe an experienced nurse providing telephone triage for at least 16 hours. There are devices available that enable two people to listen to the conversation at the same time.
- Provide supervised telephone triage for at least 24 hours.
- In a group setting, review and discuss examples of both calls that are well done and calls that could be improved. Play a recording of the call if available.
- Attend conferences, workshops, and continuing education seminars to increase your competency in telephone triage assessment and communication skills.

---

**Through Direct Listening and Observation the Nurse Will Learn How to:**
- elicit the caller's concern to select the appropriate protocol.
- recognize serious symptoms that should be directed to an urgent/emergent disposition.
- ask appropriate assessment questions to reach an appropriate disposition.

- review home care instructions to help callers manage their problems at home or before going to the doctor or ED.
- advise the caller when to call back or seek treatment.
- assure caller understanding and agreement with the advice and plan and what action the caller will take. If not in agreement, reassess.
- document the call.

## Strategies to Help Ensure a Quality Telephone Triage System

- The top priority should always be patient safety.
- Use the medically approved protocols to establish a standard of care. Do not deviate from the protocols unless changes are made in writing and approved by the appropriate medical authority.
- Orient and train staff in telephone triage protocols, policies, and procedures; telephone encounter techniques; dealing with difficult callers; and documentation. See page (537) for a sample training outline and pages (538–541) for training exercises.
- Develop a mechanism to regularly review documentation and advice for consistency, accuracy, and quality. (See page (536) for documentation review form.)
- Measure outcomes. Follow up promptly on problems and quality issues. (See page (543) for a skills assessment tool.)
- Use telephone triage to improve access to care, not to impede it. Follow up on all complaints concerning limited access to care.
- Follow up and review calls where staff fail to use protocols and rely only on nursing knowledge. Review caller concern, advice given, reason for deviating from a protocol, and outcome.
- Know your State Board of Nursing laws regarding medication advice. Laws vary from state to state.
- Research and review current events, such as local outbreaks of communicable diseases like pertussis, influenza, and meningitis. Callers may hear about them on the news and have questions or be worried that they have been exposed. Telephone triage nurses can be the first to recognize an outbreak from the frequency and types of calls received.

# Appendix D1: Community Resources Telephone List

**Emergency Services:**

Ambulance _____ or 911

Fire _____ or 911

Police _____ or 911

County Sheriff _____

State Police Patrol _____

Poison Control _____

Local Hospitals _____

_____

_____

_____

_____

Public Health Clinic _____

Immunization Clinic _____

STD Clinics _____

Other Clinics _____

_____

Local Pharmacies _____

_____

_____

_____

_____

Rape Crisis _____

STD Hotline _____

AIDS Hotline _____

Mental Health Crisis Line _____

Drug and Alcohol Crisis Line _____

Detox _____

Alcohol and Drug Treatment _____

Child Protective Services _____

Women's Shelter _____

**Resources:**

Animal Control _____

Handicapped/Senior Transport _____

Home Health _____

Medical Equipment Rental _____

Crutch Rental _____

Planned Parenthood _____

Mental Health Center _____

Physician Referral _____

# Appendix D2: Telephone Triage Quality Improvement Survey

| Patient Name | | Telephone # | | Date and Time of Initial Call |
|---|:---:|:---:|:---:|:---:|

| Question | Yes | No | Comments |
|---|:---:|:---:|:---:|
| 1. Was the nurse courteous and professional? | | | |
| 2. Were you comfortable with the advice given? | | | |
| 3. Did you follow the advice given? | | | |
| 4. Were you provided adequate referral information? | | | |
| 5. Would you use our service again? | | | |

Comments:

_____

_____

_____

_____

_____

_____

Follow-up:

_____

_____

_____

_____

_____

_____

| Surveyor Name | Date and Time of Call |
|---|---|

# Appendix D3: Telephone Triage Documentation Form

Date:_____ Time:_____ Time Returned Call: _____

Name of patient: _____ Phone: _____

Name of caller: _____ Relationship: _____

Age of patient: _____Sex: _____ Physician: _____

Has patient tried to contact physician? Yes_____ No_____

Presenting Problem/Symptoms:

_____

_____

_____

_____

Protocol used (list source, protocol name, and page number):

1. _____ Page #_____

2. _____ Page #_____

3. _____ Page #_____

4. Other: _____

Problem Emergent_____Urgent_____Semiurgent_____Nonurgent_____

       (immediately)    (2 to 4 hours)  (within 24 hours)  (make appointment/home care)

1. Call 911 or ambulance for transport to nearest hospital.

2. Go to ED.

3. Call own physician; if unavailable, follow-up with ED or Urgent Care Clinic.

4. See physician within 24 to 48 hours.

5. Call Mental Health Crisis Line @_____now.

6. Contact Health Department @_____

7. Follow home care instructions:

_____

_____

_____

Additional Comments: _____

_____

_____

_____

Does caller agree with action taken? (circle) Yes    No

Told caller to call back or be seen if problem worsens Yes    No

Please review this taped conversation

Please call this person back for follow-up_____

Signature:_____

# Appendix D4: Telephone Triage Log

| Date and Time of Call | Patient Name/ Age/Sex | Symptom or Concern and Onset | Protocol Used | Advice Given | Disposition and Caller Agreement | Nurse Name |
|---|---|---|---|---|---|---|
| | | | | | | |
| | | | | | | |
| | | | | | | |
| | | | | | | |
| | | | | | | |
| | | | | | | |
| | | | | | | |
| | | | | | | |
| | | | | | | |

# Appendix D5: Telephone Triage "Call Back" Log

| Date of Call | Time of Call | Name | Phone #1 | c/o | Treatment Location | Current Health Status | | | | Signature | Date/Time |
|---|---|---|---|---|---|---|---|---|---|---|---|
| | | | | | | I | S | W | Other | | |
| | | | | | | | | | | | |
| | | | | | | | | | | | |
| | | | | | | | | | | | |
| | | | | | | | | | | | |
| | | | | | | | | | | | |
| | | | | | | | | | | | |
| | | | | | | | | | | | |
| | | | | | | | | | | | |
| | | | | | | | | | | | |
| | | | | | | | | | | | |
| | | | | | | | | | | | |

Key: c/o, complaint; I, improved; S, same; W, worse.

535

# Appendix D6: Call Documentation Review

Name of Consulting Nurse:_____ Date and Time of Call:_____

Name of Reviewer:_____ Date of Review:_____

| | Yes | No | N/A |
|---|---|---|---|
| Signature of consulting nurse on form? | | | |
| Date and time of call recorded? | | | |
| Did RN record time call returned? | | | |
| Did RN record patient's name? | | | |
| Did RN record caller's telephone number? | | | |
| Did RN record relationship of patient to caller? | | | |
| Did RN record name of patient's PCP? | | | |
| Did RN record whether caller had attempted to contact PCP? | | | |
| Did RN record present problem/symptoms? | | | |
| Did RN record protocol used? | | | |
| Did RN record whether problem was urgent, emergent, or nonurgent? | | | |
| Did RN record action taken? | | | |
| Did RN record whether caller agreed with information given? | | | |
| Did RN record whether caller was instructed to call back prn? | | | |

Comments: _____

_____

_____

_____

_____

_____

_____

# Appendix D7: Telephone Triage Training Outline

I. Overview
   1. Program description
   2. Evolution of telephone triage
   3. Role of telephone triage in health care today
   4. Medicolegal considerations
II. Operational Considerations
   1. Policy and procedure review
   2. Introduction to telephone triage program
   3. Components of a call
   4. Documentation
   5. Call management
   6. Community resources
III. Communication Skills
   1. Uniqueness of telephone triage and management
   2. Establishing rapport with the caller
   3. Dealing with difficult calls
IV. Protocol Review and Practice
   1. Review most common protocols
   2. Review additional resources
   3. Form triads to practice with scenarios
   4. Written scavenger protocol hunt
V. Quality Improvement Process
   1. Review QI process and forms
   2. Practice listening to actual calls
VI. Summary and Evaluation

# Appendix D8: Guidelines for Scenario Practice

This exercise contains 10 different scenarios. There are no right or wrong answers. There are several different protocols that can be used to address the problems described in the scenarios. In general, it is best to choose a protocol that most closely matches the caller's greatest concern. This is strictly a learning experience to introduce you to the protocols and practice assessment and documentation of the telephone triage encounter. Read each scenario and indicate in the space provided:

- the protocol name and page number
- any additional information you want to know
- your disposition decision

In addition, practice documenting the call using the documentation tools (Appendix D3 and Appendix D4) or your own organization's documentation tool.

1. Spend only about 5 to 6 minutes per scenario, as if you were on the phone talking with the caller. This includes looking up the protocol and providing advice and all necessary documentation.) This exercise should take about an hour to complete.

2. Document the protocol used and page number on both the scenario and documentation form.

3. In the space provided for each scenario, describe additional information that would be important to manage the call appropriately. Not all scenarios provide adequate information to thoroughly assess the problem and to reach a disposition. Use this section to identify other questions that you would ask to complete a thorough assessment and choose an appropriate protocol. Based on the information provided, indicate your disposition decision.

4. Complete all 10 scenarios. Your supervisor will review your worksheets with you after you have completed this exercise. Remember, this is a learning opportunity. This exercise is designed to help you feel more comfortable with the protocols, applying your assessment skills and documenting the encounter.

## Scenario Practice

1. Call received at 23:40 and returned at 23:50 hours. Mary Smith called regarding her daughter Linda. Phone number is 404-444-0202. Linda is 10 years old and a patient of Dr. Allen, who was not called prior to this call. Mary states that her daughter has a wasp sting to the forearm that is badly swollen and is warm and painful to the touch. She has pain in her arm and shoulder. There is no stinger. She has applied Benadryl lotion to the area. The incident occurred at 18:00 hours today. Mom states there is no difficulty breathing, chest pain, rash, or other problems. She wants to know what else can be done or if she should take her daughter to the ED.

**Protocol Name/Page #** _____

**Additional Information Desired** (what else is important to know in reaching a disposition):

**Disposition Decision:**

538

2. Call received at 20:20 hours. Patty Sing, a 16-year-old female, is concerned about abdominal cramping and vaginal bleeding. Her phone number is 505-555-6767. Her PCP is Dr. Smitt, whom she has not tried to contact. She states that she is 1½ months' pregnant and has abdominal cramping in her lower abdomen. She denies any other pain. She began having vaginal bleeding yesterday and has not passed any clots or tissue. She has saturated 2 to 3 pads this afternoon. She wants to know if she should be seen, because she is afraid she will lose her baby.

**Protocol Name/Page #**_____

**Additional Information Desired** (what else is important to know in reaching a disposition):

**Disposition Decision:**

3. Call received at 17:30 hours and returned at 18:05 hours. Lisa Kennedy, is calling about her daughter Mandy who has abdominal pain and vomiting. Her phone number is 808-845-2002. Dr. Shelby, her PCP, was not called because his office is closed. She states that Mandy has had severe abdominal pain since noon today. The discomfort started as heavy bloating, then vomiting about 15 times this afternoon. No diarrhea or gas noted, but light-headed and dizzy for the past 45 minutes. She describes her pain as 8/10, with no relief after vomiting. Mom is asking what she can do at home. She does not want to go to the ER because she thinks that their health-care plan discourages ED use.

**Protocol Name/Page #**_____

**Additional Information Desired** (what else is important to know in reaching a disposition):

**Disposition Decision:**

4. Call received at 02:00 hours and returned at 02:05 hours. The caller is concerned about her 18-year-old daughter living away from home and attending a university. Her daughter's name is Marie Mason, and the caller's name is Jane Nelson. The phone number where she can be reached is 707-777-4242. Her daughter has no PCP. The mother states that her daughter has been sweating off and on since yesterday and has a cough. She developed small water blisters all over her body today and is nauseated. She has had a headache for 4 days and has been dizzy. She describes her rash as 20 to 30 red spots that are fleabite size with blisters in the middle. Some of the spots itch. She does not know if she has a fever, because she does not have a thermometer. There are no scabs. Mom cannot remember if this daughter ever had chickenpox. The daughter wants to know if she has chickenpox, if she should go home rather than continue at school, and if she should make an appointment to see a doctor.

**Protocol Name/Page #**_____

**Additional Information Desired** (what else is important to know in reaching a disposition):

**Disposition Decision:**

5. Call received at 12:00 hours and returned immediately. The caller's name is Paul, and he refuses to give his last name. He states that he does not have a phone, and he is calling from a friend's house and does not want to give out the number. He does not have a PCP because he does not have insurance, and he is unemployed at this time. Paul is 17 years old. He states that he was in a fight about 3 to 4 days ago. Now, his lower right arm is swollen and very sore. The other guy bit him twice just below the elbow. He has a reddened area about 3 × 6 that is very painful to the touch. There is pus in two areas, with fever of 102°F for 2 days. He describes the area on his arm as very warm to the touch and very painful.

**Protocol Name/Page #**_____

**Additional Information Desired** (what else is important to know in reaching a disposition):

**Disposition Decision:**

6. Call received at 02:00 hours. The caller's name is Barry Haines. He is calling about his 2-year-old daughter Rebecca. His phone number is 404-444-7272. Rebecca's PCP is Dr. Kneehigh, but he did not call him because he did not want to wake up the doctor. His daughter woke up at 01:00 hours, crying with ear pain. Barry gave her Tylenol 15 minutes ago and is asking what else he can do. His daughter is not crying at this time, but is lying on the couch holding her ear.

**Protocol Name/Page #**_____

**Additional Information Desired** (what else is important to know in reaching a disposition):

**Disposition Decision:**

7. Call received at 18:50 hours and returned at 19:03 hours. Peter Hammer is calling about his 3-year-old son, Derek Hammer. The phone number is 808-848-8080. The child does not have a PCP. The father stated that his son was running and fell, striking his head on a coffee table, and has a large abrasion to the forehead, approximately 1½″ × 3″. The accident occurred about 30 minutes ago. Peter states that there was no loss of consciousness, and the child cried right away for a few minutes. His son is now playing quietly. The father is worried about a potential head injury and wants to know what he should do or observe.

**Protocol Name/Page #**_____

**Additional Information Desired** (what else is important to know in reaching a disposition):

**Disposition Decision:**

8. Call received at 20:20 hours and returned at 20:50 hours. Sue Shepard is calling about her niece Amanda, who is 2 months old. Her phone number is 444-454-0044. The child's PCP is Dr. Jollet, but she has not been called. The aunt states that the child has a fever of 102.5°F rectally and has not been eating or

drinking much. She has a runny nose and cough. Further questioning reveals a very fussy baby who had a long nap earlier today. Sue cannot describe any other problems. The fever started last night. The child has been taking Tylenol every 4 to 6 hours, and the last dose was at 20:00 hours. Sue wants to know if she should take her niece to the ER or what else can be done.

**Protocol Name/Page #**_____

**Additional Information Desired** (what else is important to know in reaching a disposition):

**Disposition Decision:**

9. Call received at 18:42 hours and returned at 19:03. The caller's name is Jane Lambo, who is calling about her 6-month-old daughter, Jolyn Bosner. Her home phone number is 404-435-6789. The child does not have a pediatrician. The child has had a fever of up to 102°F for 2 days. Now the temperature is 102.4°F. Mom gave Tylenol at 7:30 this morning. The child is vomiting, "sleeping all the time today," and only waking up to cry or vomit. She has thrown up 6 times since noon and has had diarrhea 4 times. Her last wet diaper was around 11:00, but it was not very wet. Mom states that the child will not eat or drink anything. When questioned further, Mom states that Jolyn only drank 2 ounces of Pedialyte today and will not drink formula. Mom is concerned and wants to know what to do.

**Protocol Name/Page #**_____

**Additional Information Desired** (what else is important to know in reaching a disposition):

**Disposition Decision:**

10. Call received at 23:00 hours and returned at 23:40 hours. Jack Schmidt is calling about his son, John Simms, age 5. He states that his phone number is 310-444-5678 and that they are on vacation in Washington. He does not know his son's pediatrician's (Dr. Band) phone number by memory, so he has not called him. He states that his son has had a bad headache and a high fever. His temperature is now 102.6°F. Tylenol was given 1 hour ago. The child vomited once an hour ago and slept all day today, in addition to last night. Dad states that his son is lying on the couch holding his head. He has had a cold for the past few days with a runny nose. When asked, the child is unwilling to touch his chin to his chest when his dad shows him how and states that "it hurts too much." The dad is concerned and wants to know what he should do.

**Protocol Name/Page #**_____

**Additional Information Desired** (what else is important to know in reaching a disposition):

**Disposition Decision:**

# Appendix D9: Quality Improvement Program

1. **Triage Skills Assessment Form - Appendix D9**—This form is versatile and can be used in a variety of ways to measure quality and competency.
   - Initial competency review during training
   - Competency performance review
   - Ongoing quality review of adherence to standards and opportunities for improvement and education
   - Training exercises

2. **For ongoing competency review and quality see the following:**
   - Telephone Triage Quality Improvement Survey—Appendix D2
   - Telephone Triage Documentation Form—Appendix D3 and Appendix D4
   - Call Documentation Review—Appendix D6
   - Telephone Triage Skills Assessment Form—Appendix D9

3. **Mystery Caller Practice Exercise**

This exercise is designed to help the telephone nurse to gain experience with and insight into call management, and to explore potential problems in soliciting accurate information to determine the appropriate disposition of a call.

It involves calling a telephone nurse within your organization or another facility (if the two facilities have agreed to participate). Staff should be notified that a mystery caller might be calling. You should participate as both the mystery caller and the telephone nurse receiving a call from the mystery caller.

1. Use the scenarios in Appendix D8 as a basis for your mystery call. Make up your own scenario if you feel it is more relevant to your practice. Write down the primary information before making the call. It helps to keep you on track and prevents the nurse from leading you down a different path than you had intended.

2. Use the "Telephone Triage Skills Assessment" form during the call to provide feedback to the telephone nurse. The mystery caller will use the same form to provide you with feedback during your practice calls.

3. At the completion of the call, inform the nurse that you are a mystery caller and thank the nurse for her or his participation. Feedback can be provided either at that time or in a review session at a later time.

4. Practice making and receiving 3 to 5 telephone calls.

5. Keep in mind that it is important to understand what it feels like to be a caller as well as the nurse receiving the call, to gain some understanding of the perceptions a caller may have of your telephone encounter.

## Telephone Triage Skills Assessment Form

| Greeting | Call Time: | | | All Time: | | |
|---|---|---|---|---|---|---|
| | Yes | No | N/A | Yes | No | N/A |
| • Greets caller courteously. | | | | | | |
| • Utilizes proper opening script (identifies self, services, RN, recorded line). | | | | | | |
| • Clarifies accurately the type of call (triage, health info, other). | | | | | | |
| • Gathers appropriate demographic data. | | | | | | |
| • Comments: | | | | | | |
| **Protocol Utilization** | | | | | | |
| • Identifies emergency signs and symptoms. | | | | | | |
| • Selects appropriate protocol. | | | | | | |
| • Gathers appropriate patient history. | | | | | | |
| • Upgrades caller to higher level of urgency as needed (child, confused adult, foreign speaking). | | | | | | |
| • Makes acceptable recommendation and/or referral for care and time frame. | | | | | | |
| • Offers appropriate medication recommendations/protocol. | | | | | | |
| • Offers and documents interim care measures if not emergent. | | | | | | |
| • Request caller feedback to evaluate understanding of information provided. | | | | | | |
| • Documents appropriately, including assessment, advice given, protocol used, caller agreement with plan, and warning. | | | | | | |
| • Comments: | | | | | | |
| **Communication Skills** | | | | | | |
| • Conveys a positive image of organization. | | | | | | |
| • Maintains a courteous, calm, professional demeanor. | | | | | | |
| • Exhibits ability to adapt to different personalities and emotions. | | | | | | |
| • Assumes control of call: Listens attentively, interjects appropriately, and elicits necessary information. | | | | | | |
| • Takes time with caller when appropriate; efficient without compromising quality. | | | | | | |
| • Uses simple, direct language that caller understands. | | | | | | |
| • Does not interrupt or interject for caller. | | | | | | |

| | | | | | | |
|---|---|---|---|---|---|---|
| • Speaks at a moderate rate with expressive modulation of tone. | | | | | | |
| • Maintains control of call. | | | | | | |
| • Comments: | | | | | | |
| **Closing Speech** | | | | | | |
| • Ends call efficiently. | | | | | | |
| • Offers instructions to call back or seek medical care if condition worsens, new symptoms develop, or concern regarding condition. | | | | | | |
| • Reviews recommendations and requests feedback to evaluate caller understanding and agreement with advice. | | | | | | |
| • Disconnects last. | | | | | | |
| • Comments: | | | | | | |

# Appendix E: Temperature Conversion Chart

| CELSIUS | FAHRENHEIT |
|---------|------------|
| 43.0 | 109.4 |
| 42.0 | 107.6 |
| 41.0 | 105.8 |
| 40.5 | 104.9 |
| 40.0 | 104.0 |
| 39.5 | 103.1 |
| 39.0 | 102.2 |
| 38.5 | 101.3 |
| 38.0 | 100.4 |
| 37.5 | 99.5 |
| 37.0 | 98.6 |
| 36.5 | 97.7 |
| 36.0 | 96.8 |
| 35.0 | 95.0 |
| 34.0 | 93.2 |
| 33.0 | 91.4 |
| 32.0 | 89.6 |
| 31.0 | 87.8 |
| 30.0 | 86.0 |
| 29.0 | 84.2 |
| 28.0 | 82.4 |
| 27.0 | 80.6 |
| 26.0 | 78.8 |
| 25.0 | 77.0 |
| 24.0 | 75.2 |
| 23.0 | 73.4 |
| 22.0 | 71.6 |
| 21.0 | 69.8 |
| 20.0 | 68.0 |
| 19.0 | 66.2 |
| 18.0 | 64.4 |

Formula for Fahrenheit to Celsius: $(1.8 \times \text{Celsius reading}) + 32 =$ \_\_\_\_
Formula for Celsius to Fahrenheit: $0.55 \times (\text{Fahrenheit reading} - 32) =$ \_\_\_\_

# Appendix F: Weight Conversion Chart

| POUND | KILOGRAM |
|-------|----------|
| 1 | 0.45 |
| 2 | 0.5 |
| 3 | 1.35 |
| 4 | 1.8 |
| 5 | 2.25 |
| 6 | 2.7 |
| 8 | 3.6 |
| 10 | 4.5 |
| 11 | 5 |
| 22 | 10 |
| 33 | 15 |
| 44 | 20 |
| 55 | 25 |
| 66 | 30 |
| 77 | 35 |
| 88 | 40 |
| 99 | 45 |
| 110 | 50 |
| 121 | 55 |
| 132 | 60 |
| 143 | 65 |
| 154 | 70 |
| 165 | 75 |
| 176 | 80 |
| 187 | 85 |
| 198 | 90 |
| 209 | 95 |
| 220 | 100 |

| POUND | KILOGRAM |
|-------|----------|
| 231 | 105 |
| 242 | 110 |
| 253 | 115 |
| 264 | 120 |
| 275 | 125 |
| 286 | 130 |
| 297 | 135 |

# Appendix G: Teaching Self-Assessment

| | INSTRUCTION | QUESTION |
|---|---|---|
| **Ankle swelling** | Using one finger, press over the bony part of the ankle for 2 seconds. Count 1001, 1002, and release. | Does the skin remain depressed or spring back into place? |
| **Circulation** | Squeeze the nail bed of your left middle finger between the first finger and thumb of your right hand. Count 1001, 1002, and release. | Does the color of the nail bed return immediately or is it sluggish? Repeat the action, and tell me the number of seconds it takes to return to normal. Count 1001, 1002, 1003, etc. |
| **Dehydration** | Pinch the skin over the top of the hand for 5 seconds. Count 1001, 1002, 1003, 1004, 1005, and release. | Does the skin remain raised like a tent, or does it spring back into place? |
| **Extremity circulation** | Expose both limbs (hands, feet, arms, legs). Using four fingers of one hand, touch the affected area for 2 seconds. Count 1001, 1002. Now touch the same area on the unaffected limb and count 1001, 1002. | Does one area feel cooler to touch than the area on the other limb? Is there a difference in color? |
| **Extremity injury** | Expose both limbs (hands, feet, arms, legs). Observe the area for swelling, discoloration, bone protrusion through the skin, or deformity. | Does one extremity look different from the other? |
| **Infection** | Using four fingers of one hand, touch the affected area for 2 seconds. Count 1001, 1002. Then move the hand and touch unaffected skin for 2 seconds. Observe the area and compare to surrounding skin. | Does one area feel warmer to touch than the other? Is the area red or swollen? Is there drainage? Are there red streaks? Is the area painful to touch? |
| **Joint mobility** | Bend and extend the affected joint to the extent possible. Move the joints above and below the affected area. | Does the movement cause or increase the pain? Is there difficulty moving the part? |

| | INSTRUCTION | QUESTION |
|---|---|---|
| **Pain** | Point to the location of the pain. Press on the painful area. | Describe the location of the pain. Can you locate the pain with one finger (localized pain)? Is the painful area larger than one finger? Describe the size of the painful area, i.e., size of a fist, one hand, or two hands (diffuse pain). Describe your pain on a scale of 1 to 10, 1 being minimal, and 10 being severe. Is the pain worse or the same when you press on the area? Does anything make the pain better or worse? |
| **Postural** | While in the presence of another adult, stand up from a sitting position. | Did any dizziness or light-headedness occur? |
| **Pulse** | Place two fingers (do not use your thumb) over the inner side of the wrist just below the base of the thumb. Feel the pulse. Count the number of beats for 30 seconds. Start counting when I say start and stop when I say stop. | How many beats did you feel? Did the beats feel even or regular? |
| **Respirations** | Remove clothing covering the chest. Observe the chest rising and falling. Count the number of times the chest rises for 15 seconds. Start counting when I say start and stop when I say stop. | Look at the fingernail beds, lips, earlobes, and skin. How many chest rises did you count? Are the respirations noisy? Is there a blue or gray discoloration in the fingernail beds, lips, or earlobes? Is the skin hot, cold, or moist? Is there excessive drooling in a child? Will the child eat or drink? What color is the sputum? |
| **Swelling** | Expose both limbs (hand, feet, arms, legs). Compare the limbs. | Is one area larger than the other? |

# Appendix H: Resources

**Internet Resources by Topic**

Anxiety
http://www.nimh.nih.gov/health/topics/anxiety-disorders/index.shtml

Bites, Animal
http://emedicine.medscape.com/article/768875-overview
http://www.cdc.gov/rabies/

Bites, Bedbug
http://emedicine.medscape.com/article/1088931-overview

Bites, Human
http://emedicine.medscape.com/article/768978-overview

Bites, Insect
http://www.cdc.gov/niosh/topics/insects/
http://emedicine.medscape.com/article/769067-overview

Bites, Snake
http://www.emedicine.com/med/topic2143.htm

Common Cold Symptoms; Congestion, Avian Flu, Influenza
http://www.cdc.gov/flu/about/disease.htm

Diarrhea
Food Poisoning, Suspected
http://www.foodsafety.gov/poisoning/index.html
http://emedicine.medscape.com/article/175569-overview

Hepatitis
http://www.cdc.gov/ncidod/diseases/hepatitis/index/htm

Immunizations
www.cdc.gov/vaccines

Influenza
http://www.cdc.gov/flu/about/disease.htm

Lice
http://www.cdc.gov/parasites/lice/head/

Meningitis
http://www.cdc.gov/meningitis/about/faq.html

Mental Health Topics
http://health.nih.gov/

Neurologic Disorders and Stroke
http://www.ninds.nih.gov/

Overdose; Poisoning, Suspected (Link to Poison Control Centers)
http://www.aapcc.org/

Scabies
http://www.cdc.gov/ncidod/dpd/parasites/scabies/default.htm

Sexual Assault; Sexually Transmitted Disease
http://www.cdc.gov/std/general/
http://www.cdc.gov/ViolencePrevention/sexualviolence/index.html

Stye
http://www.emedicinehealth.com

Suicide Attempt, Threat
http://emedicine.medscape.com/article/288598-overview

## Standards and Professional Organizations

American Academy of Ambulatory Care Nursing. (2004). *Telehealth nursing practice administration and practice standards* (3rd ed.). Pitman, NJ: Anthony J. Jannetti.

American Accreditation Healthcare Commission. (2002). *Health call center standards V.3.* Washington, DC. Retrieved from www.urac.org

American Academy of Ambulatory Care Nursing. (2016). Retrieved from www.aaacn.org

# Bibliography

American Academy of Ambulatory Nursing. (1997). *Telephone nursing practice administration and practice standards*. Pitman, NJ: Anthony J. Jannetti.

American Health Consultants. (2000, March). Bite wounds: Don't let patients leave with the wrong impression. *ED Legal Letter, 2*(3), 21–32.

American Health Consultants. (2005, March). Are elderly patients undertriaged? Don't miss life-threatening conditions. *ED Nursing*, 49.

American Health Consultants. (2005, March). Tips to teach nurses to do neuro assessments. *ED Nursing*, 54.

American Health Consultants. (2005, October). Sickle cell: Learn how to help patients in severe pain. *ED Nursing*, 136.

American Health Consultants. (2005, October). Use this protocol for sickle cell patients in your ED. *ED Nursing*, 137.

American Health Consultants. (2005, September). EDs aren't following heart attack guidelines: Revamp protocols now. *ED Nursing, 8*(11), 121.

American Heart Association. (2006). *Healthcare provider's manual for basic life support*. Dallas, TX: Author.

Antoon, J., Potisek, N. & Lohr, J. (2015). Pediatric fever of unknown origin. *Pediatrics in Review, 36*, 380–390.

Ball, J., Bindler, R., & Cowen, K. (2015). *Principles of Pediatric Nursing: Caring for Children* (6th ed.). Boston, MA: Pearson Education, Inc.

Barrueto, F. Jr., Gattu, R. & Mazer-Amirshahi, M. (2013). Updates in the general approach to the pediatric poisoned patient. *Pediatric Clinics of North America, 60*, 1203–1220.

Beaulieu, R. & Humphreys, J. (2008). Evaluation of a telephone advice nurse in a nursing faculty managed pediatric community clinic. *Journal of Pediatric Health Care, 22*, 175–181.

Berger, W., Granet, D. & Kabat, A. (2017). Diagnosis and management of allergic conjunctivitis in pediatric patients. *Allergy and Asthma Proceedings, 38*, 16–27.

Blank, L., Coster, J., O'Cathain, A., Knowles, E., Tosh, J., Turner, J. & Nicholl, J. (2012). The appropriateness of, and compliance with, telephone triage decisions: A systematic review and narrative synthesis. *Journal of Advanced Nursing, 68*, 2610–2621.

Boyle, K. & Rosenbaum, C. (2014). Oxycodone overdose in the pediatric population: Case files of the University of Massachusetts Medical Toxicology Fellowship. *Journal of Medical Toxicology, 10*, 280–285.

Brennan, M. (1992). Nursing process in telephone advice. *Nursing Management, 23*(5), 62–66.

Briggs, J. (2016). *Telephone Triage Protocols for Nurses* (5th ed.). Philadelphia, PA: Wolters Kluwer.

Briggs, J., & Grossman, V. (2005). *Emergency nursing: 5-tier triage protocols*. Philadelphia, PA: Lippincott Williams & Wilkins.

Broides, A., Bereza, O., Lavi-Givon, N., Fruchtman, Y., Gazala, E. & Leibovitz, E. (2016). Parental acceptability of the watchful waiting approach in pediatric acute otitis media. *World Journal of Clinical Pediatrics, 5*, 198–205.

Brown, J. L. (2005). *Pediatric telephone medicine: Principles, triage, and advice* (2nd ed.). Philadelphia, PA: Lippincott Williams & Wilkins.

Buppert, C. (2009). Guidelines for telephone triage. *Dermatology Nursing, 21*(1), 40–41.

Calello, D. & Henretig, F. (2014). Pediatric toxicology: Specialized approach to the poisoned child. *Emergency Medicine Clinics of North America*, 29–52.

Clayman, C. B., & Curry, R. H. (1992). *The American Medical Association guide to your family's symptoms*. New York, NY: Random House.

Davis, M. A. (1999). *Signs and symptoms in emergency medicine*. St. Louis, MO: Mosby.

Domino, F. J., Balder, R. A., Golding, J., & Grimes, A. (2014). *The 5-minute clinical consult standard*. Philadelphia, PA: Wolters Kluwer.

Dunn, J. (1985, August). Giving telephone advice is hazardous to your professional health. *Nursing, 85*, 41.

Editors of Prevention. (2002). *The doctor's book of home remedies*. New York, NY: Rodale Books.

Ellis, M.J., Ritchie, L.J., McDonald, P.J., Cordingley, D., Reimer, K., Nijjar, S. … Russell, K. (2017). Multidisciplinary management of pediatric sports-related concussion. *The Canadian Journal of Neurological Sciences, 44*, 24–34.

Eriksson, E., Sandelius, S. &Wahlberg, A. (2015). Telephone advice nursing: Parents' experiences of monitoring calls in children with gastroenteritis. *Scandinavian Journal of Caring Sciences, 29*, 333–339.

Ferri, F. F. (2004). *Ferri's clinical advisor: Instant diagnosis and treatment*. St. Louis, MO: Mosby-Year Book.

Gorbach, S. L., Fatagas, M., Mylonakis, E., & Stone, D. R. (2001). *The 5-minute infectious disease consultant*. Philadelphia, PA: Lippincott Williams & Wilkins.

Gray, D. & Wilkie, P. (2015). Patient perspectives on telephone triage in general practice. *Lancet, 385*, 687–688.

Greensher, A., Roemer, H., & Siemering, K. (1984). *Ambulatory protocols for emergency care.* Bowie, MD: Robert J. Brady.

Griffith, W. H. (1985). *Complete guide to symptoms, illness, and surgery.* Los Angeles, CA: The Body Press.

Grossman, V. G. A. (2003). *Quick reference to triage* (2nd ed.). Philadelphia, PA: Lippincott Williams & Wilkins.

Group Health Cooperative of Puget Sound. (1984). *Nurses' guide to telephone triage and health care.* Pacific Palisades, CA: Nurseco.

Harper, R., Temkin, T. & Bhargava, R. (2015). Optimizing the use of telephone nursing advice for upper respiratory infection symptoms. *The American Journal of Managed Care, 21*, 264–270.

Hoare, K., Lacoste, J., Haro, K., & Conyers, C. (1999, October). Exploring indicators of telephone nursing quality. *Journal of Nursing Care Quality, 14*(1), 38–46.

Howell, T. (2016). ED utilization by uninsured and Medicaid patients after availability of telephone triage. *Journal of Emergency Nursing, 42*, 120–124.

Huibers, L., Keizer, E., Giesen, P., Grol, R. & Wensing, M. (2012). Nurse telephone triage: Good quality associated with appropriate decisions. *Family Practice, 29*, 547–552.

Hunter, J. (2015). An intervention to improve the comfort and satisfaction of nurses in the telephone triage of child maltreatment calls. *Pediatric Nursing, 41*, 296–300.

Jenkins, J. L., & Loscalzo, J. (1990). *Manual of emergency medicine.* Boston, MA: Little, Brown and Company.

Katz, H. P. (1990). *Telephone medicine triage and training.* Philadelphia, PA: F. A. Davis.

Kemper, D. W. (1995). *Healthwise handbook: A self-care manual* (12th ed.). Boise, ID: Healthwise Publications.

Kleinman, R. E., & Greer, F. R. (2013). *Pediatric nutrition* (7th ed.). Elk Grove Village, IL: American Academy of Pediatrics.

Langdon, R. & DiSabella, M. (2017). Pediatric headache: An overview. *Current Problems in Pediatric and Adolescent Health Care, 47*, 44–65.

Leppänen, V. (2010). Power in telephone-advice nursing. *Nursing Inquiry, 17*, 15–22.

Long, V. C., & McMullen, P. C. (2010). *Telephone triage for obstetrics & gynecology* (2nd ed.). Philadelphia, PA: Wolters Kluwer/Lippincott Williams & Wilkins.

Maimburg, R., Olsen, J. & Sun, Y. (2016). Neonatal hyperbilirubinemia and the risk of febrile seizures and childhood epilepsy. *Epilepsy Research, 124*, 67–72.

Mayo, A. M. (1998, November/December). The role of the telephone advice/triage nurse. *AAACN Viewpoint, 20*(6), 9.

McGear, R., & Price-Simms, J. (1988). *Telephone triage and management: A nursing process approach.* Philadelphia, PA: WB Saunders.

Meadows-Oliver, M. (2014). *Pediatric nursing made incredibly easy* (2nd ed.). Philadelphia, PA: Wolters Kluwer/Lippincott Williams & Wilkins.

Miller, H. S., McEvers, J., & Griffith, J. A. (1997). *Instructions for obstetric and gynecologic patients* (2nd ed.). Philadelphia, PA: WB Saunders.

Moss, E. (2014). "Just a telephone call away": Transforming the nursing profession with telecare and telephone nursing triage. *Nursing Forum, 49*, 233–239.

Murdoch, J., Varley, A., Fletcher, E., Britten, N., Price, L., Calitri, R. … Campbell, J. (2015). Implementing telephone triage in general practice: A process evaluation of a cluster randomised controlled trial. *BMC Family Practice, 16*, 47.

Murdoch, J., Barnes, R., Pooler, J., Lattimer, V., Fletcher, E. & Campbell, J. (2015). The impact of using computer decision-support software in primary care nurse-led telephone triage: Interactional dilemmas and conversational consequences. *Social Science & Medicine, 126*, 36–44.

Narayan, M. C., Tennant, J. K., Benedict, L., Morrison, K. L., & Peyton C. (1998). *Telephone triage for home care.* Gaithersburg, MD: Aspen.

Navratil-Strawn, J., Hawkins, K., Hartley, S., Wells, T., Ozminkowski, R., Migliori, R. & Yeh, C. (2016). Using propensity to succeed modeling to increase utilization and adherence in a nurse HealthLine Telephone Triage Program. *The Journal of Ambulatory Care Management, 39*, 186–198.

Navratil-Strawn, J., Ozminkowski, R. & Hartley, S. (2014). An economic analysis of a nurse-led telephone triage service. *Journal of Telemedicine and Telecare, 20*, 330–338.

Pasini, A., Rigon, G. & Vaona, A. (2015). A cross-sectional study of the quality of telephone triage in a primary care out-of-hours service. *Journal of Telemedicine and Telecare, 21*, 68–72.

Patel, N., Maddalozzo, J. & Billings, K. (2014). An update on management of pediatric epistaxis. *International Journal of Pediatric Otorhinolaryngology, 78*, 1400–1404.

Payne, L., Jatana, K., Elmaraghy, C. & Justice, L. (2016). Standardization of the telephone triage process in an ambulatory pediatric otolaryngology setting. *Head and Neck Nursing, 34*, 15–17.

Perlman, M. D., & Tintinalli, J. E. (Eds.). (1998). *Emergency care of the woman.* New York, NY: McGraw-Hill.

Perry, K. (1993, January). Answering the phone: Risks and rewards. *Nursing Management, 24*(1), 77–79.

Physicians' Desk Reference. (1996). *Physicians' desk reference for nonprescription drugs.* Montvale, NJ: Medical Economics.

Pool, S. R. (2004). *The complete guide: Providing telephone triage and advice in a family practice—During office hours and/or after hours.* Elk Grove Village, IL: American Academy of Pediatrics.

Proehl, J. A., & Jones, L. M. (1998). *Mosby's emergency department patient teaching guide.* St. Louis, MO: C. V. Mosby.

Protocols help staff give appropriate telephone advice. (1994, January). *ED Management*, 8–12.

Purc-Stephenson, R. & Thrasher, C. (2010). Nurses' experiences with telephone triage and advice: a meta-ethnography. *Journal of Advanced Nursing, 66*, 482–489.

Purc-Stephenson, R. & Thrasher, C. (2012). Patient compliance with telephone triage recommendations: a meta-analytic review. *Patient Education and Counseling, 87*, 135–142.

Reinhardt, A. (2010). The impact of work environment on telephone advice nursing. *Clinical Nursing Research, 19*, 289–301.

Reisinger, P. B. (1997, September/October). Telephone triage and child abuse assessment. *AAACN Viewpoint, 19*(5), 16–17.

Robinson, D. L., Anderson, M., & Eipenbeck, P. (1997, March). Telephone advice: New solutions for old problems. *Nurse Practitioner, 22*(3), 170–192.

Rosenthal, B. (Ed.). (2000). A comprehensive resource guide to medical call centers: Players, implementation, and strategies. In *Directory of medical call centers.* New York, NY: Falkner & Gray.

Rouzier, P. (1999). *The sports medicine patient advisor.* San Francisco, CA: SportsMedPress.

Rutenberg, C. (2000, March). Telephone triage: When the only thing connecting you to your patient is the telephone. *American Journal of Nursing, 100*(3), 77–81.

Schaider, J. J., Hayden, S. R., Wolfe, R. E., Barkin, R. M., & Rosen, P. (2007). *Rosen and Barkin's 5-minute emergency medicine consult* (3rd ed.). Philadelphia, PA: Lippincott Williams & Wilkins.

Schwartz, W. M. (Ed.). (2005). *The 5-minute pediatric consult* (4th ed.). Philadelphia, PA: Lippincott Williams & Wilkins.

Schweitzer, P. B. (2000, March/April). Depression in primary care: The personal and social consequences of under treatment. *AAACN Viewpoint, 22*(2), 1.

Shaikh, N., Mattoo, T., Keren, R., Ivanova, A., Cui, G., Moxey-Mims, M. … Hoberman, A. (2016). Early antibiotic treatment for pediatric febrile urinary tract infection and renal scarring. *JAMA Pediatrics, 170*, 848–854.

Shealy, C. N. (2002). *The illustrated encyclopedia of healing remedies.* Boston, MA: Thorsons/Element.

Sheehy, S. B., & Lenehan, G. P. (1999). *Manual of emergency care* (5th ed.). St. Louis, MO: Mosby.

Soxman, J. (2016). The pediatric dental patient. *Texas Dental Journal, 133*, 144.

Springhouse. (1999). *Nursing '99 drug handbook.* Springhouse, PA: Author.

Szlam, S. & Meredith, M. (2013). Shake, rattle, and roll: An update on pediatric seizures. *Pediatric Emergency Care, 29*, 1287–1289.

Takeyama, A., Hashimoto, K., Sato, M., Sato, T., Tomita, Y., Maeda, R. … Hosoya, M. (2014). Clinical and epidemiologic factors related to subsequent wheezing after virus-induced lower respiratory tract infections in hospitalized pediatric patients younger than 3 years. *European Journal of Pediatrics, 173*, 959–966.

Telephone advice lines: Worth the risk? (1996, April). *ED Management, 8*(4), 44–47.

Tintinalli, J. E. (Ed.) (1996). *Emergency medicine: A comprehensive study guide* (4th ed.). New York, NY: McGraw-Hill.

U.S. Department of Health and Human Services. (2006, January). *Pandemic influenza planning: A guide for individuals and families.* Retrieved from http://www.pandemicflu.gov

Vickery, D. M., & Fries, J. F. (1993). *Take care of yourself* (5th ed.). Menlo Park, CA: Addison Wesley.

Walls, A., Pierce, M., Krishnan, N., Steehler, M. & Harley, E. Jr (2015). Pediatric head and neck complications of Streptococcus pneumoniae before and after PCV7 vaccination. *Otolaryngology—Head and Neck Surgery, 152*, 336–341.

Weinstein, A. (2002). Topical treatment of common superficial tinea infections. *American Family Physician, 65*(10), 2095.

Wheeler, S. Q. (1993). *Telephone triage, theory, and protocol development.* Albany, NY: Delmar Publishers.

Wheeler, S. Q. (1994, May). Telephone triage: Sidestepping the pitfalls. *Nursing, 24*(5), 32LL–32OO.

Wheeler, S. Q. (1997). Calling all nurses: How to perform telephone triage. *Nursing, 27*(7), 37–41.

Wheeler, S. Q. (2009). *Telephone triage protocols for adult populations.* New York, NY: McGraw-Hill.

Wheeler, S., Greenberg, M., Mahlmeister, L. & Wolfe, N. (2015). Safety of clinical and non-clinical decision makers in telephone triage: A narrative review. *Journal of Telemedicine and Telecare, 21*, 305–322.

Wicking, K. H. (1999, September/October). Telephone triage: Surviving the storm. *AAACN Viewpoint, 21*(5), 12.

Woodke, D. (1995). *Telephone triage protocols for primary care centers.* Indianapolis, IN: HealthNet Community Health Centers and Methodist Hospital of Indiana.

## Internet Resources

American Academy of Academy of Pediatric Dentistry. (2017). www.aapd.org

American Academy of Pediatrics. (2015). *Anal itching in young children.* https://www.healthychildren.org/English/health-issues/conditions/skin/Pages/Anal-Itching-in-Young-Children.aspx

American Academy of Pediatrics. (2015). *Bedbug bites.* https://www.healthychildren.org/English/health-issues/conditions/from-insects-animals/Pages/Bedbug-Bites.aspx

American Academy of Pediatrics. (2015). *Birthmarks and hemangiomas.* https://www.healthychildren.org/English/health-issues/conditions/skin/Pages/Birthmarks-Hemangiomas.aspx

American Academy of Pediatrics. (2015). *Bottle feeding basics.* https://www.healthychildren.org/English/ages-stages/baby/feeding-nutrition/Pages/Bottle-Feeding-How-Its-Done.aspx

American Academy of Pediatrics. (2015). *Breastfeeding.* https://www.healthychildren.org/English/ages-stages/baby/breastfeeding/Pages/default.aspx

American Academy of Pediatrics. (2015). *Circumcision.* https://www.healthychildren.org/English/ages-stages/prenatal/decisions-to-make/Pages/Circumcision.aspx

American Academy of Pediatrics. (2015). *Crying and colic*. https://www.healthychildren.org/English/ages-stages/baby/crying-colic/Pages/default.aspx

American Academy of Pediatrics. (2015). *Earaches and your child*. https://www.healthychildren.org/English/health-issues/conditions/ear-nose-throat/Pages/Earaches-and-Your-Child.aspx

American Academy of Pediatrics. (2015). *Fever*. https://www.healthychildren.org/English/health-issues/conditions/fever/Pages/default.aspx

American Academy of Pediatrics. (2015). *Headaches*. https://www.healthychildren.org/English/health-issues/conditions/head-neck-nervous-system/Pages/Headaches.aspx

American Academy of Pediatrics. (2015). *Hives*. https://www.healthychildren.org/English/health-issues/conditions/skin/Pages/Hives.aspx

American Academy of Pediatrics. (2015). *Identifying insect bites and stings*. https://www.healthychildren.org/English/health-issues/conditions/from-insects-animals/Pages/Identifying-Insect-Bites-and-Stings.aspx

American Academy of Pediatrics. (2015). *Impetigo*. https://www.healthychildren.org/English/health-issues/conditions/skin/Pages/Impetigo.aspx

American Academy of Pediatrics. (2015). *Jaundice*. https://www.healthychildren.org/English/ages-stages/baby/Pages/Jaundice.aspx

American Academy of Pediatrics. (2015). *Molluscum Contagiosum*. https://www.healthychildren.org/English/health-issues/conditions/skin/Pages/Molluscum-Contagiosum.aspx

American Academy of Pediatrics. (2015). *Pinkeye (Conjunctivitis)*. https://www.healthychildren.org/English/health-issues/conditions/eyes/Pages/PinkEye-Conjunctivitis.aspx

American Academy of Pediatrics. (2015). *Pinworms*. https://www.healthychildren.org/English/health-issues/conditions/skin/Pages/Pinworms.aspx

American Academy of Pediatrics. (2015). *Roseola infantum*. https://www.healthychildren.org/English/health-issues/conditions/skin/Pages/Roseola-Infantum.aspx

American Academy of Pediatrics. (2015). *Scabies*. https://www.healthychildren.org/English/health-issues/conditions/skin/Pages/Scabies.aspx

American Academy of Pediatrics. (2015). *Sports-related concussion: Understanding the risks, signs, and symptoms*. https://www.healthychildren.org/English/health-issues/injuries-emergencies/sports-injuries/Pages/Sports-Related-Concussion-Understanding-the-Risks-Signs-Symptoms.aspx

American Academy of Pediatrics. (2015). *Sunburn treatment and prevention*. https://www.healthychildren.org/English/health-issues/conditions/skin/Pages/Sunburn-Treatment-and-Prevention.aspx

American Academy of Pediatrics. (2015). *Teething and tooth care*. https://www.healthychildren.org/English/ages-stages/baby/teething-tooth-care/Pages/default.aspx

American Academy of Pediatrics. (2015). *Tinea infections*. https://www.healthychildren.org/English/health-issues/conditions/skin/Pages/Tinea-Infections-Ringworm-Athletes-Foot-Jock-Itch.aspx

American Academy of Pediatrics. (2015). *Umbilical cord care*. https://www.healthychildren.org/English/ages-stages/baby/bathing-skin-care/Pages/Umbilical-Cord-Care.aspx

American Academy of Pediatrics. (2015). *Warts*. https://www.healthychildren.org/English/health-issues/conditions/skin/Pages/Warts.aspx

American Academy of Pediatrics. (2015). *What causes acne?* https://www.healthychildren.org/English/health-issues/conditions/skin/Pages/What-Causes-Acne.aspx

American Academy of Pediatrics. (2017). www.aap.org

American Association of Poison Control Centers. (2017). http://www.aapcc.org/

American Lung Association. (2011). Retrieved from http://www.lungusa.org

American Lung Association. (2017). www.lung.org

Body Piercing Aftercare Guidelines. (2011). Retrieved from http://www.safepiercing.org

Centers for Disease Control and Prevention. (2011). *Acute public health consequences of methamphetamine laboratories*. Retrieved from http://www.cdc.gov/mmwr/preview/mmwrhtml/mm5414a3.htm

Centers for Disease Control and Prevention. (2011). *Avian flu*. Retrieved from http://www.cdc.gov/flu/avian/index.htm; http://id_center.apic.org/cidrap/content/influenza/avianflu/biofacts/avflu_human.html

Centers for Disease Control and Prevention. (2011). *Influenza*. Retrieved from http://www.cdc.gov/flu

Centers for Disease Control and Prevention. (2011). *Swine flu (H1N1 virus)*. Retrieved from http://www.cdc.gov/h1n1flu

Centers for Disease Control and Prevention. (2011). *West Nile virus*. Retrieved from http://www.cdc.gov/ncidod/dvbid/westnile/

Centers for Disease Control and Prevention. (2014). *Pertussis*. Retrieved from www.cdc.gov/pertussis/index.html

Centers for Disease Control and Prevention. (2014). *Vaccines homepage for vaccines & immunizations*. Retrieved from http://www.cdc.gov/vaccines

Centers for Disease Control and Prevention. (2015). *Pertussis*. https://www.cdc.gov/vaccines/pubs/pinkbook/pert.html

Centers for Disease Control and Prevention. (2015). *Rubella*. https://www.cdc.gov/vaccines/pubs/pinkbook/rubella.html

Centers for Disease Control and Prevention. (2015). *Varicella*. https://www.cdc.gov/vaccines/pubs/pinkbook/varicella.html

Centers for Disease Control and Prevention. (2015). *West Nile Virus: Information for health care providers*. https://www.cdc.gov/westnile/healthcareproviders/index.html

Centers for Disease Control and Prevention. (2016). *Key facts about influenza*. https://www.cdc.gov/flu/keyfacts.htm

Centers for Disease Control and Prevention. (2016). *Measles.* https://www.cdc.gov/vaccines/pubs/pinkbook/meas.html

Centers for Disease Control and Prevention. (2016). *Mumps.* https://www.cdc.gov/vaccines/pubs/pinkbook/mumps.html

Centers for Disease Control and Prevention. (2017). *Zika virus: For health care providers.* https://www.cdc.gov/zika/hc-providers/index.html

Conditions. (2014). Retrieved from http://www.medicinenet.com

Cooper, M. A. (2014). Lightning injuries. *eMedicine.* Retrieved from http://www.emedicine.com/emerg/topic299.htm

Dehydration. (2014). Retrieved from http://www.emedicine health.com/dehydration_in_adults/article_em.htm

Dryden-Edwards, R. (2014). *Anxiety.* Retrieved from http://www.emedicinehealth.com/anxiety-health/article_em.htm

Frostbite. (2014). Retrieved from http://www.webmd.com/first-aid/frostbite-treatment

National Association of Pediatric Nurse Practitioners. (2017). www.napnap.org

National Heart Lung and Blood Institute. (2014). *Asthma.* Retrieved from http://www.nhlbi.nih.gov/health/public/lung/index.htm#asthma

National Institute of Allergy and Infectious Diseases. (2014). Retrieved from http://www.niaid.nih.gov

North American Society for Pediatric and Adolescent Gynecology. (2017). http://www.naspag.org/

Ringworm. (2011). Retrieved from http://www.nlm.nih.gov/medlineplus/ency/article/001439.htm

Society of Pediatric Nurses. (2017). www.pedsnurse.org

U.S. Drug Enforcement Administration: Methamphetamine. (2011). Retrieved from http://www.dea.gov/pubs/pressrel/methfact03.html

U.S. National Library of Medicine. *Piercing and tattoos.* (2017). https://medlineplus.gov/piercingandtattoos.html

Webmd.com. Retrieved from http://www.webmd.com/

# Index